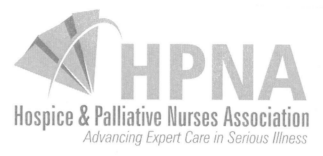

Hospice & Palliative Nurses Association
Advancing Expert Care in Serious Illness

Core Curriculum for the Advanced Practice Hospice and Palliative Registered Nurse

Second Edition

Volume II

Editors:

Constance M. Dahlin, APRN-BC, ACHPN®, FPCN®, FAAN
Palliative Care Specialist
North Shore Medical Center
Salem, MA

Maureen T. Lynch, MS, ANP-BC, AOCN, ACHPN®, FPCN®
Nurse Practitioner
Dana Farber Cancer Institute
Boston, MA

Hospice and Palliative Nurses Association
One Penn Center West, Suite 425
Pittsburgh, PA 15276-0109
www.AdvancingExpertCare.org/

HPNA Mission Statement:

To advance expert care in serious illness.

TABLE OF CONTENTS

CONTRIBUTORS

Marie Bakitas, DNSc, APRN, ACHPN®, AOCN
Clinical Researcher, Nurse Practitioner
Dartmouth-Hitchcock Medical Center
Lebanon, NH

Leslie Blatt, MBA, MSN, APRN®
Coordinator, Palliative Care
Yale New Haven Hospital
New Haven, CT

Pam Binnie, MS, ANP
Staff Nurse
Hospice of the North Shore & Greater Boston
Danvers, MA

Tami Borneman, RN, MSN, CNS, FPCN
Senior Research Specialist
City of Hope
Duarte, CA

Sterling R Bouxman, RRT, RN, ACNP-BC, MSN
Palliative Care Nurse Practitioner
Old Colony Hospice
Randolph, MA

Margaret L. Campbell, PhD, RN, FPCN
Director
Detroit Receiving Hospital
Assistant Professor
Wayne State University College of Nursing
Detroit, MI

Heather A. Carlson, BSN, APN-BC, ACHPN®
Palliative Care Nurse Practitioner
North Shore Medical Center
Salem, MA

Garret K. Chan, PhD, APRN, FPCN, FAEN, FAAN
Lead Advanced Practice Nurse & Associate Clinical Director
Stanford Hospital & Clinic
Stanford, CA

Nessa Coyle, NP, PhD, ACHPN®, FAAN
Nurse Practitioner
Memorial Sloan-Kettering Cancer Center
New York, NY

Constance M. Dahlin, APRN-BC, ACHPN®, FPCN, FAAN
Palliative Care Specialist
North Shore Medical Center
Salem, MA

Sheila M. Davis, DNP, ANP-BC, FAAN
Adult Nurse Practitioner
MGH Institute of Health Professions
Partners® Healthcare
Boston, MA

Susan Derby, MA, GNP-BC, ACHPN®
Nurse Practitioner, Pain & Palliative Care Service
Memorial Sloan-Kettering Cancer Center
New York, NY

Carma Erickson-Hurt, APRN, ACHPN®
Adjunct Faculty
Grand Canyon University
Phoenix, AZ

Kelli Gershon, FNP-BC, ACHPN®
Nurse Practitioner
Symptom Management Consultant (SMC)
The Woodlands, TX

Linda Gorman, RN, MN, PMHCNS-BC, CHPN®, OCN, FPCN
Palliative Care Clinical Nurse Specialist
Cedars-Sinai Medical Center
Los Angeles, CA

Marian Grant, RN, CRNP, ACHPN®, DNP
Assistant Professor
University of Maryland School of Nursing
Baltimore, MD

Linda Hadden, DNP, CANP, CPNP
Palliative Consultant
Unity Hospital
Fridley, MN

Rebecca Hawkins, MSN, ANP, ACHPN®
Palliative Care Nurse Practitioner/Coordinator
Providence St. Mary Medical Center
Walla Walla, WA

Ann Hughes, RN, PhD, ACHPN®, FAAN
Advanced Practice Palliative Care Nurse
Laguna Honda Hospital/San Francisco
    Department of Public Health
San Francisco, CA

Mary Layman-Goldstein, RN, MS, ANP-BC, ACHPN®
Nurse Practitioner, Pain & Palliative Care
    Service
Memorial Sloan-Kettering Cancer Center
New York, NY

Judy Lentz, RN, MSN, NHA
Oncology Palliative Care Doula
Moon Township, PA

Marijo Letizia, PhD, APN/ANP-BC, FAANP
Professor & Associate Dean, MSN & DNP
    Programs
Loyola University Chicago
Maywood, IL

Maureen T. Lynch, MS, APRN-BC, ACHPN®, AOCN, FPCN
Nurse Practitioner, Adult Palliative Care
Dana Farber Cancer Institute
Boston, MA

Carol Mathews, MSN, APRN, ACHPN®
Advanced Practice Palliative Care Nurse
Lake Health/University Hospitals Seidman
    Cancer Center
Mentor, OH

Marlene E. McHugh, DNP, DCC, FNP-BC
Associate Director of Palliative Care
Montefiore Medical Center
Assistant Professor of Clinical Nursing
Columbia University School of Nursing
New York, NY

Joan Panke, MA, RN, ACHPN®
Palliative Care NP/Palliative Care Consultant
Arlington, VA

Victor Phantumavnit, PharmD, BCPS, BCOP
Clinical Pharmacy Specialist in Palliative
    Care
Dana-Farber Cancer Institute
Boston, MA

Therese Rochon, MSN, MA, RNP, ACHPN®
Palliative Care Coordinator
Home & Hospice Care of Rhode Island
Providence, RI

Marguerite M. Russo, MS, CRNP-F, ACHPN®
Palliative Care Nurse Practitioner
University of Maryland Medical Center
Baltimore, MD

Mary Beth Singer, MS, ANP-BC, AOCN, ACHPN®
Oncology Nurse Practitioner and Patient
    Program Manager
Tufts Medical Center Cancer Center
Boston, MA

Robert Smeltz, RN, MA, NP, ACHPN®
Palliative Care NP/Clinical Coordinator
NYU School of Medicine
New York, NY

Lisa Stephens, MSN, APRN, ACHPN®
Nurse Practitioner, Palliative Medicine
Dartmouth-Hitchcock Medical Center
Lebanon, NH

Joetta Descartes Wallace, MSN, NP-C, CHPPN®, CPON
Program Coordinator, Pediatric Supportive &
    Palliative Care Service
Miller Children's Hospital Long Beach
Long Beach, CA

Debra L. Wiegand, RN, MBE, PhD, CCRN, CHPN®, FAHA, FAAN
Assistant Professor
University of Maryland School of Nursing
Baltimore, MD

Margery A. Wilson, MSN, FNP, ACHPN®
Coordinator & Nurse Practitioner, Advanced
    Illness Consultants/Palliative Care Team
Wellmont Bristol Regional Medical Center
Bristol, TN

Sarah Wilson, PhD, RN
Emeritus Associate Professor
Shorewood, WI

REVIEWERS

Anne Marie Barron, PhD, RN, PMHCNS-BC
Clinical Nurse Specialist
Associate Dean, Undergraduate Curriculum
and Student Affairs, School of Nursing
and Health Sciences, Simmons College
Inpatient Oncology and Bone Marrow
Transplant Unit,Massachusetts General
Hospital
Boston, MA

Vanessa Batista, RN, MS, CPNP, CCRC
Pediatric Advanced Care Team
Children's Hospital of Philadelphia
Chestnut Hill, MA

Therese Cortez, NP, MSN, ACHPN®
Palliative Care Program Manager
Veteran Affairs VISN 3
New York, NY

**Patrick J. Coyne, MSN, APRN, ACHPN®,
ACNS-BC, FAAN, FPCN**
Clinical Director, Thomas Palliative Care
Program
VCU/Massey Cancer Center
Richmond, VA

**Constance M. Dahlin, APRN-BC, ACHPN®,
FPCN, FAAN**
Palliative Care Specialist
North Shore Medical Center
Salem, MA

Vivian Donahue, RN, MS, ACNS-BC, CCRN
Nursing Director
Massachusetts General Hospital
Boston, MA

**Susan Gibson, RN, MSN, FNP-BC,
ACHPN®**
Program Coordinator, Community Palliative
Care
Visiting Nurse and Hospice Care
Santa Barbara, CA

Joan Panke, MA, RN, ACHPN®
Palliative Care NP/Palliative Care Consultant
Arlington, VA

Martha Jurchak, RN, PhD
Executive Director, Ethics Service
Brigham and Women's Hospital
Boston, MA

**Kathryn M. Lanz, DNP, ANP-BC, GNP-BC,
ACHPN®**
Director of Geriatric Services & Palliative
Education
UPMC Palliative & Supportive Institute
Pittsburgh, PA

**Maureen T. Lynch, MS, APRN-BC,
ACHPN®, AOCN, FPCN**
Nurse Practitioner, Adult Palliative Care
Dana Farber Cancer Institute
Boston, MA

**Carol Matthews, CNS, APRN, MSN,
ACHPN®**
Advanced Practice Palliative Care Nurse
Lake Health/University Hospitals Seidman
Cancer Center
Mentor, OH

Petique Oeflein, RN, NP-C
Western Reserve Navigator Team Leader
Hospice of the Western Reserve
Cleveland, OH

Sheila Poswolsky, MSN, APRN, ACHPN®
Nurse Practitioner, Palliative Care Consult
Team
Veteran Affairs Boston Health Care System
Boston, MA

Deanna Schneider, MSN, RN, CPNP
Pediatric Nurse Practitioner, Supportive Care
Program
Children's Hospital of Pittsburgh of UPMC
Pittsburgh, PA

Dena Jean Sutermaster, RN, MSN, CHPN®
Director, Education Products
Hospice and Palliative Nurses Association
Pittsburgh, PA

Sally Welsh, MSN, RN, NEA-BC
Chief Executive Officer
Hospice and Palliative Nurses Association
Pittsburgh, PA

**Christine Westphal, NP, MSN, ACNS-BC,
ACHPN®, CCRN**
Director/Nurse Practitioner
Oakwood Healthcare System
Dearborn, MI

DISCLAIMER

The Hospice and Palliative Nurses Association (HPNA), its officers and directors, and the authors and reviewers of this core curriculum make no claims that buying or studying it will guarantee a passing score on the ACHPN® certification examination.

HPNA will not be held liable or responsible for individual treatments, specific plans of care, or patient and family outcomes. This core curriculum is intended for professional education purposes only.

INTRODUCTION

Over the last fifteen years, the role of the advanced practice registered nurse (APRN) in palliative and hospice care has evolved. The APRN role is essential in the interdisciplinary process of palliative care. Since 1998, palliative care programs have been developing at a rapid pace. APRNs have had a major presence in many of these programs as clinicians and leaders, and have fostered clinical excellence in hospices. Changes in reimbursement regulations have contributed to the expanding presence of the APRN in hospice and palliative care programs. APRNs provide efficient, high quality, cost effective care, while improving access to palliative care.

The history of advanced practice nursing is rich. In 1998, the Peaceful Death Competencies[1] were developed by the American Association of Colleges of Nursing, delineating recommendations for incorporating end of life care in undergraduate nursing curriculum. In 1999, Ferrell and colleagues published *Strengthening Nursing Education to Improve End-of-Life Care,*[2] which identified gaps in end-of-life content in nursing textbooks, curriculum and licensing exams with a call to nursing educators to improve education on end of life care. In 2001, a group of nursing leaders met to discuss the role of the advanced practice nurse in palliative care. From that meeting the Advanced Practice Nurses Role in Palliative Care—A Position Statement from American Nursing Leaders[3] was developed. This document discussed the role of the APRN and made recommendations to healthcare leaders, nurse educators, healthcare organizations, healthcare payers and public policy actions to promote, develop and advocate for the role. Simultaneously, a monograph *Advanced Practice Nursing: Pioneering Practices in Palliative Care*[4] was produced to offer various models of the role.

With the growth of APRN roles in hospice and palliative care, the National Board for Certification of Hospice and Palliative Nursing (NBCHPN®), in a partnership with the American Nurses Credentialing Center, initiated specialty certification for the advanced practice nurse in 2001. The first examination was offered in the spring of 2002. In January, 2005, NBCHPN® became full proprietor of this exam.

In 2002, ANA and HPNA developed the title *Scope and Standards of Hospice and Palliative Nursing Practice*[5], which included standards for advanced practice nursing. These were updated in 2007 and 2013. A companion document, *Competencies for Advanced Practice Hospice and Palliative Care Nurses*[6] was also produced.

In 2004, the National Consensus Project produced *Clinical Practice Guidelines for Quality Palliative Care,*[7] which set the standard for all programs that deliver palliative care. These were revised in 2009 to reflect the changing heath care environment. The third edition will appear in 2013. In 2006, the Clinical Guidelines were endorsed by the National Quality Forum in the document: *A Framework for Hospice and Palliative care with Preferred Practices: A Consensus Statement.*[8] Certification for palliative care programs is available from The Joint Commission.[9] All of these quality measures include the provisions that palliative care clinicians should keep current in the field and attain certification as available.

There is a synergy in this responsibility and the mission of the Hospice and Palliative Nurses Association (HPNA) to promote excellence in end-of-life nursing. To support the quality of care required by the HPNA scope and standards, competencies, and NBCHPN® certification, HPNA has provided educational products to support consistent, expert practice for both novice and experienced clinicians as well as mid-career APRNs entering the specialty. In keeping with that goal, the first edition of the *Core Curriculum for the Advanced Practice Hospice and Palliative Nurse*[10] was published in 2007.

Just as it is the responsibility of the APRN to stay abreast of the state of the science and the developing evidence in palliative care, *the Core Curriculum for the Advanced Practice Hospice and Palliative Registered Nurse, Second Edition,* also must present the current knowledge in advanced hospice and palliative nursing. This revision reflects the expertise of APRNs from throughout the field who serve in a variety of settings.

As editors, our effort of this revision has been a labor of love for the work, commitment to quality, and passion for education. We have worked diligently with the authors to assure the most up to date knowledge in the various topics.

The goal of the curriculum is to provide a foundation of knowledge from which APRNs can practice palliative care. In the last decade, the evidence base for palliative care has expanded. The chapters in this Curriculum reflect the current evidence. To meet the rapidly changing needs of the APRN, the *Core Curriculum* has been reorganized. The first section, *Issues in Palliative Nursing*, presents an overview of the role and practice concerns. The second section, *Dimensions of Care*, reviews common symptoms, and psycho-social-spiritual aspects of care. The third section, *Management of Common Serious or Life-Threatening Illnesses*, describes various conditions, including the pathophysiology and the specific management to that condition. New in this edition are 2 sections: a section devoted on vulnerable and special populations and an expanded resources to include a pharmacological quick reference, a review of oxygen therapy, and useful references.

Our hope is that it will be useful to APRNs who are new to palliative nursing and to those who are more experienced. We have strived to incorporate the state of the science and the state of the art of palliative nursing. Knowing that you are committed to excellence in practice, we feel certain that you will have comments, feedback and requests for changes in future edition that reflect the evolution of practice and knowledge.

Constance M. Dahlin, APRN-BC, ACHPN®, FPCN, FAAN

Maureen T. Lynch, MS, ANP-BC, AOCN, ACHPN®, FPCN

REFERENCES

1. American Association of Colleges of Nursing. *Peaceful death: Recommended competencies and curricular guidelines for end-of-life nursing care.* American Association of Colleges of Nursing/Robert Wood Johnson Foundation; 1998.
2. Ferrell BR, Grant M, Virani R. *Strengthening Nursing Education to Improve End-of-Life Care. Nurs Outlook.* 1999;47(6):252-256.
3. American Nursing Leaders. *Advanced Practice Nurses Role in Palliative Care—A Position Statement.* 2002. Available at: www.promotingexcellence.org/apn/. Accessed June 10, 2012.
4. *Advanced Practice Nursing: Pioneering Practices in Palliative Care.* 2002. Available at www.promotingexcellence.org/apn/. Accessed June 10, 2012.
5. Hospice and Palliative Nurses Association; American Nurses Association. *Hospice and Palliative Nursing: Scope and Standards of Practice.* Silver Spring, MD: American Nurses Association; 2007.
6. Sherman D, Abbott, P, Ryan M, Dahlin C, Sheehan, DK, Derby S. *Competencies for Advance Practice Hospice and Palliative Care Nurses.* Pittsburgh, PA: Hospice and Palliative Nurses Association; 2002.
7. National Consensus Project for Quality Palliative Care. *Clinical Practice Guidelines for Quality Palliative Care.* 3rd ed. Pittsburgh: PA: National Consensus Project for Quality Palliative Care; 2013. *Available at:* www.nationalconsensusproject.org.
8. National Quality Forum: *A National Framework and Preferred Practices for Palliative and Hospice Care Quality.* Washington, DC: National Quality Forum; 2006.
9. The Joint Commission. *Palliative Care Manual –Standards, Elements of Performance, Scoring, and Certification Policies.* Oakbrook, IL: The Joint Commission; 2012.
10. Perley, MJ, Dahlin CM, eds. *Core Curriculum for the Advance Practice Hospice and Palliative Care Nurse.* Pittsburgh, PA: Hospice and Palliative Nurses Association; 2007.

PART IV

CONSIDERATIONS FOR SPECIAL POPULATIONS

CHAPTER 27

PALLIATIVE CARE IN THE EMERGENCY DEPARTMENT AND CRITICAL CARE UNIT

Garrett K. Chan, PhD, APRN, FPCN, FAEN, FAAN

I. INTRODUCTION

A. Since the beginning of the palliative care movement, experts have advocated that palliative care should be integrated with disease-modifying care from the time of diagnosis.[1,2] Historically, palliative care has focused on long-term chronic illness. However, there is now an emphasis on palliative care for patients with trauma and acute illness. The care of these patients necessitates that multiple specialties be involved in the planning and provision of care. Decision-making about patient care is complicated by diverse multi-specialty perspectives on directions and options for care, as well as the distress of families struggling to cope with a healthcare crisis.

B. Living with illness or injury can often result in severe, unexpected exacerbations or complications. In the case of emergencies, however, a sudden illness or traumatic injury may be the first encounter with the healthcare system.[3] Patients, in both scenarios, experience serious and possibly life-threatening situations. In the United States, there is culture focused on rescue and saving lives no matter the cost, consequences, or potential impact on quality of life.[3] Clinicians in emergency department and intensive care units are confronted with this societal expectation and must carefully balance likely outcomes and patient and family wishes. Patients, families, and clinicians may find themselves challenged, not only by the management of the illness or injury, but by the associated physical, psychological, social, and spiritual distress.

C. Role of Palliative APRN—palliative APRNs are essential to assisting patients, families, and staff to navigate through these difficult situations, and in the management of the resultant symptoms. Careful exploration of life goals, patient and family hopes, and expectations of care will help identify which interventions may be appropriate.

D. This chapter describes 2 care settings—the emergency department (ED) and the intensive care unit (ICU). The rationale for combining ED and ICU into one chapter is that many patients with advanced illness or injuries require critical or intensive care regardless of the practice setting. Although there are some unique attributes to each settings that will be described, the disease processes, skills, and interventions for palliative care in the critical illness phase can be applied in both the ED and ICU settings.

E. This chapter is divided into 3 sections—Care of the Patient; Special Topics Regarding Families; and Care for the Clinicians. Common life-threatening with high mortality rates are discussed along with the unique aspects of palliative care. Palliative care interventions that support proxy decision-making as well as reduce anxiety and posttraumatic stress are presented. Debriefing and self-care activities to prevent burnout are reviewed.

II. OVERVIEW

A. The Emergency Department (ED)

The ED is a fast-paced, high-stress environment where clinicians often make clinical decisions with sub-optimal information.[3] A core concept of emergency medicine and nursing is to diagnose illness and injury and initiate treatment in an effort to cure. Patients present to the ED with

1. New and sudden illness or injury (e.g., acute myocardial infarction, severe laceration, fracture)

2. Life-threatening injuries related to a catastrophic event (e.g., automobile accident)

3. Exacerbations of a chronic illness (e.g., chronic pulmonary disease with onset of acute respiratory distress syndrome).

The ED is a place of transition, not a destination. Patients are transferred to inpatient units, other hospitals, or discharged to another facility, or venue of care.

Palliative care, ideally, is a larger construct than just the end-of-life care. However, understanding the various trajectories of approaching death is important for clinicians to discern which clinical situations call for intensive palliative care. This understanding can elucidate which of the trajectories could benefit from anticipatory planning. There are seven trajectories of approaching death in the emergency department—1) dead on arrival; 2) prehospital resuscitation with subsequent ED death; 3) prehospital resuscitation with survival until admission; 4) terminal illness necessitating ED care for symptom management; 5) frail and hovering near death; 6) alive and interactive on arrival, but arrests in the ED; and 7) potentially preventable death by omission or commission.[4]

B. The Intensive Care Unit (ICU)

ICUs were created to sustain the use of the advances and improvements in medical knowledge, technology, and pharmacology, such as mechanical ventilation and cardiac monitoring, as well the need for prolonged monitoring following complex surgeries.[5] The ICU is a setting where low nurse-to-patient ratios allow close observation and intervention to respond rapidly to the changing health status of patients and the psychosocial needs of families. There is often more time and more resources that can be dedicated to patients and families in the ICU. The resulting benefits of time and resources can aid in the incorporation of palliative care principles in the ICU.

In both the ED and ICU, there is a heavy emphasis on technology and procedures as cornerstones of healthcare. Technology helps provide vital information to determine the severity of illness, treat underlying pathology, and assess the response to treatment. This also means there are more choices about when to use technology, more potential interventions for patients and the need for education and advocacy in a treatment focused environment. There is a risk for the patient to be lost in the bed while clinicians pay attention to the technology.

III. CARE OF THE PATIENT

A. Illnesses and conditions with high mortality rates

1. Infection—microbial phenomenon characterized by an inflammatory response to the presence of microorganisms or the invasion of normally sterile host

27

tissue by those organisms. Common advanced-illness presentations in critical care include sepsis from severe pneumonia, bacterial endocarditis, viral infections (e.g., myocarditis), necrotizing fasciitis, meningitis/encephalitis, intra-abdominal pathogens (e.g., intra-abdominal abscesses, peritonitis, toxic megacolon), line infection in an immunosuppressed host, and urosepsis.

a) Advanced comorbid conditions predispose patients to infections and reduce host immune response placing the patient at higher risk for mortality when a pathogen is present.

b) Sociocultural

   i. Elders and persons who are marginally housed or live at poverty level are at high risk due to impaired host defenses

c) Healthcare-associated infection (HAI) is the most common in the critical care environment. Predisposition to HAI increases with acuity, age, stress, transplant, chemotherapy, and an immunocompromised host. HAI can be caused by endogenous and/or exogenous sources.[6]

   i. Endogenous sources are body sites, such as the skin, nose, mouth, gastrointestinal (GI) tract, or vagina that are normally inhabited by microorganisms.

   ii. Exogenous sources are those external to the patient, such as patient care personnel, visitors, patient care equipment, medical devices, or the facility environment.

d) Causes

   i. Pneumonia

      (a) Ventilator associated pneumonia (VAP)[7]

         (i) Definition—pneumonia in people who have a device to continuously assist with or control respiration through a tracheostomy, or by endotracheal intubation within 48 hours before the onset of infection, inclusive of the weaning period.

         (ii) Causes—tracheostomy or endotracheal tubes (ETT) bypass natural defense mechanisms such as cough and mucociliary clearance. The tracheostomy or ETT is non-sterile and is colonized with endogenous or exogenous pathogens that can travel directly into the lungs causing VAP.

         (iii) Epidemiology—VAP accounts for 25% of all ICU infections. Estimated rate is 2 cases per 1,000 ventilator days.

         (iv) Mortality—8-15%

      (b) Catheter-related blood stream infections (CR-BSI)[8]

         (i) Definition—known (i.e., positive blood 0r catheter cultures) or suspected infection related to a short-term or long-term blood stream catheter such as peripheral IV, peripherally inserted central venous catheter (PICC), central venous catheter (CVC), or arterial line.

27

(ii) Causes—pathogens (e.g., bacteria, fungi) are introduced into the blood stream at the insertion site, hubs, or via intravenous solutions.

(iii) Epidemiology—an estimated 80,000 cases/year in the ICU.

(iv) Serious soft tissue infections could present in a variety of forms including cellulitis (especially necrotizing fasciitis), pressure ulcer infections, surgical site infections, and infected burns. The etiology, prevalence, and mortality vary depending on the organism and the host defenses.

2. Systemic inflammatory response, sepsis, and multisystem organ dysfunction syndrome (MODS)

   a) Septicemia is the 11th cause of death in the United States with 34,843 deaths.[9]

   b) Poor prognosis

      i.   700,000 per year die of either septic shock or bacteremia.

      ii. Septic shock is the leading cause of death in non-coronary intensive care units.

      iii. MODS mortality rates are 50%-60% when two organs involved.

   c) Systemic inflammatory response syndrome (SIRS). Diagnosis of SIRS is made when at least 2 of the 4 conditions below present.[10]

      i.   Temperature above 38°C or below 36°C

      ii. Heart rate above 90 beats/minute

      iii. Respiratory rate above 20 breaths/minute or Pco_2 below 32 mmHg

      iv. White blood cell (WBC) count > 12,000 mm^3 or below 4000mm^3 or > 10% immature band forms

   d) Sepsis—at least two of the four SIRS criteria in addition to a known or suspected infection (e.g., bacterial, viral, fungal).

      i.   Often associated with history of immunosuppression, malnutrition, alcohol use, acute illness, chronic disease or prolonged intensive care unit stay with intubation longer than 48 hours

      ii. Gram negative bacteria most common cause

      iii. Gram positive invasive lines such as PICC lines contribute to this bacteremia

      iv. Pathophysiology of sepsis includes 3 major concepts—inflammation, a procoagulant response (i.e., increased coagulation), and inhibited fibrinolysis. These 3 mechanisms cause widespread thromboses that can lead to endovascular injury and organ impairment/dysfunction depending on the severity. The clinical signs of multi-organ dysfunction are listed below.

   e) Septic shock—sepsis induced state with at least one organ dysfunction, which includes the following conditions

      i.   Hypotension (BP < 90 mmHg or systolic drop > 40 mmHg) despite fluid resuscitation

27

    ii.   Lactic acidosis

    iii. Oliguria

    iv. Mental status deterioration

    v.   Tachycardia (> 90 bpm)

    vi. Pulmonary artery findings—as measured below

        (a) Cardiac output (> 7 L/min)

        (b) Systemic vascular resistance (< 900 dynes/second/cm)

        (c) Pulmonary wedge pressure below 6 mmHg

  f) Multi-organ dysfunction syndrome (MODS)—Sepsis with involvement of three or more organs

    i.   Pulmonary failure—acute respiratory distress syndrome (ARDS)

    ii.   Central nervous system—acute mental deterioration

    iii. Renal—rise in serum creatinine, oliguria

    iv. Hematologic—disseminated intravascular coagulation (DIC)—D-dimer > 3 mcg/mL, thrombocytopenia, platelet drop

    v.   Hepatic—elevated enzymes/coagulation findings to twice their normal levels

    vi. Gastrointestinal—paralytic ileus

3. Acute lung injury (ALI)/acute respiratory distress syndrome (ARDS)[11]

  a) ALI is defined as a syndrome of inflammation and increased permeability of alveoli that may or may not coexist with left atrial or pulmonary capillary hypertension to differentiate the syndrome from pulmonary edema secondary to heart failure.[11] Causes of ALI and ARDS include sepsis, primary pneumonia, aspiration pneumonia, trauma, massive transfusions, fat embolism, cardiopulmonary bypass, and pancreatitis. The defining characteristics of ALI includes the following

    i.   Timing—acute onset

    ii.   Oxygenation—Pao_2/Fio_2 ratio $\leq$ 300 mmHg (regardless of positive end-expiratory pressure [PEEP] level)

    iii. Chest radiograph—bilateral infiltrates seen on frontal chest radiograph

    iv. Pulmonary artery wedge pressure— $\leq$ 18 mmHg when measure or no clinical evidence of left arterial hypertension.

  b) ARDS is the most extreme form of ALI resulting in severe respiratory failure. The defining characteristics of ARDS include all of the following

    i.   Timing—acute onset

    ii.   Oxygenation—Pao_2/Fio_2 ratio $\leq$ 200 mmHg (regardless of PEEP level)

    iii. Chest radiograph—bilateral infiltrates seen on frontal chest radiograph

27

iv. Pulmonary artery wedge pressure— ≤ 18 mmHg when measure or no clinical evidence of left arterial hypertension

c) Pathophysiology

i. Site of injury is the alveolar-capillary membrane where there is a disruption, which alters permeability.

ii. Caused by direct injury (e.g., aspiration, inhalation of toxins, pulmonary contusion)

iii. Indirect injury (e.g., shock, head injury, pancreatitis, diabetic coma)

iv. Changes lead to leaky membrane and accumulation of protein-rich fluid in the interstitial and intra-alveolar spaces, which interferes with gas exchange.

v. Edema, hemorrhage, and atelectasis occur.

vi. Ventilation-perfusion mismatch with eventual increase in dead space.

vii. Decreased lung surfactant leads to decreased compliance and increased lung stiffness.

viii. Resistance of blood flow through lungs leads to narrowing of pulmonary vessels.

d) Prognosis

i. ARDS is often fatal with mortality rate of 60%.

ii. Highest mortality is for those presenting with sepsis.

iii. Lung repair can take up to 6 months with 50% of patients having no significant lung damage after that time.[7]

4. Traumatic injuries

a) Unintentional tramatic injuries are the 5th leading cause of death in the United States.[12] Traumatic injuries that are associated with high mortality rates include traumatic brain injury (e.g., subdural hemorrhage, subarachnoid hemorrhage, diffuse axonal injury), thoracic trauma (e.g., cardiac tamponade, open thorax, tracheobronchial tree injuries, great vessel disruption), abdominal trauma (e.g., mesenteric ischemia, liver injury, splenic injury), and orthopedic fractures (e.g., pelvic ring disruption, long bone fractures).

b) Severity of injury is reported as the Injury Severity Score (ISS).[13] The ISS is a composite score with a range of 0-75. An ISS of 15 or greater indicates severe trauma and is associated with high mortality rates.

c) Traumatic injuries also have high morbidity rates and often require prolonged rehabilitation, which places a psychological, emotional, and financial burden on the patient and family.

5. Acute renal failure (ARF) (See Chapter 21, *Renal Conditions*)

a) Acute renal failure is characterized by the loss of ability to excrete waste products and to regulate fluid and electrolytes and acid-base balance as described below.

27

b) Pre-renal failure—caused by a physiologic state causing decreased renal perfusion resulting from decreased renal arterial pressures and filtration

c) Intrarenal failure—problems that involve the renal tissue

   i. Common type is acute tubular necrosis.

   ii. Accounts for 75% of acute renal failure.

   iii. Caused by decreased perfusion to renal tissue over period of time associated with

     (a) Hypotension

     (b) Hypovolemia secondary to general hemorrhage or dehydration

     (c) Burns, trauma

   iv. Other causes include

     (a) Radiographic contrast

     (b) Nonsteroidal anti-inflammatory drugs (NSAIDs)

     (c) Antibiotics

     (d) Transfusion reaction

     (e) Infection

d) Post renal failure—caused by obstruction preventing urine output.

   i. Calculi, clot, neurogenic bladder, abscess, prostate hypertrophy, tumor

   ii. Acute tubular necrosis (ATN)

e) Renal replacement therapies—acute treatment that uses a highly porous filter and an extracorporal blood circuit for the purpose of removing intravascular fluids and solute.

   i. Hemodialysis—traditional means of providing ultrafiltration by principles of osmosis, diffusion, and convection.

     (a) Removes large volumes of blood.

     (b) Requires heparin for circuits in most cases.

   ii. Continuous veno-venous hemodialysis (CVVH) provides ultrafiltration in patients who are hemodynamically compromised and would not tolerate the large volume shifts associated with hemodialysis. Patients on CVVH should be considered as having advanced illness and therefore may be an indicator for a palliative care consult.

     (a) Most common renal replacement therapy in critical care environment.

     (b) Does not depend on a heparinized circuit to manage dialysis.

     (c) May be managed by critical care personnel rather than hemodialysis team.

27

        iii.   Peritoneal dialysis—means of filtration through peritoneal cavity via an access device 4-5 times a day. This method is for patients who cannot tolerate rapid fluid volume or glucose variations.

            (a)   A complication includes peritonitis if catheter malfunctions.

            (b)   Managed by patient and family so instruction and adherence to sterile technique is important to preventing infection.

    f)   Prognosis

        i.   50% mortality rate occurs in oliguria with acute renal failure.

        ii.   70% mortality rate in ARF occurring 24 hours following cardiogenic shock from myocardial infection.

6.   Palliative care considerations for acute presentations

    a)   The APRN should initiate discussions of likely outcomes, goals of care and benefits/burdens and risks of care in collaboration with the critical care team or the attending team as requested by consultation.

    b)   The APRN can initiate early family meetings to explain seriousness of condition, risks and benefits of therapies, possible outcomes, end-of-life values when necessary, determine proxy decision makers and advance care planning, and to update family regarding current status, changing prognosis, and need to consider therapeutic options. (See Chapter 5, *Communication*)

    c)   The APRN can assist in or initiate possible discussions regarding withholding or withdrawing care and non-beneficial (futile) care.

    d)   The APRN can explain and document discussions to not escalate care (e.g., transfer to the intensive care unit) but still treat reversible conditions.

    e)   The APRN can advocate for aggressive symptom management for dyspnea, fever, pain, and delirium.

    f)   The APRN can suggest transfer to a lesser-acuity unit to support changing goals of care as appropriate that match the goals and facilitate smooth transfer with information and continuity of care.

    g)   The APRN can consult social work and chaplaincy to support family in the setting of poor prognosis conditions.

B.   Patient Symptoms in Advanced Illness[14]

1.   Pain—there are many barriers that exist to providing optimum pain management for critically ill patients. Identified barriers include provider and patient knowledge deficits, inadequate ordering of pain medications, personal and cultural biases of clinicians, and communication difficulties.[15] Education of clinicians is important to remove these barriers. One challenge for the ED or ICU is that patients may be on long-term opioids at home. There are barriers of oligoanalgesia (under treatment of pain) in the ED related to multiple factors such as poor communication, inadequate education of providers, physicians concern that accurate diagnosis cannot be made when analgesia is provided, concern of encouraging drug-seeking behavior, lack of time to reassess pain and analgesic interventions in a busy setting.[16,17] The role of the palliative APRN is to help educate and recommend resuming the outpatient medication

27

regimen and/or providing appropriate doses of medication to meet the pain crisis needs of the patient. (See Chapter 6, *Pain*)

a) Assessment—assessment may be difficult due to inability of the patient to self-report the pain due to pathology or medications. Pain assessment tools for the nonverbal patient include behavioral observations as well as physiological parameters, but none of the current assessment tools are considered the standard measure of pain.[18] Pain assessment tools for the non-verbal patient include the Behavioral Pain Rating Scale,[19] PAIN Algorithm,[20] Behavioral Pain Scale,[21] Nonverbal Pain Scale,[22] Pain Behavior Assessment Tool,[23] and the Critical Care Pain Observation Tool.[24]

b) Anticipation of painful procedures and interventions—proactive intervention with analgesics before a procedure or intervention is essential in managing pain.[14] Painful procedures and interventions can include, but are not limited to, repositioning, suctioning, range of motion exercises, blood monitoring (e.g., arterial blood gases), dressing changes, and invasive procedures (e.g., indwelling catheter placement).

c) Daily goals for pain control should be discussed and high-dose analgesics, in conjunction with adjuvant therapies, may be required for some pain syndromes. Careful balance of dosing with adverse side effects require frequent re-assessment.

d) The palliative APRN can collaborate with critical care and emergency department leaders to develop educational tools (e.g., pocket cards) or policies for appropriate pain management during pain crises.

e) It may also be advantageous for ED and ICU collaboration to create policies for difficult pain crises and the use of various intravenous medications and consultation with anesthesia based pain services.

2. Dyspnea—there are many pathologies that cause dyspnea ranging from cardiac, pulmonary, oncology, trauma, or metabolic in addition to iatrogenic causes such as intubation. Anxiety can also exacerbate the sensation of breathlessness. (See Chapter 7, *Dyspnea*)

a) As with other symptoms, clinicians rely on patient self-report in order to understand the intensity and quality of dyspnea. However, in critical care settings, patients may be unable to report their dyspnea. A proposed model, Respiratory Distress Observation Scale (RDOS), incorporates physiological measures (e.g., heart rate, respiratory rate), behavioral observations (e.g., restlessness, paradoxic breathing pattern), accessory muscle use, nasal flaring, and the look of fear on the face of the patient to arrive at a composite score to rate dyspnea.[25] (See Chapter 20, *Pulmonary Conditions*)

b) The American College of Chest Physicians (ACCP) published their recommendations for the management of dyspnea in advanced cardiac and pulmonary diseases.[26] The recommendations include an ethical responsibility to treat dyspnea, collaborating with patients, individualized care plan to address dyspnea, dosing and titrating opioids to relieve dyspnea, and frequent reassessment to assure that treatments are serving the goal of palliating dyspnea without causing adverse effects, and communicating about palliative and end-of-life care with patients.

27

c) The American Thoracic Society (ATS) issued an official clinical policy statement recommending palliative care for patients with respiratory diseases in critical illness.[27] ATS asserts that all patients with serious or life-threatening diseases, particularly those with critical illness or advanced respiratory diseases, regardless of age or social circumstances, should have access to palliative care. In addition, health professionals should have an appropriate level of competence in palliative care and should seek consultation from palliative care experts as needed.

d) Treatment for dyspnea is indicated during disease-modifying therapies. Concurrent disease-modifying therapies can include

   i. Invasive airways (e.g., endotracheal intubation or advanced surgical airways such as a tracheostomy)

   ii. Non-invasive positive pressure ventilation (NPPV) such as BiPAP, nasal CPAP

   iii. Medications to reverse pathology such as beta agonists (e.g., albuterol), anticholinergics (e.g., ipratropium), steroids, antibiotics, nitric oxide/oxygen blends, among others.

e) Treatment of dyspnea during ventilator weaning or withdrawal is indicated. In the ED, when patients sustain a devastating injury or when an advance directive has indicated that intubation is not desired, patients can and should be extubated. In the ICU, patients are routinely extubated depending on resolution of their pathology or if the patient/family desires extubation in an end-of-life situation.

3. Delirium—common symptom of critically ill patients. The characteristics of delirium include acutely changing or fluctuating mental status, inattention, disorganized thinking and an altered level of consciousness that may or may not be accompanied by agitation.[28] Delirium is commonly divided into three types—hyperactive, hypoactive, and mixed. Hyperactive delirium is characterized by delirium with agitation or combative behavior. Hypoactive delirium is characterized with psychomotor slowing. Hypoactive delirium is difficult to differentiate from over sedation. Mixed delirium has agitation and psychomotor slowing. Some contributing factors to delirium in critical care include underlying pathology, medications (e.g., sedatives), and sleep deprivation.[29] (See Chapter 12, *Delirium*)

   a) Assessment—6 assessment tools exist for ICU patients—Cognitive Test for Delirium (CTD), abbreviated CTD, Confusion Assessment Method-ICU (CAM-ICU), Intensive Care Delirium Screening Checklist, NEECHAM Scale, and the Delirium Detection Score.[28]

   b) Treatment

      i. As with all symptoms, removal or reduction of the underlying etiology is essential.

      ii. Medications to manage delirium can include typical and atypical antipsychotics (e.g., haloperidol, ziprasidone, quetiapine) except for alcohol related delirium in which benzodiazepines are used.[29]

   c) Palliative care considerations include

27

      i.   Early identification and recognition of differential diagnosis from pain and other symptoms.

      ii.   Aggressive treatment and management of underlying etiology as appropriate to goals of care.

      iii.   Initiation of systematic screening for delirium.

      iv.   Interdisciplinary staff and family education.

C. Patient Decision-Making and Communication (See Chapter 4, *Ethical Considerations* and Chapter 5, *Communication*)

1. A patient's decision-making capacity is a vital determinate of care.[14] In the emergency and critical care settings, it is important to establish if the patient has decision-making capacity to match the beneficial interventions with his/her wishes.[30] Often, the advanced stage of illness or injury and severity of the underlying pathology impairs decision-making capacity. If the patient does not have decision-making capacity, it is imperative to identify a proxy decision maker for healthcare.

2. There are 4 elements that comprise decision-making capacity—ability to communicate choice, ability to understand the information needed to make the decision, ability to escribe the consequences of the decision, and ability to reason and deliberate the choice being made.[31] Although not a substitute for a full assessment of decision-making capacity,[32] the MacArthur Competence Assessment Tool for Treatment (MacCAT-T) can help assess decision-making capacity especially in the setting of a concurrent mental illness.[33] The MacCAT-T helps clinicians assess if the patient has decision-making capacity after conducting an interview following the MacCAT-T procedure. This may need to be conducted by psychiatry or psychology.

    a) Documentation of decision-making capacity should be in the medical record.

    b) Re-assessment and documentation should be done with changes in patient condition.

3. Understanding the impact of cultural/spiritual/religious backgrounds on the patient's decision-making is important. Who needs to be involved in decision-making? In the ED and ICU, social workers, chaplains, nurses, and any other healthcare providers can ask the family how critical decisions are made in the family.

4. Decisions and plans of care should be communicated to other healthcare providers as well as the patient and family and should be documented in the medical record in a timely manner.[14] It is best if this is done by all team members.

5. Psychosocial support using an interdisciplinary team should be offered to patients, families, and possibly even staff to mitigate against traumatic stress.

6. Challenges specific to the critical care settings.[3]

    a) Lack of availability of and/or clarity in advance directives

    b) Lack of clarity of an appropriate proxy decision-maker if patient lacks capacity

27

c) Fear of litigation

d) Quickly establishment new relationships with patients and families can lead to possible mistrust or misunderstanding of values and goals since a full assessment of family dynamics, relationships, and understandings of severity of illness may not occur. Therefore, building trusting relationships is vitally important.

e) Need for emergent decisions to be made during this time of crisis.

f) Ethical dilemmas are common due to the lack of communication and understanding from both the healthcare staff as well as patients/families.

g) Decisions to withdraw life-sustaining technology in intensive care for unconscious patients necessitate supportive/palliative care measures.

   i. Complex decisions made concerning benefit of critical care with respect to functional outcome versus medical futility.

      (a) Decisions about escalation of aggressive care and outcomes are often not able to be made by patient.

      (b) The presence of advance directives, when available, guide the hospital staff in identifying the patient's surrogate decision maker and assist in determining the level of care desired.

      (c) Two standards for surrogate decision-making.[9] (See Chapter 4, *Ethical Considerations*)

         (i) Substituted judgment

         (ii) Best interests of the patient

      (d) Social service involvement may assist with the identification and management of surrogate decision-maker and family dynamics.

         (i) Withdrawal or withholding of technology may be initiated by the patient, family, or the critical care team.

   ii. Quality of life decisions need to be discussed at family meetings attended by physician, nurse, and/or social worker and chaplain.

      (a) Shared decision-making among the patient, family, and healthcare providers drives the process.

      (b) Families exhibit certain common behaviors when moving through the process of withdrawal of technology. They include

         (i) A willingness to admit that recovery of the patient is not likely.

         (ii) Acknowledgement that the patient would not have wanted to continue treatment that will not reverse condition.

         (iii) Struggling with the conviction that they are doing the right thing.

      (c) Palliative care intensifies when decisions of withdrawal of technology are contemplated.

      (d) Families need support and validation that these are difficult decisions.

27

    iii. Preparation for withdrawal of technology includes

        (a) A pre–event clinical team meeting to prepare for the process with time to review medications, concerns, and support for process.

        (b) Assessment of spiritual, religious, and cultural rituals and practices that need to be addressed and facilitated by the team. Address contacting spiritual leaders, dressing in religious garments and/or honoring rituals if possible.

        (c) The removal of extraneous equipment such as transducer, ventilator, or blood equipment from bedside to allow family access to the patient.

        (d) The placement of chairs, tissues, etc. in room to promote comfort. Place bed in low position, side rails down to allow access to patient. Provide chairs for comfort, favorite music etc. to promote healing environment.

        (e) Pre-medicate the patient with appropriate medications for comfort such as pain, dyspnea, seizures, and agitation.

        (f) Make sure to clamp arterial lines, central lines etc. Discontinue unnecessary medications, IVs, tubes such as nasogastric tube (NGT) or oral gastric tubes again to make patient look as normal as possible.

        (g) Cover patient with blanket, leaving arms out to provide family with opportunity to hold patient's hand.

        (h) Turn off monitor screens in room to prevent distraction. This allows family to concentrate on patient, not monitoring screen.

        (i) Provide basic hygiene, clean and moisturize mouth to promote respectful care of the body.

        (j) Remove ETT—if family members are present conceal tube removal with towel or pad.

7. The role of the palliative APRN is to support the family and staff during crisis and traumatic stress of withdrawal of technological support in critical care settings. This is best done in collaboration with fellow team members and determining who can support whom. Several conditions that are difficult include

    a) Brain death—established criteria that recognizes brain death as death. This may be difficult for families as the patient still has physiological functioning and can seem to still be "alive" yet the higher brain functions are no longer present. (See Chapter 23, *Neurological Conditions*)

        i. Uniform Determination of Death Act of 1980[34]

            (a) Model for state legislation, definition of death.

            (b) Defines death as

                (i) Irreversible cessation of circulatory and respiratory functions.

27

      (ii) Irreversible cessation of all brain functions, including the brain stem.

  ii. Criteria commonly used

    (a) Known cause or condition causing decline.

    (b) Absence of medication, which could interfere with exam.

    (c) Temperature greater than 32°C

    (d) Requires two neurologic exams; one by a qualified physician (preferably one in neuroscience specialty) 6 hours apart. Exam establishes unresponsiveness, in particular

      (i) No brainstem reflexes (function)

      (ii) Apnea testing

    (e) If barbiturates have been used, then criteria may be established by radionuclide brain perfusion imaging secondary to diagnosis of no cerebral blood flow.[8] Effects of barbiturates may mimic a depressed neurologic exam and the half-life can be long. Therefore, this study may help in determining whether the cerebral blood flow has been catastrophically altered throughout the entire brain.

    (f) Other ancillary testing—these tests will help understand if there is organized electrical activity of the brain (required for purposeful movement or organized thinking) and to understand if catastrophic blood flow interruption has occurred.

      (i) Electroencephalography (EEG)

      (ii) Transcranial Doppler

      (iii) Cerebral angiography

      (iv) Somatosensory and brain stem auditory evoked potentials

  iii. The APRN should model family support behaviors that can be offered by nurses (bedside and charge nurses), social workers, and/or chaplains in the ED and ICU.

    (a) There must be ongoing family meetings throughout hospitalization with focus on the preparation of the family for a grave prognosis. Strategies include

      (i) Learning about the patient's life, family dynamics as first steps in relationship building.

      (ii) Explaining the process of withdrawal. Assessment of important social, cultural, or religious rituals.

      (iii) Asking family who they want present to support them.

      (iv) Clarifying and answering questions while determining understanding of concept of grave prognosis, ICU care, and, when appropriate, brain death.

      (v) If brain death is established, the family should be told that the patient has been declared dead and provided with

27

explanations for continued heart beat and other autonomic functions.

(vi) It is vital that the discussion of brain death is always separate from discussion of organ donation. Organ donation must be done by authorized Organ Procurement Organization (OPO) representative.

(vii) If organ donation is not an option, a timely plan is made for removal of the ETT and ventilator with the family.

    a.   The family should be reminded that the patient is dead and assured that therefore the patient is not experiencing discomfort and/or suffering. The ETT is removed after such discussions.

    b.   Provide the family access to the patient during this process, if they want to and are able.

    c.   Allow for as much time at the bedside as possible before and after process.

    d.   Discussion with family about process of withdrawal of ETT, including their presence at the bedside if desired.

        i)   Describe what the process may look like including observed phenomena; explanation of movements that may occur as oxygen leaves muscle which may be misinterpreted as purposeful movement. Since patient has been declared dead by virtue of brain death, avoid referral to dying process.

        ii)   Assess and implement cultural or religious rituals that may be a comfort during the process.

    e.   Review the patient's inability to feel pain or distress as the brain is no longer working.

    f.   Describe the process of post-withdrawal care so family knows what to expect and they can choose whether to perform these tasks with assistance from nurses.

i.   Healthcare chaplaincy and social work should be present for all meetings if possible and during the actual withdrawal process.

    (a)   Considerations in withdrawal of mechanical ventilation. (See Chapters 20, *Pulmonary Conditions* and Chapter 35, *Oxygen: From Supplemental Therapy to Mechanical Ventilation*)

        (i)   Immediate removal of endotracheal tube versus terminal weaning.

            a.   Removal of ETT may help decrease the time to asystole but increase the possibility of respiratory stridor.

            b.   Patient looks more natural with tubes removed from face and may be able to communicate with loved ones.

        (i)   Terminal wean—may increase time to asystole.

27

      a. Keeping the ETT in place while turning down the ventilator may increase comfort by decreasing stridor.

      b. Consideration should be given to the reason for ETT tube, impairment of the integrity of the tracheal region versus respiratory failure.

      c. Pre-assessment of the potential for stridor once the ETT is removed should be done. Institutions have many various protocols for ETT removal as there is no definitive process or research to show evidence of one way over another.

      d. Most situations of withdrawal are unpredictable. So proactive planning should be in place for acute stridor including opioids, benzodiazepines, or even epinephrine.

      e. Premedication with morphine or other opioid for pain and dyspnea before tube removal.

(a) Anticipatory dosing of medication opioid and benzodiazepine regimen depending on symptoms and patient's current symptom management plan.

(b) Withdrawal of hemodynamic support discontinuance of fluid volume and/or vasopressor support.

(c) Use of physiologic signs such as tachypnea, tachycardia, distressed breathing patterns to make decisions for titration in nonresponsive patients.

   (i) For opioid naïve patients, morphine 2.5-5 mg IV boluses every 5-10 minutes as needed. This provides rapid onset within a few minutes. An opioid infusion may also be appropriate with dosing titrated to prevent discomfort from respiratory distress and pain. Dosages to be adjusted for chronic use. Also hydromorphone may be needed in renal patients. Avoid fentanyl as the efficacy has not been established in the literature.

   (ii) Anxiolytics

      a. Lorazepam or midazolam is shorter acting and preferred. Dosing 0.5-2 mg IV every 10-15 minutes as needed for respiratory distress or other discomfort. After reaching stable dosing, consider round-the-clock (RTC) dosing every 2-4 hours. Thereafter can bolus every 2-4 hours with boluses or infusions per institution policy.

      b. Diazepam 2-10 mg IV or PR may need every 1-2 hours for distress.

   (iii) Anticholinergics for secretion control

      a. Scopolamine 0.4 mg IV every hour as needed. It should be noted that patches are inappropriate as they take 4 hours to reach peak effect.

  b. Glycopyrrolate IV 0.2-0.4 mg every 4-6 hours or nebulizer 0.8 3/day. The heart rate may increase as a side effect of the medication. It is not intended to resuscitate the patient.

  c. Hyoscyamine 0.2 mg sublingually every 6 hours.

  d. If hospice is involved, they may be allowed to use atropine ophthalmic solution. However, many hospital pharmacies will not allow because this is not an FDA approved usage of the medication.

 (iv) Neuroleptics for delirium if present. Haloperidol 0.5-2 mg IV every 2-4 hours. If patient may survive longer term, considerations to the cardiac effects of haloperidol need to be considered. Check the QTc interval on an electrocardiogram (ECG) as haloperidol can increase the QTc interval and pre-dispose a patient to torsades de pointes.

 (v) Antipyretics

  a. Acetaminophen 650-1000 mg orally or via gastrostomy tube every 6-8 hours; 600-1200 mg by rectum every 6-8 hours, 650-1000 mg IV every 4-6 hours. Not to exceed 4 gm in 24 hours.

  b. Can also consider the use of IV ketorolac for 15-30 mg every 8 hours. Avoid in renal failure or in bleeding disorders.

(a) Family—essential to provide support after death occurs.

 (i) Provide information for social work follow-up, support groups, and grief counseling. This includes community resources such as hospice bereavement support.

b) Organ donation

 i. Families facing the brain death of a loved one, or death from other causes may find comfort in being able to help others through the offer of organ donation.

 (a) Combination of two medical advances that have promoted the practice of transplant medicine.

 (b) Immunosuppression

 (c) Brain death criteria established by Uniform Determination of Death Act of 1980.[34]

 ii. Organs that may be donated

 (a) In the critical care setting, organs that may be donated include the heart, liver, lungs, pancreas, liver, and bowel.

 (b) Organ procurement criteria are ever changing. Prompt referral to organ procurement organizations in the face of an imminently dying patient is mandated so that designated requestors can talk about donation with families.[35]

27

(c) Eyes, skin, bone, heart valves, cornea may be donated post mortem.

iii. Organ procurement organizations (OPO) are available on referral to assist patient, family through organ donation process.

(a) Need to inform families that organ donation can only occur in critical care setting. This may affect potential transfer or referral to hospice.

(b) Changing criteria requires a referral to help in determination of patient's eligibility for donation.

(i) Health Care Financing Administration (HCFA) regulations include mandated revisions—these are conditions of participation in Medicare and Medicaid[35]

c. All deaths must be reported to OPO.

d. OPO must determine medical suitability.

e. Only OPO trained expert requestors present donation options to the family.

(ii) Early referral to OPO concerning impending brain death or donation after cardiac death enhances ability to explore patient's suitability for donation.

(iii) If patient is considered a possible donor candidate, the healthcare team and OPO representative collaborate to create a plan for presenting the OPO to the family for the consent process.

f. Decision by the family about withdrawal of medical support is made before consent sought.

g. Family may independently request OPO consult.

iv. Policies and process are different at each institution though the Joint Commission regulations are universal.

v. Brain death donation[36]

(a) Early referral to OPO

(b) Family asked for consent after brain death declared.

(c) Consent granted and recipient matching process is started by OPO.

(d) Healthcare team continues support and education to the family.

(e) Patient's body supported until operating room ready and recipient found.

(f) OPO informs family of successful transplantation and recipient status.

vi. Donation after cardiac death.

(a) Referral made when poor prognosis is evident.

(i) Chart reviewed by OPO for possible donor status.

27

        (ii) If not eligible, no further action needed.

        (iii) If eligible, a collaborative plan for presenting donation to the family is made.

  (b) Donation after cardiac death is described as a donation of organs after a patient has had medical support withdrawn and becomes asystolic in 60-90 minutes depending upon the organ to be donated. The duration of asystole before declaration of death is anywhere from 3-8 minutes depends on institutional protocols.[37]

        (i) Organs include kidney, pancreas, liver, with possibility of lung.

            a. Eligibility criteria are determined by OPO.

            b. If family consents, plans are made to withdraw support in the operating room.

        (ii) Requires coordination with OPO, ICU, operating room staff.

        (iii) Family must be educated about entire process with cultural sensitivity and with respect to specific institutional policies. Concerns include the following

            a. Whether family will be able to be present with patient in the operating room for withdrawal.

            b. Whether family taken to the operating room and dressed in operating room attire (scrubs)

        (iv) Healthcare provider accompanies patient and actively withdraws support.

            a. Patient is managed as a he/she would be in ICU environment with medications that ensure comfort.

            b. Family may stay with patient only until asystole and then escorted out by OPO family counselor.

        (v) If patient does not reach asystole within prescribed time he/she is taken back to the intensive care to a palliative care bed depending on availability and institutional policy.

        (vi) Support is needed for the family as they may now be disappointed that donation could not take place in the face of their loved ones death. Referral to bereavement programs, including hospice may be appropriate.

        (vii) Social worker, OPO, and palliative APRN provide help in coordinating care and follow up support to the family after the patient's death.

III. SPECIAL TOPICS REGARDING FAMILIES

  A. Family meetings—family meetings are usually initiated by healthcare providers and are used to explain to the family the patient's condition and to discuss the plan of care. This is an incredibly stressful time for families. The goal of the family meeting should be discussed among all healthcare providers and specialties before meeting with the family. There should be one single message from all healthcare providers. Specific steps for conducting a family meeting and providing support to families before and after the family meeting have been proposed below.[38]

1. As the ED is designed to identify the medical issues and create a disposition plan, the family meeting can help determine the course of care throughout the hospital stay and at discharge. Family meetings in the ED are difficult due to the sense of urgency and limited time.[2] Meetings should have a singular focus such as resolving a question, understanding patient values and wishes, communicating a patient's status and prognosis, or establishing goals of care. Many of the following principles for an ICU family conference apply to the family conference in the ED.[2]

2. Preparing for a family conference about end-of-life care.

    a) Review of previous knowledge of the patient and/or family.

    b) Review of previous knowledge of the family's attitudes and reactions.

    c) Review of one's own knowledge of the disease including prognosis, treatment options.

    d) Examination of one's own personal feelings in terms of attitudes, biases, and related grief.

    e) A plan of the specifics of location and setting—a quiet, private place.

    f) Discussion with the family in advance about both health professional and family members who will be present at the meeting.

    g) Clarification of decision-makers such as surrogate decision-maker, power of attorney for healthcare, guardian, etc.

3. Holding a family conference about end-of-life care.

    a) Introduce everyone present.

    b) If appropriate, set the tone in a nonthreatening way: "This is a conversation we have with all families…"

    c) Discuss the goals of the specific conference. Elicit concerns of family.

    d) Find out what the family understands.

    e) Review what has happened and what is happening to the patient.

    f) Discuss prognosis frankly in a way that is meaningful to the family.

    g) Acknowledge uncertainty in the prognosis.

    h) Review the principle of substituted judgment—"What would the patient want?"

    i) Support the family's decision.

    j) Do not discourage all hope; consider redirecting hope toward a comfortable death with dignity if appropriate.

    k) Avoid temptation to give too much medical detail.

    l) Make it clear that withholding life-sustaining treatment is not withholding caring.

27

    m) Make explicit what care will be provided including symptom management, where the care will be delivered, and the family's access to the patient.

    n) If life-sustaining treatments will be withheld or withdrawn, with request or permission of family, offer explanation of the possible dying process.

    o) Use repetition to show that you understand what the patient or family is saying.

    p) Acknowledge strong emotions and use reflection to encourage patients or families to talk about these emotions.

    q) Tolerate silence.

4. Finishing an ICU family conference about end-of-life care.

    a) Achieve common understanding of the disease and treatment issues.

    b) Make a recommendation about treatment.

    c) Ask if there are any questions.

    d) Ensure basic follow-up plan and make sure the family knows how to reach you for questions.

5. Talking with families before the family conference.

    a) Invite the family to include other essential members of the patient's family such as friends or clergy.

    b) Tell the family what to expect during their conference with the healthcare team members.

    c) Talk with the family about their spiritual or religious needs and take actions to address the unmet spiritual or religious needs.

    d) Talk with the family about specific cultural needs and take actions to address unmet cultural needs.

    e) Talk with the family about what the patient valued in life.

    f) Talk with the family about the patient's illness and treatment.

    g) Talk with the family about their feelings.

    h) Reminisce with the family about the patient.

    i) Tell the family it is all right to talk to and touch their loved one.

    j) Discuss with the family what the patient might have wanted if he/she were able to participate in the treatment decision-making process.

    k) Locate a private place or room to allow the family to talk among themselves.

6. After the conference

    a) Talk with the family about how the conference went.

    b) Talk with any other healthcare team members who were present at the conference about how the conference went.

    c) Ask the family if they had any questions following the conference.

27

d) Talk with the family about their feelings.

e) Talk with the family about any disagreement among the family concerning the plan of care.

f) Talk with the family about changes in the patient's plan of care as a result of the conference.

g) Support the decisions the family made during the conference.

h) Assure the family that the patient will be kept comfortable.

i) Tell the family it is all right to talk to and touch their loved one.

j) Locate a private place or room for the family to talk among themselves.

B. Family presence during resuscitation (FPR)—the option for family to be present during resuscitation has been demonstrated to help in the bereavement of survivors during a cardiopulmonary arrest.[39] Components of a successful program to integrate FPR include the following[40]

1. Assessing whether FPR is appropriate in the situation. Talking with the resuscitation providers, assessing the family's coping strategies, and giving appropriate information are important.

2. Having a facilitator who is trained to assess families and understands the functioning of the medical team accompany the family into the room, and provide support during and after resuscitation. This may be a designated person from ED or a palliative care provider.

3. Limit the number of family present during resuscitation to 1 or 2 to ensure adequate support for them.

4. Preparing the family with "ground rules" such as where they will stand, how long they will remain, how to ask questions, what the patient will look like, and cautions about disrupting medical personnel.

5. Surrogate decision-making—the facilitator may be the liaison to support the family in making decisions regarding continued resuscitation depending on local laws about who can make proxy decisions.

6. Post-event family support—debriefing the family after the resuscitation is an important aspect in their coping and grief.

IV. CARE FOR THE CAREGIVER

A. Caregiver Stress—professional caregivers in critical care areas are challenged with preparing for both survival and death as possible outcomes simultaneously.[41] This tension of trying to provide curative or disease-modifying care while also being thoughtful that the care may not be successful. It may lead to great uncertainty and potential moral distress among clinicians and families.

B. Additional stressors include role conflict, overload, and strain; caring for brain-dead patients; communication problems with other healthcare professionals; and communication problems with patients and family members.[41]

C. In the ED, clinicians have reported challenges in providing palliative care such as equating palliative care with end-of-life care; disagreement about the feasibility and desirability of providing palliative care in the ED; patients for whom a palliative

27

approach has been established often visit the ED because family members are distressed by end-of-life symptoms; lack of communication between outpatient and ED providers leads to undesirable outcomes (e.g., resuscitation of patients with a do-not-resuscitate order); conflict around withholding life-prolonging treatment is common (e.g., between patient's family and written advance directives); and training in pain management is inadequate.[42]

D. Some coping behaviors of clinicians may include distancing; depersonalization or avoidance of patients or families; feelings of grief, guilt, or helplessness.[41]

E. Palliative care clinicians can help support critical care clinicians through frequent debriefings during creation of plans of care, during patient care conferences, as well as after a patient death.[29] This is particularly true for difficult or 'bad' deaths.

F. One format for formal debriefing can include[43]

1. Welcome and introductions.

2. Factual information/case review regarding the circumstances of the case as seen by the various participants.

3. Grief responses by providers after the death.

4. Emotional responses about the care of the patient/family/other staff over the course of the hospitalization.

5. Acknowledgment that it is okay to experience grief and loss. This is followed by a discussion of strategies for coping with grief.

6. Review of lessons learned.

7. Acknowledgement of care provided in the spirit of beneficence and identification of resources for further help.

G. Encouraging clinicians to engage in self-care activities can help with coping and prevent burn out and compassion fatigue in the ED and ICU.[44]

1. Empower staff to be relieved from care responsibilities and take a break.

2. Encourage discussions about the experience with a colleague.

3. Promote reflection of one's feelings after the event.

4. Focus on the positive actions, and not the negative.

5. Utilization of basic health principles such as physical exercise, meditation, humor, music, eating properly, and adequate rest to promote self-care as well as encourage use of earned time.

V. CONCLUSION

A. Emergency and ICU settings are high-stress, fast-paced environments that require quick decision-making.

B. Constant tension between providing disease-modifying treatments with the possibility that these treatments may not be working.

C. Assessment of symptoms in a population that may not be able to self-report is difficult and therefore symptom directed treatments may be under-utilized.

D. Families may experience traumatic stress so communication is vital and shared decision-making is imperative.

E. Care of the caregiver is also important to relieve accumulated stress and prevent compassion fatigue.

F. The APRN has a vital role in communicating with all of the internal and external healthcare teams. They have a perspective of the holistic view of the patient and the situation in the critical care arena. They can help guide the process triaging the patient in the ED and advocating for aggressive ICU care or promoting comfort in the ICU. She/he can promote early consultation to a hospice team to collaborate on the care plan. The APRN can provide continuity in following the patient and family from the ED to the intensive care area. The APRN is essential to provide communication across transitions of care. Finally, she/he can advocate the wishes of the patient in terms of values, preferences, and beliefs and initiate interdisciplinary care.

CITED REFERENCES

1. Ferrell BR, Dahlin C, Campbell ML, Paice JA, Malloy P, Virani R. End-of-Life Nursing Education Consortium (ELNEC) training program: improving palliative care in critical care. *Crit Care Nurs Q.* 2007;30(3):206-212.

2. Emanuel L, Quest T, eds. *The Education in Palliative and End-of-Life Care for Emergency Medicine.* Chicago, IL: The EPEC™ Project; 2007.

3. Chan GK. End-of-life care models and emergency department care. *Academic Emergency Medicine.* 2004;11(1):79-86.

4. Chan GK. Trajectories of approaching death in the emergency department: clinician narratives of patient transitions to the end of life. *J Pain Symptom Manage.* 2011;42(6):864-881.

5. Kaplow R, Relf M. Critical care nursing practice: promoting excellence through caring, competence, and commitment. In: Morton PG, Fontaine DK, eds. *Critical Care Nursing. A Holistic Approach.* 9th ed. Philadelphia, PA: Wolters Kluwer Health/Lippincott Williams & Wilkins; 2009:3-17.

6. Horan TC, Andrus M, Dudeck MA. CDC/NHSN surveillance definition of health care-associated infection and criteria for specific types of infections in the acute care setting. *Am. J. Infect. Control.* 2008;36(5):309-332.

7. Ashraf M, Ostrosky-Zeichner L. Ventilator-associated pneumonia: a review. *Hosp Pract (Minneap).* 2012;40(1):93-105.

8. Mermel LA, Allon M, Bouza E, et al. Clinical practice guidelines for the diagnosis and management of intravascular catheter-related infection: 2009 update by the Infectious Diseases Society of America. *Clin Infect Dis.* 2009;49(1):1-45.

9. Kochanek KD, Xu J, Murphy SL, Miniño AM, Kung HC. Deaths: Preliminary data for 2009. National Vital Statistics Reports. Hyattsville, MD: National Center for Health Statistics. 2011;59(4):1-51. Available at: www.cdc.gov/nchs/data/nvsr/nvsr59/nvsr59_04.pdf. Accessed September 4, 2012.

10. Levy MM, Fink MP, Marshall JC, et al. 2001 SCCM/ESICM/ACCP/ATS/SIS International Sepsis Definitions Conference. *Crit Care Med.* 2003;31(4):1250-1256.

11. Bernard GR, Artigas A, Brigham KL, et al. The American-European Consensus Conference on ARDS. Definitions, mechanisms, relevant outcomes, and clinical trial coordination. *Am J Respir Crit Care Med.* 1994;149(3 Pt 1):818-824.

12. Centers for Disease Control. *Leading Causes of Death.* 2012. Available at: www.cdc.gov/nchs/fastats/lcod.htm. Accessed March 20, 2012.

13. Baker SP, O'Neill B, Haddon W, Long WB. The injury severity score: a method for describing patients with multiple injuries and evaluating emergency care. *J Trauma.* 1974;14(3):187-196.

14. Mularski RA, Curtis JR, Billings JA, et al. Proposed quality measures for palliative care in the critically ill: a consensus from the Robert Wood Johnson Foundation Critical Care Workgroup. *Crit Care Med.* 2006;34(11 Suppl):S404-411.

15. Pasero C, Puntillo K, Li D, et al. Structured approaches to pain management in the ICU. *Chest.* 2009;135(6):1665-1672.

16. Stalnikowicz R, Mahamid R, Kaspi S, Brezis M. Undertreatment of acute pain in the emergency department: a challenge. *Int J Qual Health Care.* 2005;17(2):173-176.

17. Puntillo K, Neighbor M, Chan GK, Garbez R. The influence of chief complaint on opioid use in the emergency department. *J Opioid Manage.* 2006;2(4):228-235.

27

18. Li D, Puntillo K, Miaskowski C. A review of objective pain measures for use with critical care adult patients unable to self-report. *J Pain.* 2008;9(1):2-10.

19. Mateo OM, Krenzischek DA. A pilot study to assess the relationship between behavioral manifestations and self-report of pain in postanesthesia care unit patients. *J Post Anesth Nurs.* 1992;7(1):15-21.

20. Puntillo KA, Miaskowski C, Kehrle K, Stannard D, Gleeson S, Nye P. Relationship between behavioral and physiological indicators of pain, critical care patients' self-reports of pain, and opioid administration. *Crit Care Med.* 1997;25(7):1159-1166.

21. Payen JF, Bru O, Bosson JL, et al. Assessing pain in critically ill sedated patients by using a behavioral pain scale. *Crit Care Med.* 2001;29(12):2258-2263.

22. Odhner M, Wegman D, Freeland N, Steinmetz A, Ingersoll GL. Assessing pain control in nonverbal critically ill adults. *Dimen Crit Care Nurs.* 2003;22(6):260-267.

23. Puntillo KA, Morris AB, Thompson CL, Stanik-Hutt J, White CA, Wild LR. Pain behaviors observed during six common procedures: results from Thunder Project II. *Crit Care Med.* 2004;32(2):421-427.

24. Gelinas C, Fillion L, Puntillo KA, Viens C, Fortier M. Validation of the critical-care pain observation tool in adult patients. *Am J Crit Care.* 2006;15(4):420-427.

25. Campbell ML. Assessing respiratory distress when the patient cannot report dyspnea. *Nurs Clin North Am.* 2010;45(3):363-373.

26. Mahler DA, Selecky PA, Harrod CG, et al. American College of Chest Physicians consensus statement on the management of dyspnea in patients with advanced lung or heart disease. *Chest.* 2010;137(3):674-691.

27. Lanken PN, Terry PB, Delisser HM, et al. An official American Thoracic Society clinical policy statement: palliative care for patients with respiratory diseases and critical illnesses. *Am J Respir Crit Care Med.* 2008;177(8):912-927.

28. Devlin JW, Fong JJ, Fraser GL, Riker RR. Delirium assessment in the critically ill. *Intensive Care Med.* 2007;33(6):929-940.

29. Frontera JA. Delirium and sedation in the ICU. *Neurocrit Care.* 2011;14(3):463-474.

30. Magauran BG, Jr. Risk management for the emergency physician: competency and decision-making capacity, informed consent, and refusal of care against medical advice. *Emerg Med Clin North Am.* 2009;27(4):605-614, viii.

31. President's Commission for the Study of Ethical Problems in Medicine and Biomedical and Behavioral Research. *The Ethical and Legal Implications of Informed Consent in the Patient-Practitioner Relationship. Making Health Care Decisions.* Vol. 1. Washington, DC: US Government Printing Office; 1982.

32. Appelbaum PS. Clinical practice. Assessment of patients' competence to consent to treatment. *NEJM.* 2007;357(18):1834-1840.

33. Raymont V, Bingley W, Buchanan A, et al. Prevalence of mental incapacity in medical inpatients and associated risk factors: cross-sectional study. *Lancet.* 2004;364(9443):1421-1427.

34. National Conference of Commissioners on Uniform State Laws. *Uniform Determination of Death Act.* 1980. Available at: www.law.upenn.edu/bll/archives/ulc/fnact99/1980s/udda80.htm. Accessed May 8, 2012.

35. Centers for Medicare and Medicaid Services, Department of Health and Human Services. *Section 482.45 Condition of Participation: Organ, Tissue and Eye Procurement.* 2009. Available at: www.gpo.gov/fdsys/search/pagedetails.action?browsePath=Title+42%2FChapter+IV%2FSubchapter+G%2FPart+482%2FSubpart+C%2FSection+482.45&granuleId=CFR-2009-title42-vol5-sec482-45&packageId=CFR-2009-title42-vol5&collapse=true&bread=true. Accessed June 22, 2011.

36. Joint Commission. *Revisions to Standard LD.3.110.* 2006. Available at: www.sharenj.org/.../JCAHO%20Standard%20LD%203%20110.pdf. Accessed May 8, 2012.

37. Steinbrook R. Organ donation after cardiac death. *NEJM.* 2007;357(3):209–213.

38. Curtis JR, Patrick DL, Shannon SE, Treece PD, Engelberg RA, Rubenfeld GD. The family conference as a focus to improve communication about end-of-life care in the intensive care unit: opportunities for improvement. *Crit Care Med.* 2001;29(2 Suppl):N26-33.

39. Egging D, Crowley M, Arruda T, et al. Emergency nursing resource: family presence during invasive procedures and resuscitation in the emergency department. *J Emerg Nurs.* 2011;37(5):469-473.

40. Bradley C, Lensky M, Brasel K. Implementation of a family presence during resuscitation protocol #233. *J Palliat Med.* 2011;14(1):98-99.

41. Block SD. Helping the clinician cope with death in the ICU. In: Curtis JR, Rubenfeld GD, eds. *Managing Death in the Intensive Care Unit.* New York, NY: Oxford University Press; 2001:183-191.

42. Smith AK, Fisher J, Schonberg MA, et al. Am I doing the right thing? Provider perspectives on improving palliative care in the emergency department. *Ann Emerg Med.* 2009;54(1):86-93, 93 e81.

43. Keene EA, Hutton N, Hall B, Rushton C. Bereavement debriefing sessions: an intervention to support health care professionals in managing their grief after the death of a patient. *Pediatr. Nurs.* 2010;36(4):185-189; quiz 190.

44. Badger JM. Understanding secondary traumatic stress. *Am J Nurs.* 2001;101(7):26-32.

27

ADDITIONAL RESOURCES

Aslakson RA, Wyskiel R, Thornton I, et al. Nurse-perceived barriers to effective communication regarding prognosis and optimal end-of-life care for surgical ICU patients: a qualitative exploration. *J Palliat Med.* 2012;15(8):910-915.

Bradley C, Lensky M, Brasel K. Family presence during resuscitation #232. *J Palliat Med.* 2011;14(1):97-98.

Brandt DS, Shinkunas LA, Gehlbach TG, Kaldjian LC. Understanding goals of care statements and preferences among patients and their surrogates in the medical ICU. *J Hosp Palliat Nurs.* 2012;14(2):126-132.

Chou KT, Chen CS, Su KC, et al. Hospital outcomes for patients with stage III and IV lung cancer admitted to the intensive care unit for sepsis-related acute respiratory failure. *J Palliat Med.* July 2012, ahead of print.

Lamba S, Nagurka R, Walther S, Murphy P. Emergency-department-initiated palliative care consults: a descriptive analysis. *J Palliat Med.* 2012;15(6):633-636.

Lamba S, Quest TE, Weissman DE. Emergency department management of hospice patients #246. *J Palliat Med.* 2011,14(12):1345-1346.

Lamba S, Quest TE, Weissman DE. Initiating a hospice referral from the emergency department #247. *J Palliat Med.* 2011;14(12):1346-1347.

Lewis SL. Critical reflection as a facilitator of palliative care in the neonatal intensive care unit: a concept clarification. *J Hosp Palliat Nurs.* 2012;14(6):405-413.

McKeown A, Booth MG, Strachan L, Calder A, Keeley PW. Unsuitable for the intensive care unit: what happens next? *J Palliat Med.* 2011;14(8):899-903.

Nelson JE, Cortez TB, Curtis JR, et al. Integrating palliative care in the icu: the nurse in a leading role. *J Hosp Palliat Nurs.* 2011;13(2):89-94.

Nelson P, ed. *Withdrawal of Life-Sustaining Therapies.* Pittsburgh, PA: Hospice and Palliative Nurses Association; 2010.

Richards CT, Gisondi MA, Chang CH, et al. Palliative care symptom assessment for patients with cancer in the emergency department: validation of the screen for palliative and end-of-life care needs in the emergency department instrument. *J Palliat Med.* 2011;14(6):757-764.

Smith TJ, Vota S, Patel S et al. Organ donation after cardiac death from withdrawal of life support in patients with amyotrophic lateral sclerosis. Journal of Palliative Medicine. 2012;15(1):16-19.

Waugh DG. Palliative care project in the emergency department. *J Palliat Med.* 2010;13(8):936-936.

Zomorodi M, Bowen GL. Value-behavior congruency when providing end-of-life care in the intensive care unit. *J Hosp Palliat Nurs.* 2010;12(5):295-302.

CHAPTER 28

PEDIATRICS

Joetta Descartes Wallace, RN, MSN, NP-C, CPON, CHPPN®

I. INTRODUCTION

The art and science of providing palliative and hospice care to infants, children, and adolescents with serious or life-threatening conditions requires special considerations by the APRN.

A. While the general principles of APRN practice remain consistent between adult and pediatric populations, the provision of palliative care for pediatrics is different in many aspects.

1. A recent multicenter cohort study found that most pediatric palliative care patients are still alive for more than a year after the initiation of palliative care. This relates to earlier referral in the disease trajectory than has typically been seen in adult populations, and the wide range of complex, chronic conditions that may precipitate referrals.[1]

2. Clinical models of care delivery, methods of communication, ethical issues, management concerns, education goals, reimbursement issues, and research foci, vary greatly depending on the child's age, developmental level, diagnosis, and family-specific circumstances.[2]

3. There are many other aspects of palliative care for pediatrics that are significantly different from adults. (see Table 1)

B. The National Hospice and Palliative Care Organization put forth *Standards of Practice for Pediatric Palliative Care and Hospice,* which serve as the foundation for optimal care for children with serious or life-threatening conditions.[3,4]

28

Table 1: Highlights of Pediatric Palliative Care[1,3-6]

Principles of Care	Therapies
• Various developmental and cognitive levels along course of illness • Developmental level may regress during stressful times • Concept of illness & death varies along developmental continuum • Widely variable time course of illness • Prognostication is very difficult[7] • Multiple subspecialists actively involved in care for treatment and evaluation • Hospice and palliative interdisciplinary approach to care • Diagnoses with genetic component • Legal issues regarding consent & assent • Family issues more pronounced, especially siblings • Reimbursement issues when pediatric patients fail to meet adult standards[3,4]	• Symptom assessment is more difficult • Healthier organs overall versus multi-organ system involvement • Palliation may include more aggressive therapies (e.g., surgery, parenteral nutrition, chemotherapy, monitors) • Lack of FDA approval for many meds • Nutrition • Dosing of medications based on weight, which can change significantly over course of illness • Expressive therapies highly utilized (e.g., child life, music/art therapy)

C. In 2003, the Institute of Medicine (IOM) Committee on Palliative and End-of-Life Care for Children and Their Families published the report, *When Children Die: Improving Palliative and End-of-Life Care for Children and their Families.* This document delineated a new philosophy and recommended specific practices including having children and families participate in treatment decision-making, communication with families, accessing necessary organizations and services, creating support programs, providing appropriate education, and managing financial issues of healthcare.[5] The IOM report emphasized the development of programs, which would not require families to choose between palliative care services and continued approaches toward a cure. It spurred the initiation of the Children's Hospice and Palliative Care Coalition focusing on improving the care of children with life-threatening conditions.

D. Families and healthcare providers recognized that children benefit greatly when hospice teams become involved in the management of physical, social, and spiritual aspects of care, but realized that established criteria for beginning hospice were difficult for children to meet.

E. The need to accept a less than 6-month life expectancy and to forego all approaches to the underlying disease resulted in families being offered and opting for hospice benefits only very near the death of their child. This minimized the comfort the child might have received if accepted earlier, such as at diagnosis. The 2010 Patient Protection and Affordable Care Act (PPACA) included a small provision, which assured that terminally ill children enrolled in a Medicaid or state Children's Health Insurance Plan hospice benefit could receive curative approaches to their terminal health condition while simultaneously receiving palliative care.[8] Many hospices have not been prepared to meet the needs of this highly specialized clientele because there have been very few hospices staffed with pediatric clinicians. Today, programs are being initiated throughout the United States for concurrent hospice services for pediatric patients while disease based approaches to care are still being undertaken.[8]

II. PRINCIPLES OF PEDIATRIC PALLIATIVE CARE

A. Pediatric Palliative Care—there are several definitions of pediatric palliative care. According to the World Health Organization (WHO) definition, pediatric-specific palliative care should[9]

1. Include active total care of the child's body, mind, and spirit, and provision of support to the entire family.

2. Begin with diagnosis and continue whether or not the child is receiving treatment directed at the disease.

3. Demand evaluation and alleviation of physical, psychological, and social distress by healthcare providers.

4. Require a broad interdisciplinary approach.

5. Include the family and utilize community resources, recognizing resources may be limited.

6. Be provided in extended care facilities, group homes, acute and intensive care hospital units, and at home.

7. Be developmentally appropriate and in-line with the family's cultural and personal values.[9]

28

Some programs may organize themselves according to the National Consensus Project For Quality Palliative Care, *Clinical Practice Guidelines for Quality Palliative Care,* which serve all populations, both adult and pediatrics.[10]

B.   Demographics of Childhood Death in the United States

All children who die do not receive palliative care. Conversely, all children who receive palliative care will not die while receiving palliative care. National mortality figures are helpful in looking at the scope of conditions and diseases in children. Key findings from the Linked Birth/Infant Death Data Set and Preliminary Mortality Data File of the Center for Disease Control revealed[11]

1.   The U.S. infant mortality rate did not decline from 2000 to 2005 and declined only 2% from 2005 to 2006.

2.   The U.S. infant mortality rate is higher than those in most other developed countries, and the gap between the U.S. infant mortality rate and the rates for the countries with the lowest infant mortality appears to be widening. (see Table 2)

3.   Increases in preterm birth and preterm-related infant mortality account for much of the lack of decline in the United States infant mortality rate from 2000 to 2005.

C.   Describing the Pediatric Palliative Care Population

Children with complex chronic conditions (CCC) are appropriate for pediatric palliative care services. A CCC is defined as a medical condition that

1.   Can reasonably be expected to last at least 12 months unless death intervenes.

2.   Involves either several organ systems or one organ system severely enough to require subspecialty pediatric care with a likelihood of some period in a tertiary care center.[2]

Survey data showed 13.9% of the 10.2 million U.S. children under the age of 17 have special healthcare needs. While not always considered for palliative care services, 24% have conditions that affect their daily activities.[2]

As a result of advances in pediatric technology, the number of children living with serious or life-threatening conditions requiring complex healthcare

28

Table 2: Infant mortality rate: United States, 2000-2005 and 2006 preliminary[11]

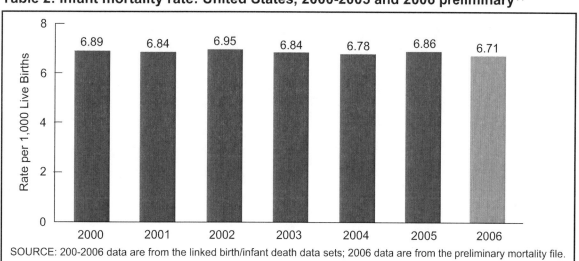

SOURCE: 200-2006 data are from the linked birth/infant death data sets; 2006 data are from the preliminary mortality file.

services is increasing as is the lifespan of these children. While it is recognized that children with these conditions could benefit from palliative care services, a Canadian study review of pediatric palliative care caseloads in 8 different centers found that only 5-12% of these children received services from established programs.[12] It is estimated that over 400,000 children suffer from life-long struggles with complex, chronic illnesses.[13] These children could benefit from and are appropriate referrals to pediatric palliative care services.[14] (see Table 3)

Between the ages of 1-19 years, the death rate is 32.2 per 100,000. This number has decreased by 5% since 2000, with the causes of death in 2005 being most often related to (in decreasing order) accidents, assault, malignancy, suicide, congenital malformations, chromosomal anomalies, and heart disease (see Table 4).[2] The leading causes of death varies within the age groups, and can be further categorized as death related to complications of a specific CCC. For example, in infancy the primary causes of death are congenital malformations and prematurity, but these infants can also be grouped with those who die from cardiovascular, respiratory, or neuromuscular conditions.[2] (see Table 4)

The Children's Project on Palliative/Hospice Services (previously known as Children's International Project on Palliative/Hospice Services [ChiPPS])

Table 3: Conditions Appropriate for Pediatric Palliative Care Referrals[14]

• Cancer • Chromosomal disorders (trisomy 5, 13, 16, 18) • Congenital defects or anomalies (anencephaly) • Hematological abnormalities (aplastic anemia) • HIV/AIDS • Inoperative cardiac conditions, lethal cardiac defects and hypoplastic lungs • Metabolic disorders (mitochondrial disorders, cystic fibrosis) • Multiple major medical problems, which together are life threatening (after trauma, complications of prematurity)	• Neurodegenerative disorders (adrenoleukodystrophy, mucopolysaccharidosis) • Neuromuscular degenerative conditions (Duchene's muscular dystrophy, spinal muscular atrophy) • Organ transplantation-before, during, and after • Perinatal hospice indicators—prenatal potentially lethal diagnosis & family chooses to continue pregnancy • Static encephalopathy

Table 4: Leading Causes of Death in Infants and Children[2]

	Leading Causes of Death	Complex Chronic Conditions
Infants— in utero-1 year	• Congenital malformations (19.5%) • Short gestation/LBW (16.5%) • Sudden Infant Death Syndrome (7.4%) • Maternal complications (6.3%) • Complications of placenta, cord, or membranes (4%) • Accidents/unintentional injury (4%)	• Cardiovascular (32%) • Congenital/genetic (26%) • Respiratory (17%) • Neuromuscular (14%)
Children— 1-19 years	• Accidents • Assault • Cancer • Suicide • Congenital abnormalities (malformations, deformations) • Chromosomal anomalies • Heart disease • Cerebrovascular diseases	• Malignancy (43%) • Neuromuscular (23%) • Cardiovascular (17%)

Used with permission: Friebert S. *NHPCO Facts and Figures: Pediatric Palliative and Hospice Care in America.* Alexandria, VA: National Hospice and Palliative Care Organization. 2009.

estimated that 53,000 children under the age of 14 years die annually in the United States.[2,5] Close to 50% of these children will die unexpectedly from trauma, birth defects or sudden infant death syndrome (SIDS), but the other half will die of prolonged chronic conditions. However, only 5,000 of the 53,000 who will die will receive hospice services.[2,5]

In 2008, Feudtner et. al. did a study to describe the demographics and clinical characteristics of 515 pediatric patients who received hospital-based palliative care consultations. The results of this 'snap-shot' look at pediatrics receiving palliative care are in Table 5.[15]

D. Site of death

Studies have shown 70% of families would prefer for their child to die at home.[2] The availability of technology and reimbursement patterns has made home care possible for even very complex conditions previously requiring hospitalization. This has resulted in an estimated 15-20% increase in the number of children dying at home of CCC.[2] This choice is predicated on many factors including support systems available to them, family conditions, and child/family choices. While home deaths have increased, children continue to die primarily in the hospital; usually in intensive care settings.[2] Families and children with CCCs

Table 5: Characteristics of Pediatric Palliative Care Recipients[15]

Gender	• Male—54%	• Female—46%
Age	• Not yet born to < 1 month—4.7% • 1-11 months—12.4% • 1-9 years—37.5%	• 10-18 years—30% • 19 years and older—15.5%
Race & ethnicity	• White—69.5% • Black—8.9% • Asian—36% • Native population—1.8%	• Mixed—4.7% • Other & not indicated—8.2% • Hispanic—7.4%
Living arrangements	• With both parents—60.4% • Only/mostly with mother—21.9%	• Institutional facility/foster care/only father/alone or with spouse/hospitalized since birth/not yet born—17.7%
Condition • 55% of the children had > 1 diagnosis	• Genetic/congenital—40.8% • Neuromuscular—39.2% • Hematologic cancer—7.0% • Solid tumor—7.0% • Brain tumor—5.6% • Hematologic and solid tumors—0.1% • Respiratory—12.8%	• Other—10.7% • Gastrointestinal—9.9% • Cardiovascular—8.3% • Metabolic—7.2% • Renal—2.7% • Immunology—2.6%
Use of medical technology	• None—20.4% • Any feeding tubes—59.6% • Gastrostomy tube—48.5% • Nasogastric tube—9.9% • Jejunostomy tube—9.7% • Central venous catheter—22.3%	• Tracheostomy—10.1% • Noninvasive ventilation—9.5% • Ventilator-dependent—8.5% • Wheelchair—4.1% • Ventroperitoneal/ventriculojugular shunt—2.9%
Other	• Cognitive impairment—47.2% • Experienced pain—30.9% • Average number of medications each child was taking—9.1 • Average time from consultation to death—107 days • Children who died during the 12-month follow-up period—30.3%	

28

may perceive the hospital as a second home and desire the familiar support of the hospital at end of life. More important than where they die is where the family would choose for them to die, and whether the child died in the location of their family's choice.[2]

E. Gaps to Provision of Excellent Pediatric Palliative Care

There are continued barriers to providing excellent palliative care for children. Adult providers may not be wholly prepared for the special nature of pediatric patients, their conditions, and the significant differences in effective pain and symptom management. The following is a brief summary of unmet needs of this vulnerable population.[2]

1. Financial issues—families with young children with CCCs are financially affected by their child's condition in 3 categories—insurance, missed work, and out-of-pocket expenses. Many may have limited income and insurance coverage. High costs of insurance can be prohibitive—especially for young families, resulting in 38% of this population being uninsured or underinsured.[6] Providing for a child with CCC usually requires one parent to remain at home, limiting potential financial earnings. Appointments and travel may necessitate missed work. Many families may have to travel significant distances from home to receive care at a specialized pediatric facility, especially if child has a rare disease. This means often expensive travel, more time missed from work and being away from the supportive environment at home. Out-of-pocket expenses assumed by the family are considerable as they may include childcare for siblings during medical appointments and hospitalizations, a special vehicle for transportation, individualized wheelchair, meals and lodging away from home, as well as equipment and services not covered by the insurance plan.[1] Medications may be expensive with tiered copayments, or need to pay out of pocket for uncovered drugs. Families also may need to pay out of pocket for some extra skilled care or custodial coverage in the home. Financial costs become particularly challenging for adolescents over the age of eighteen years who may not be eligible for coverage under their parents' plan. It should be noted, however, that the PPACA (Patient Protection Affordable Care Act) may provide some additional assistance

   a) Children with preexisting conditions must be eligible for insurance

   b) Young adults are covered under their parents insurance until age 26 and may continue to receive benefits

2. Transition services—in the past, children with CCC (i.e., cystic fibrosis, heart failure) often died prior to adolescence, but now live into adulthood. Adult services are usually ill-prepared to care for adolescents/young adults with these conditions. For example, there are different rules to provide confidential care to the patient as an adult. Due to desired privacy, the young adult may not want family to be present during testing procedures, overnight hospital stays, etc. in adult care settings. However, many healthcare settings are focusing on patient and family-centered care and will try to provide assistance for family presence if desired. Additionally, there may be changes in available services such as extra nursing care in the home. These crucial services that aid the family may significantly reduce when the child turns 21 years.

3. Mechanisms to address continuity of care—communication across the multiple subspecialties and health settings is difficult. Potential areas for problems exist when a child's condition changes, hospitalization occurs, or

28

the family's goals of care change. Access to collaborative care across the spectrum and/or portability of care is needed. However, it may be helpful to suggest to families that they keep a list of current medications and ask for copies of test reports or the most recent discharge summaries to promote information and communication.

4. Affordable care in the home—longer disease courses, earlier referrals, and use of aggressive supportive therapies (e.g., home ventilators, parenteral feedings, expensive chemotherapies, antifungals, antibiotics) can be cost-prohibitive and time-consuming to provide in the home. When technology occurs in the home, families may require longer and more frequent home visits to provide parental and sibling support, along with the increased time needed to coordinate care as well as hire and train pediatric specialized nursing assistants, and social workers.

F. Family Centered Care

In the broad society, a child is expected to outlive its parents. Therefore, the serious or life-threatening illness and death of a child is against this natural order of life and can represent the loss of future for a family. The loss of a child is considered to be one of the most devastating human experiences.[5] The child's death is expected to permanently change the family structure and function. Each family member will be affected differently as he/she tries to accept this "new normal" of life without the child.

1. Child—children are a part of a family system in whatever way the family is structured, organized, or defined. The ill child requires developmentally appropriate information and interventions. It is possible that children understand more than is acknowledged by the adults around them.[16]

2. Siblings—if present, are usually not the central focus in the care of a sick child; however, it essential to bring them into the circle of care. A brother or sister may feel alone, displaced, or guilty throughout a sibling's disease course and eventual time of death. A sister or brother may become resentful of the attention and presents given to their ill sibling. Well siblings especially need dedicated private time with their parents to continue their natural growth and development. Information about the ill child should be given using clear, honest, age-appropriate language. Moreover, siblings should be encouraged to participate in caring for the ill child in whatever age-appropriate capacity possible and agreed upon by the family. Attendance at death rituals such as saying good-bye, bathing, or funerals should be offered to siblings. With developmentally appropriate preparation for what to expect, and an accompanying adult to provide additional support, no child is considered too young to attend such rituals.[16]

3. Parents—often proceed upon 2 simultaneous paths when caring for a child diagnosed with CCC. On one hand, they attempt to maintain some normalcy in the everyday life of the child, hoping or pursuing a cure or a miracle while concurrently striving for comfort and quality of life. A primary concern parents with child dying with cancer reported was the need to be perceived as a 'good parent' when considering end-of-life decisions. They define being a good parent as making informed, unselfish decisions in the child's best interest, being at the child's side, showing the child that she/he is cherished, teaching the child to make good decisions, advocating for the child, and promoting the child's health.[17]

28

4. Grandparents—may suffer the dual burden of processing their grief for their dying grandchild as well as supporting their child, who is the grieving parent. They may provide significant amount of care and support to siblings, if needed. At this stage of their lives, they may also be experiencing the death of lifelong friends or spouses, compounding their grief.[16]

5. School/community—maintaining consistency in schedules and activities is essential for children. Therefore, attending school is not only an integral and essential part of a child's life and identity; it is a legal right for all children regardless of physical condition.[18] In difficult economic times, reduced school budgets may mean schools are challenged to adapt schedules, learning opportunities, classroom environment, and staffing to accommodate needs of the child with complex medical conditions, or provide tutors for children at home and at school. Online schooling or courses may be an alternative to the traditional classroom setting. The child or adolescent should be encouraged to continue to participate in sports teams, clubs, church groups, and other social groups as much as desired and appropriate. Pediatric palliative APRNs can participate in educating and supporting the community, the child, and the family for their continued involvement.

III. MANAGEMENT OF SYMPTOMS

A. Overview

Children with serious or life-threatening or chronic, complex conditions suffer from symptoms that may cause distress and challenge the quality of their life. Dr. Eric Cassel's description of suffering as, "a specific state of distress that occurs when the intactness or integrity of the person is threatened or disrupted,"[19, p.32] is applicable to children and to their families along the trajectory of these conditions. A key goal of the APRN in providing palliative care to the pediatric population is to ease suffering in any of the 4 domains of quality of life, whether it is physical, social, psychological, or spiritual.[20] In her Quality of Life Model, Dr. Betty Ferrell reveals that any physical symptoms of distress may cause distress and disruption in daily activities, impacting the quality of life for the child and family.[20] Adequate management of the symptom can have positive outcomes in each of these domains.[20] While there are diseases and conditions for which no cure may be available, relief from distressing symptoms can be achieved with evidence-based practices.

B. Assessment

Continual assessments are needed for all potentially distressing symptoms of serious, life-threatening, or chronic, complex conditions. Each symptom can be distressing enough by itself, but symptoms rarely exist alone. In adults, symptom clusters, where more than one distressing symptom occurs simultaneously, may severely affect quality of life. This is being investigated in the pediatric populations. Symptoms should be alleviated as appropriate to goals of care in order to assure the best quality of life possible for the child. For instance, one child may endure more pain to be more alert, while another may chose sedation over anxiety. Appropriate symptom assessment tools for children include The Memorial Symptom Assessment Scale (MSAS), Edmonton Symptom Assessment Scale (ESAS), and the Pediatric Quality of Life Scale (PedsQL).[21] While the Karnofsky Performance Scale is helpful for determining an adult or older child's ability to perform activities of daily living (ADL), the Lansky Play Performance

Scale is helpful for quantifying a child's tolerance to activity and play.[22] The scale can be found in Chapter 37, *Performance and Prognostic Tools.*

C. Management of Common Symptoms

See Appendix 28-A at the end of this chapter for pediatric-specific aspects of symptom etiology, assessment, and treatment.

1. Pain

Children and their parents frequently identify pain as the most frightening and difficult aspects of their condition.[23] Children's pain experience is affected by the child's age, developmental level, temperament, parental style, disease process, and previous experiences.[23] Providers may lack adequate knowledge and resources to assess and treat pain in children resulting in pain being undertreated. A frequently referenced study found that 89% of parents who had had a child die of cancer felt their child had suffered a great deal, with pain being one of the 3 most commonly reported symptoms.[24] Of those children who were treated for their pain, relief was achieved only 27% of the time.[24] The potential for and interventions to address pain can be different depending on the underlying cause, culture, beliefs, previous pain experiences, etc. The assessment for pain in children also requires additional tools due to differences in cognitive development. (see Table 6)

2. Common myths related to pain management in children[30]

a) Children playing or sleeping are not in pain—children have unique ways of coping with their pain and may distract themselves or escape to sleep when pain is unbearable.

b) Children's nervous systems are immature and are unable to perceive and experience pain the same way as adults—it has been shown that the anatomical and neurochemical capabilities for complete nociception are completed between 16-26 weeks gestation.[31]

c) Children can cope with their pain better than adults—younger children actually experience higher levels of pain and pain tolerance increases with age.[30]

d) Opioid pain control leads to addiction—as discussed elsewhere in this publication, addiction is a neurobiological disease with genetic and environmental influences. Children have an even less risk of addiction than adults.[30]

e) Early opioid use leaves no future options—again, as with adults, there is no established ceiling dose for opioids. There are multiple opioid options available for children.

f) Children are unable to tell us they have pain—it is our challenge to recognize their behavior and symptoms indicative of pain. This is done via cognitively and behaviorally appropriate tools. (see Table 6)

3. Barriers to pain relief

In addition to dispelling common myths regarding pain control in children, it is necessary for the APRN to also recognize and overcome certain challenges to pain relief.[30]

a) The child may not understand words used by others related to pain and need 'translation' to words used by their family, such as "boo boo" or "owie."

28

Table 6: Tools for Pediatric Pain and Related Symptom Assessment

Tool	Age Group	How administered
CRIES (Cries, Requires Oxygen, Increased Vital Signs, Expression, Sleeplessness)[25]	• 0-6 months • Procedural and post-op	• Scored from 0-2 on each measure, higher score is higher level of pain
N-PASS (Neonatal Pain, Agitation and Sedation Scale)[26,27]	• Neonatal	• Score -2 to 2 for cry, irritability, behavior state, facial expression, extremity tone, and vital signs • Negative scores indicate sedation, positive scores indicate agitated &/or pain
COMFORT[28]	• Neonate – 3 years	• Measures alertness, calmness/agitation, respiratory response, physical movement, blood pressure, heart rate, muscle tone, facial tension • Possible 5 points each for max of 80
FLACC (Face, Legs, Activity, Cry, Consolability)[29]	• 2 months – 7 years • Non-communicative patient	• Five point observation scale with each point graded 0-2
Wong-Baker Faces	• 3+ years	• Patient chooses one of 6 faces depicting how pain makes them feel
Oucher	• 3-12 years	• 6 photographs varying between 'no hurt' & 'biggest hurt' • Ethnically based
PCT (Poker Chip Tool)[25]	• 3-5 years	• 4 poker chips placed in horizontal row • Child picks how many 'pieces of hurt' being experienced
VAS (Visual Analog Scale)[25]	• Preschool	• Horizontal line similar to Likert scale indicating no pain to worst pain
NPS (Numeric Pain Scale)[25]	• School aged & older	• Pain is scored from 1-10 with 10 being the most

b) A child may fear that reporting pain will cause distress for their family and be eager to "show a happy face." They may fear that reporting pain will result in a trip to the clinic or hospital, or that it will be followed by unpleasant medications or restriction from desired activities.

c) Older children and adolescents may fear addiction and may have a "Say no to drugs" philosophy, which could be in conflict with the need for opioids to treat their pain.

d) The parents and families of children receiving palliative care services may fear that reporting pain heralds the return of the underlying condition, or that it is a sign that the disease is accelerating and that death is imminent.

e) Families may also fear addiction, with use of opioids having a negative connotation and raising concerns regarding the impact they may have made on the lives of others in their family or community. Many clinicians have changed their terminology from "narcotic" to "opioid" or simply, 'pain medication' to help differentiate the therapeutic role of these agents.

f) Healthcare professionals, even hospice professionals, are not always adequately trained in providing pain management to children.

g) Pain assessment tools are not always used consistently and correctly.

28

h)   The fear of respiratory suppression and the misunderstanding of the pharmacokinetics of pain medications are common.

i)   The healthcare system does not always adequately reimburse for pain therapies, especially nonpharmacological methods. Additional services for specialists from other disciplines such as anesthesia, child life, physical therapy, and psychiatry are not always covered for palliative or hospice patients.

j)   More evidence-based direction regarding pain control is necessary in the pediatric palliative care discipline. Although greatly improved over the last decade, it remains difficult to conduct research with children and there is still a need for more studies and development of consistent, valid, and accurate assessment tools.

4.   Pain assessment

When assessing a child's pain, it is important to consider the cognitive and developmental level of the child versus the chronological age. The following provides general considerations for each developmental period. Validated tools for assessing pain appropriate to developmental stages are found in Table 6.

a)   Neonate—pain experienced during the neonatal period may cause children to be more fearful of pain during childhood than their peers.[31] It has also been found that infants spending at least 40 days in neonatal intensive care units display more profound nerve responses to noxious stimuli than their gestational age-corrected peers.[32] Exposure to frequent noxious stimuli can have a profound impact on the child due to the plasticity of the developing neonate's brain.[33] Studies such as these have led to changes in neonatal intensive care units with greater attention to[34]

   i.   Environment—noise and light reductions and rest time between interventions

   ii. Nursing behavior—swaddling of the baby and use of sugar-dipped pacifiers

   iii. Pharmacological—appropriate use of anesthetics, analgesics, and anxiolytics

One model of care derived from a consensus document encourages consistency in the approach to caring for newborns with serious or life-threatening illness.[34] Included in this model are—a description of education; community and tertiary center relationships; supporting a neonatal death; care of the family while respecting cultural, spiritual, and practical differences; pain and symptom management; ventilator withdrawal; family follow-up and staff support.[34]

The palliative APRN must be aware of physiologic issues when prescribing medications for neonates. Since a neonate or premature infant's organs are still maturing, their metabolism may be decreased, requiring lower starting doses of opioids.[34]

b)   Infants—while the majority of people would recognize an infant's cry as indicative of pain, the most consistent indicator of pain is their facial expression. Older infants can physically resist, refuse to lie still, or try to

28

move away from painful stimuli. Other behaviors indicative of pain in infants could be

    i.   Not using an affected extremity

    ii.   Decrease in appetite

    iii.   Decrease in activity

    iv.   Inconsolability—however, pain may continue even after a child stops crying, requiring continued soothing and pain control measures

c)   Toddlers—ranging from 1-3 years; toddlers comprise a group with diverse cognitive and expressive abilities. Their reaction to pain is often intense, incorporates emotional distress, and is displayed with physical struggle. Their specific behavioral responses may be influenced by memory, physical restraint, parent separation, emotional reaction of others, and lack of preparation. Toddlers may become restless and overly active when in pain, which may be missed or misinterpreted by care providers.[35]

d)   Preschoolers—ranging from 3-5 years; preschoolers have a wide range of cognitive and social abilities. They begin to understand the concept of illness. However, they take words for their literal meaning; such as 'take your blood pressure' has two significant concerns; the word 'blood' is never good, and 'take' meaning—someone is taking something from me that is mine. This can lead to more fear and confusion. Explaining the process of a blood pressure as, "I'm going to give your arm a hug," may be more acceptable. Preschoolers are more receptive to preparatory explanations and distractions.

e)   School-aged children—ranging from 5-13 years; because most school-aged children are quite verbal, the APRN must also be attentive to nonverbal cues of distress. In this population, nonverbal cues include becoming quiet or uninvolved in activities. They can state when they have pain and may be capable of further describing their pain with adjectives like, "burning," or "aching," etc.[36] They frequently take an active interest in their medical condition and enjoy participating in healthcare responsibilities. Since they are beginning to understand cause and effect, school-aged children may feel guilty for being sick, especially if they attribute illness to not following parental instructions. Advanced preparation for painful procedures is very helpful for this group.

    This group of children begins to have a more realistic concept of death and disability. Children with chronic conditions may have experienced the death of a friend with a similar condition.

f)   Adolescent—ranging from 13-19 years; body image is very important for an adolescent. They also view the injury, disability, or conditions in terms of how it affects them currently versus in the future. Physical changes brought on by the condition can tremendously impact their rapidly changing body and negatively impact their need for normalcy. The developmentally appropriate desire for independence from parents can be challenged when the parent must re-assert control with the goal to protect their child but also to provide for healthcare needs. Overconfidence and pride may be displayed as the teen tries to obtain

28

and maintain self-control during painful experiences. Illness may disrupt their peer relationships, social development, school, and academic progress, as well as vocational choices. Due to a desire to appear healthy and protect family members, pain may be under-reported and behaviors such as limited movement, excessive quietness, or irritability may indicate pain.[36]

g) Nonverbal child—children with chronic complex conditions or neurologic impairment may have a limited ability to verbally express pain. Those who are intubated or sedated will be unable to verbally express pain. Any impairment in the ability to express pain requires additional APRN assessment and management skills. Parent/caregiver input can be very valuable in learning how they determine their child's discomfort; frequently through identification of behaviors unique to their child. Observation of pain behaviors such as grimacing or extremity extension may be indicative of pain. It may be appropriate to assume pain with painful procedures and to consider a trial with a pain medication to assess effect on behavior and vital signs in a nonverbal child.[29]

h) Hierarchy of Pain Assessment Techniques

Since pain is subjective, methodological approaches must be used for assessment. In the pediatric population, the Hierarchy of Pain Assessment Techniques is applied as follows[26]

i. Use of self-report, if possible and appropriate. This is usually not possible until a child is about 2 years of age due to being in the preverbal developmental level from birth until 2.

ii. Search for potential causes of pain/discomfort. If the procedure or situation could cause pain, it should always be suspected and proactively managed.

iii. Observation of child's behavior—several of the pain scales use this measure to systematically quantify the child's pain.

iv. Surrogate reporting of pain. Parents and care providers, including nursing staff, should be asked if they feel the child is in pain, or if the child is comfortable.

v. Analgesic trial—initiating a trial with appropriately dosed adjuvants or opioids should be tried if other attempts to comfort the child have been unsuccessful.[29]

5. Pain management guidelines

a) Goals—the goals for pain management for the child receiving palliative care are for the child to be

i. As pain-free as possible

ii. Active with minimal discomfort

iii. Maintain some function

iv. Free from intervention side effects

v. Able to interact with others to the extent desired by child and family[25]

b) General considerations in pediatric pain management

28

As with all practice, APRNs should consult current drug reference materials when dosing medications for pain control for children. It is strongly recommended that all first/new dosage calculations be double-checked with another healthcare professional, preferably with expertise in pediatrics, such as a nurse, physician, or pharmacist; either in person or by phone. Medications for children are dosed per kg when the child is less than 50 kg, with attention to maximum dosage.[25] For 50 kg and above, usual adult dosages are used. Premature infants and infants less than 6 months of age are dosed at approximately 25% of the per kilogram dosing calculated due to their reduced clearance of most medications secondary to the immaturity of their organs.[28]

c) Pharmacological therapies

Pain should be viewed as an urgent symptom. Complete assessment and appropriate interventions should be implemented. The key concepts of pain management in pediatrics are similar to adult. Since sedatives blunt behavioral responses to noxious stimuli without providing pain relief, pain control must be included if sedation is needed for procedures, maintaining endotracheal tubes, etc.

    i.   Routes of administration—medications used to alleviate pain come in several formulations, which facilitates using the least invasive route for children. When hospitalized, this may be the intravenous route. When at home, the oral route is preferred. However, many children with CCC have a gastrostomy tube, which can be used. Rectal, intramuscular, and subcutaneous routes of administration of medication are generally avoided in children.

    ii.   Adjuvant non-opioids—acetaminophen and ibuprofen are considered routine adjuvant, non-opioid analgesics in children. Aspirin should be avoided due to the added risk of Reye's syndrome. In the pediatric population, the maximum dose of acetaminophen (75 mg/kg/day) may be reached quickly, requiring the APRN to use caution with combination products such as acetaminophen with codeine or acetaminophen with hydrocodone.[25] Ibuprofen doses should be kept to less than 40 mg/kg/day for children less than 50 kg.[25]

    iii. Opioids—morphine and fentanyl are the most common opioids used. See Table 7 for dosage guidelines. Complications related to the use of opioids are similar in pediatrics as for adults and will not be covered in this section. (See Chapter 6, *Pain*)

d) Nonpharmacological techniques[7]

Approaches to pain control in infants and children include techniques that do not require medications. Important considerations for children should be given to the following

    i.   Parental presence and comfort, though a very anxious parent could have the opposite effect

    ii.   Family and relative presence and distraction as appropriate

    iii. Play therapy

    iv. Art therapy

28

v. Cognitive-behavioral therapies—relaxation, guided imagery, cognitive reframing

vi. Music therapy

vii. Pet therapy

viii. Pastoral counseling/prayer

ix. Physical measures—massage therapy, heat/cold, swaddling, cuddling, rocking, repositioning/bracing, acupressure, acupuncture

x. Relaxation techniques—meditation, deep breathing

xi. Biofeedback

xii. Hypnosis

Additional therapies for infants and neonates include

i. Modifying the environment to reduce noise and bright lights.

ii. Offer pacifier for non-nutritive sucking.

iii. Give 0.5-2 mL 24% sucrose solution orally 2 minutes before minor painful procedure.

iv. Blanket or hand swaddling

IV. ETHICS IN PEDIATRIC PALLIATIVE CARE

Table 7: Analgesic Doses for Children 6 months to 50 kg[25]

Drug	Parenteral Starting Dose	Oral Starting Dose
Acetaminophen (many products including APAP®, Tylenol®)	• 12.5 mg/kg IV every 4 hours (max dose 75 mg/kg/24 hour)	• 15 mg/kg every 4-6 hours • Maximum dose 75 mg/kg/24 hour
Ibuprofen (many products including Advil®, Motrin®)	• N/A	• 10-15 mg/kg every 4-6 hours
Ketorolac (Toradol®)	• 0.5 mg/kg IV not to exceed 48-72 hours in children 1 month – 2 years • Not to exceed 5 days of therapy in children 2-16 children	• N/A
Codeine	• N/A	• 0.5-1 mg/kg every 3-4 hours
Morphine	• Bolus: 0.1 mg/kg every 2-4 hours • Infusion: 0.03 mg/kg/hour	• IR: 0.3 mg/kg every 3-4 hours • SR: 20-35 kg: 10-15 mg every 12 hours • 35-50 kg: 15-30 mg every 12 hours
Oxycodone (OxyContin®)	• N/A	• 0.1-0.2 mg/kg every 3-4 hours
Methadone	• 0.1 mg/kg every 4-8 hours	• 0.2 mg/kg every 4-8 hours
Fentanyl	• Bolus: 0.5-1 mcg/kg every 1-2 hours • Infusion: 0.5-2 mcg/kg/hour	• N/A
Hydromorphone (Dilaudid®)	• Bolus: 0.02 mg/kg every 2-4 hours • Infusion: 0.006 mg/kg/hr	• 0.04 mg/kg every 3-4 hours

*Greater than 50 kg: Use adult dosing; Infants < 6 month/premature infants are dosed at 25% of above
IR: Immediate Release
SR: Sustained Release

28

A. Overview

Ethics provides values, morals, and guiding principles for actions and decisions. Healthcare providers, patients, and families may have differing perspectives on these elements. Ethical concerns may arise when there is conflict around deciding the best course of action. In particular, there may be discord about the benefit and burden of procedures and alignment with expected outcomes. When determining goals of care, it may be necessary to evaluate what makes life meaningful for the child and what burdens are acceptable to achieve those goals. A moral framework for decision-making involving children can be referred to as shared decision-making, which assumes the principles of beneficence, nonmaleficence, and respect for persons and justice.[37] Decision-making for children with complex, chronic conditions and/or children at end of life may evoke ethical issues, which can develop into ethical dilemmas. As with adults, dilemmas in pediatric care often occur when there is conflict among providers or between providers and family regarding communication of goals of care, withdrawing or withholding therapy, or opioid use for symptom control.[38] General ethical principles of justice, beneficence, nonmaleficence, and autonomy are similar for children as for adults. This section will address only aspects specific to pediatrics. (See Chapter 4, *Ethical Considerations*)

1. Balancing benefit and burden—it is logical that treatment choices should benefit the infant or child while minimizing burdens or harm produced by the therapy. Surgical procedures aimed at relief of a particular symptom must be included in this issue. While the outcome of a procedure may be beneficial, the process to get to the outcome may be burdensome. The best interests of the child are not just biological, but also developmental, functional, emotional, social, and spiritual. The balance of benefit and burden may be difficult to define in some situations. The reasonable standard may be used to weigh benefits and burdens and determine what is in the child's best interest. Society assumes that a parent or surrogate is this reasonable person.[39] As such, parents are viewed as the "experts" on the child and his/her ability to cope. They must have a clear sense of the burdens and benefits.

2. Respect for persons—this principle assumes all persons, including infants and significantly impaired children, have value and that their thoughts, experiences, and opinions matter, despite their developmental immaturity and legal status as minors. Children must be acknowledged and valued outside of their medical condition. This premise can result in conflict when parents believe their child will be harmed if informed about a diagnosis or prognosis. One study revealed that parents regretted not discussing death with their children and that those discussed death harbored no regrets.[40] Consideration of a child's developmental age and ability to understand the condition and implications of treatment can be expected to change over the course of complex, chronic conditions and require frequent re-assessments of understanding and their acceptance of plans of care. Children too young to legally make a decision and consent to therapy should be asked to assent to treatment. This indicates that they agree to proceed with a treatment plan with the approval and consent of their parent or surrogate.[40] Minors who are emancipated (state law defines age), pregnant, married, or in military services may be expected to provide consent versus assent.

28

3. Justice—demands that all patients be treated fairly and that decisions are unrelated to race, age, gender, religious beliefs, or socioeconomic situation. Decisions that will benefit individual patients must be separated from decisions related to allocation of resources. Many states are enacting pediatric palliative care benefits that assure care across the continuum. Criteria for hospice benefits are not universally applicable for children. Subsequent to the PPACA federal legislation, states are beginning to enact legislation allowing for hospice services to coincide with approaches to a cure.[41]

V. COMMUNICATION AND DECISION-MAKING IN THE PEDIATRIC POPULATION

A. General

Effective communication between a child/family unit and healthcare providers is a critical requirement for successful palliative care. A strong collaboration between members of the interdisciplinary team and the family is necessary. As discussed earlier, serious or life-threatening or complex, chronic conditions are a family experience. Communication includes imparting necessary medical information, allowing for informed decision-making, eliciting values, preferences, and concerns, as well as gaining an understanding of the illness experience for child and family. Such communication may help dispel preconceived notions/myths about illness or treatments, and promote collaborative care.

B. Communicating with the Child

When communicating with children, it is important to understand the family system and family "norms" regarding communication to children. Some families will ask the child how much information they want and others will not. While most families are open to honest communication with their children, some families are fearful and need guidance in how to communicate and address issues around illness. It is essential to respect cultural traditions/influences/ restrictions and to recognize that communication must be based on the developmental age of the child. Art, music, and play therapy may be considered safe venues for a child to communicate.[42]

The use of figurative language (anecdotes and familiar metaphors) may help with understanding and retention of information.[42] However, vague terms (e.g., going away, going home, passing) can be confusing as children do not understand the nuances and can misinterpret these terms. They may have magical thinking regarding illness and death. With exposure to cartoons, they may expect that death is temporary, because the favorite character returns in the next scene. It is appropriate to let the child know that this is not like in a cartoon or on television; that those who die will not be back tomorrow.[35,43]

C. Decision-Making

1. Shared decision-making depends upon establishing and nurturing a synergistic and reciprocal relationship between the child, family, and healthcare professionals. Decision-making may change with how much parents allow the child's involvement in the decision-making process. Desired outcomes include mutual respect, preserved integrity, understanding, shared meaning, hope balanced with honesty and realism, and mutual satisfaction with the process regardless of the outcome. This can be difficult to accomplish because providers tend to focus on the decision rather than the process needed to accomplish a shared journey with the child and family.[40]

28

a) There are many challenges to assisting a family with effective decision-making. The APRN needs to understand that many families prefer to be given all options rather than being told what is the best thing to do for their child.[38] This allows for mutual participation by the family, including the child when appropriate, in the decision being made. For children participating in decision-making, consideration must be given to the pre-existing family dynamics, culture, the child's cognitive abilities, developmental level, and familiarity with/understanding of the medical condition. However, when the patient is a teenager, he/she can be included in decision-making and treatment discussions. Parents may need support in these discussions. When the parent(s) of the child are teenagers themselves, they may need more support from their parents and community as well as more time to understand the disease, treatment, and prognosis. Many young children and adolescents with chronic conditions benefit from participating in decisions regarding continued approaches to managing the underlying condition and supportive care. However, this must be done with permission by the parents or guardians of the child. Information can be introduced by directing medical questions to the child, responding to information provided by the child, giving the child choices when possible, and asking for the child's assent to participate in planned interventions.[39] Decisions, which need to be considered and in which the child can participate, include participation in clinical trials, refractory symptom management, pain management interventions, continuation of disease-directed interventions, intensive care unit transfers, ventilator withdrawal, and preferred place of death.

2. End-of-life decision-making

Just as with adults, there are many decisions to make as the child's condition becomes progressively worse.

a) Disclosure—families and children have a right to know information regarding an illness. Providing children with information regarding their illness and proposed treatment in a developmentally-appropriate manner demonstrates respect for the person, veracity, beneficence, and is required to assure informed consent and assent. Healthcare providers may have difficulty disclosing information, especially in grim situations. This raises the question of who is protected by withholding information. Nonetheless, discussion should occur to determine which healthcare provider the family trusts to impart such difficult information with the appropriate compassion, sensitivity, and presence. Considerations of cultural and family issues must underpin these conversations.[40]

b) Forgoing life-sustaining treatment—when the possibility of a cure becomes remote, the benefit and burden of interventions intended to eradicate, reverse, or contain a pathological process must be considered, especially if the resultant quality of life would be undesirable. Although most people would perceive it easier to withhold therapy than to withdraw therapies, from an ethical perspective, there is no difference.[40] The Academy of Pediatrics recommends initiating potentially beneficial interventions but discontinuing them after a specified trial period if the therapy fails to produce desired outcomes which have been negotiated with child, family, and providers.[44]

28

c) Code status discussions—an important aspect of decision-making pertaining to life-sustaining therapies is cardiopulmonary resuscitation (CPR) and intubation. Families must receive accurate information regarding the likely outcomes of attempting CPR with special attention to the likelihood of survival after CPR with a given condition. This should include information about the use of ventilators and potential necessity of ventilator support. Furthermore, there should be discussion of the possibility of restoration to his/her previous functionality and quality of life with resuscitation to survival. CPR may be considered as only interrupting or prolonging the body's natural dying process but not altering the course of the disease. After discussion with the child as appropriate and family, clear documentation must be made of the interventions to be attempted by healthcare professionals should the child's respiratory status become compromised or heart function become impaired.[40]

d) Artificial nutrition and nutrition—although universally accepted by healthcare professionals and the legal system, withholding of artificial hydration and nutrition remains very controversial in the pediatric population. Food universally represents life and love. Since infants and children are naturally dependent on others for provision of fluids and nutrition, parents may see providing hydration and nutrition as a basic care requirement. Therefore, withholding artificial nutrition and hydration can be perceived as neglect by some families and care providers. However, continuation of artificial nutrition and hydration can lengthen the period of dying by interfering with the natural process of anorexia and decreased desire for food and fluids during the dying process. Provision of artificial nutrition and hydration can also add the challenges of increased secretions, edema, and abdominal distention leading to the child's discomfort.[40] Due to the complexity of this issue in regard to children, many institutions require ethics committee approval to withhold fluids or nutrition at end of life.

VI. CONCLUSION

The care of a child with complex, chronic conditions or a child at end of life necessitates a unique skill set for the APRN. Palliative care issues vary widely across the pediatric age groups. Management of discomforting symptoms, including pain, necessitates additional considerations with this population and varies greatly across the age groups and developmental levels.

While advances are being made, huge gaps remain between what is desired and what is available for children challenged with life-threatening or serious conditions. Accepted approaches to family-centered care inherent to pediatrics are especially demanding in this arena. In particular, pediatric palliative care requires special attention and flexibility in provision of care. Ethical issues are even more challenging and require effective communication as the APRN assists the family and healthcare team in decision-making. The role of the APRN is to assure every child and family a meaningful, peaceful existence and if necessary, a dignified, gentle death with supportive bereavement.

28

28

Appendix 28-A: Pediatric Symptom Management[45-47]

	SYMPTOM	PHARMACOLOGICAL/MEDICAL	NONPHARMACOLOGICAL/ MEDICAL	COMMENTS
Cardiovascular	Palpitations	• Antipyretic ○ Acetaminophen—PO or PR 10 mg/kg/dose every 4-6 hours if fever • Discontinue meds causing palpitation (e.g., albuterol, antihistamine) • Correct electrolyte imbalance	• Breathing into a paper bag • Deep breathing • Relaxation, guided imagery, hypnosis • Restrict caffeine	• Palpitations are usually secondary to another symptom (e.g., fever, electrolyte imbalance, metabolic abnormalities) & only require treatment if affecting child's quality of life
	Sinus bradycardia	• Atropine—IV/ET 0.02 mg/kg; max 0.5 mg/dose • Initiate CPR if indicated	• Arouse, stimulate child • Use caffeinated beverage	• If attempts to resuscitate are not indicated, prepare family for expected changes as death approaches
	Supraventricular tachycardia	• Adenosine—IV 0.05-0.1 mg/kg; max 12 mg • Propranolol: PO 0.5-1 mg/kg/day divided into every 6-12 hour dosing • May increase dose every 3 days; max 16 mg/kg/day • Oxygen if dyspneic • Synchronized cardioversion	• Ice bag on face for 1-2 seconds • Gentle rectal stimulation • Elicit cough, gag, bear down	• Usually not a symptom at EOL, but can affect quality of life in certain cardiac conditions
	Superior vena cava syndrome	• Opiate analgesic if pain or SOB • Oxygen • Anxiolytic (lorazepam, or diazepam) • Palliative radiation therapy or chemotherapy • Thrombolytic agent (low molecular weight heparin) • Stent placement	• Elevate head of bed • Fan, cool mist humidifier • Decrease fluids • Minimize activity • Relaxation/distraction • Pursed-lip breathing	

Gastrointestinal	Anorexia/ cachexia	• Appetite stimulant
		  ○ Dronabinol—PO 2.5 mg twice a day before meals (adolescents)
		  ○ Megestrol acetate—PO 0.5-10 mg/kg/day divided into up to 4 doses/day (max dose 800 mg)
		  ○ Corticosteroid—dexamethasone—IV/PO 0.1 mg/kg/day divided into 2-4 doses per day
			• Small, frequent meals, high caloric
			• Avoid noxious odors
			• Oral care
			• Encourage exercise as appetite stimulant
			• Include child in normal mealtime regimes
				• Parents may be very distressed by this symptom at end of life
				• Food is symbolic of life & love. It is necessary for sustenance, & strength
				• Reassurance is needed to explain that decreased intake does not always lead to hunger or thirst & may not need to be corrected
				• At EOL, discussions need to occur regarding goals for artificial nutrition with tube feeding, parenteral feeds, etc.

SYMPTOM	PHARMACOLOGICAL/MEDICAL	NONPHARMACOLOGICAL/ MEDICAL	COMMENTS

Constipation	• Stool softener
	  ○ Docusate sodium—PO dosed 1-4 doses/day
	    ▪ > 3 years—10-40 mg/day
	    ▪ 3-6 years—20-60 mg/day
	    ▪ 6-12 years—40-120 mg/day
	    ▪ > 12 years—50-200 mg/day
	• Laxative
	  ○ Bisacodyl—PO 5-15 mg/dose daily
	  ○ Lactulose—PO 3 times/day dosing
	    ▪ Infants—0.8-3.5 mL
	    ▪ Children—10-30 mL
	  ○ Polyethylene glycol—PO 8.5-17 gm dissolved in 120-240 mL water/juice once daily
	  ○ Senna—PO
	    ▪ 1 month-2 year—1.25-2.5 mL syrup daily
	    ▪ 2-12 years—2.5-5 mL syrup daily
	    ▪ > 12 years—1 tab daily
	• Promotility agents
	  ○ Metoclopramide— PO/IV 0.1 mg/kg/dose 1-3 times per day
	  ○ Erythromycin— PO 5 mg/kg 4 times per day
		• Diet high in fiber, as appropriate
		• Increase fluids
		• Easy access to toilet
		• Assist child with body signals shortly after meals
		• Increase activity
		• Tub bath for rectal discomfort
			• Occurs in as high as 59% of children at EOL
			• Metoclopramide has a black box warning regarding extrapyramidal effects that may occur at therapeutic dosing & must be used with caution, especially if liver impaired

Dehydration	• Discontinue medications contributing to dehydration (e.g., diuretics, antihistamines, antiemetics) • Rehydrate with oral or, if appropriate, IV fluids	• Continue mouth care with substitute saliva • Provide moisture to lips & mouth with water, ice, glycerin, frozen fruit bars • Assure comfort	• Should be treated as a symptom only if cause of discomfort in child or family

Diarrhea	• Loperamide—PO 0.03 mg/kg 3 times a day
	• Bismuth subsalicylate—PO 15-25mg/kg 5-6 times a day
	• Cholestyramine—PO
	  ○ 0-6 years—1-2 gm 2 times a day
	  ○ > 6 years—2-4 gm 2 times a day
	• Octreotide—IV/SQ 1-2 mg/kg 2-3 times per day, titrating for effect to max 10 mg/kg/dose
		• Rehydration
		• Diet high in carbohydrate, low residue (BRAT diet—bananas, rice, applesauce, toast)
		• Avoid hyperosmotic supplements
		• Easy access to toilet
		• Gently cleaning with each stool
		• Consider skin barrier if incontinent
		• Adequate ventilation, odor control measures
			• May be especially distressing to child causing physiologic & psychological discomfort
			• Frequent dressing changes from diarrhea may be as equally distressing

Gastrointestinal

28

Appendix 28-A: Pediatric Symptom Management[45-47]—*continued*

SYMPTOM	PHARMACOLOGICAL/MEDICAL	NONPHARMACOLOGICAL/ MEDICAL	COMMENTS

Hiccups/ hiccoughs (singultus)	• Simethicone for gas
	• Metoclopramide— PO/IV 0.1 mg/kg/dose 1-3 times per day
	• Baclofen—PO
	  ○ 2-7 years—10-15 mg/day given every 8 hours
	  ○ > 8 years—60 mg/day
		• Swallow 1 tsp sugar or dry bread
		• Forcibly retract tongue
		• Cause gag, sneeze, or cough reflex
		• Massage carotid artery, ocular globe, thyroid cartilage, or soft palate
			• There are many options because none consistently are effective
			• May occur even during sedation
			• If very distressing towards the end of life, may need palliative sedation

Nausea/ vomiting	• 5HT3-receptor antagonists
	  ○ Ondansetron—IV/PO/SL 0.1-0.2 mg/kg every 6-8 hours max 4-8 gm/dose
	  ○ Granisetron—IV/PO/TD 0.01-0.05 mg/kg every 8 hours max 3 mg/dose
	• D2 receptor antagonists
	  ○ Metoclopramide—IV/PO/PR 0.15-0.3 mg/kg every 6 hours max 10-15 mg
	  ○ Haloperidol—IV/PO 0.1-0.02 mg/kg every 12 hours titrate slowly to max 1-2 mg/kg or 100 mg/dose)
	  ○ Domperidone—PO/PR 0.2 -0.4 mg/kg every 4-8 hours; max 10 mg
	    ▪ Not available in U.S.
	• Histamine receptor antagonists
	  ○ Dimenhydrinate—IV 1-2 mg/kg every 8 hours PO/PR 2-5 mg/kg every 6-12 hours
	  ○ Diphenhydramine—PO 0.5-1 mg/kg every 6 hours; max 50 mg
	  ○ Scopolamine—TD 0.33-0.5 mg/24 hours every 72 hour patch
	• Dopamine/histamine/muscarinic receptor antagonists
	  ○ Chlorpromazine—IV push 0.5-2 mg/kg; IV slow infusion 0.25- 1 mg/kg
	  ○ Prochlorperazine—PO 0.1-0.2 mg/kg every 8 hours
	  ○ Aprepitant—PO
	    ▪ > 12 years—125 mg times 1, then 80 mg daily during chemo
	  ○ Dronabinol—PO 5 mg/m2 every 2-4 hours; max dose 4-6 times/day
		• Small, frequent meals
		• Acupressure bracelet for older children
		• Acupuncture or acupressure
		• Cool moist compress to forehead, neck, & wrists
		• Maintain room freshness
		• Scents—peppermint may help
			• Can be as distressing as pain
			• Requires active intervention & support
			• Wide variety of pharmacological treatment choices—shown are only examples of each category
			• D2 receptor antagonists—anticholinergic side effects
			• Dopamine/histamine/muscarinic receptor antagonists—
			• Extrapyramidal & anticholinergic side effects
			• Agranulocytosis
			• Have diphenhydramine available
			• Appropriate for chemotherapy induced nausea/vomiting
			• Dronabinol—may stimulate appetite, cause dizziness, hallucinations, dysphoria, arterial hypotension

Gastrointestinal

28

SYMPTOM	PHARMACOLOGICAL/MEDICAL	NONPHARMACOLOGICAL/ MEDICAL	COMMENTS
Hematological			
Anemia	• Transfusion of red blood cells • Oxygen for hypoxia or dyspnea • Epoetin alpha—50 units/kg IM 3 times/week	• Assure rest • Minimize required movements • Elevate head of bed • Diet high in iron & folate	• Focus is placed on symptom & impact on quality of life, not lab values • Transfusions may require return to hospital, fluid overload, & pain
Bleeding & hemorrhage	• Platelet transfusion • Aminocaproic acid—IV/PO 100-200 mg/kg loading dose • Carafate paste, thrombin, epinephrine or cocaine to visible site of bleeding	• Prevention • Continual pressure with ice on/off every 10 min • Elevate site of bleeding • Supply dark colored towels & bedding to make blood less stark • Provide appropriate wound care & dressings	• Bleeding can be a very troublesome symptom to the child & family • Even when RBCs are withheld, platelets are frequently considered if bleeding cannot be prevented & controlled
Integumentary			
Diaper dermatitis	• Silver sulfadiazine—topical to excoriated area 2 times/day • Antifungal cream if evidence of fungal elements • Ulcerative lesions—topical antacids 4 times/day • Urinary catheter to prevent skin exposure to chemotherapy agent	• Prevention • Open to air • Moisture barrier cream—zinc oxide preparation	• Important to balance need for hygiene & rest
Dry skin	• Low dose corticosteroid cream	• Apply lubricant, moisturizer • Decrease frequency of bathing • Oral hydration • Cool room temperature	• Can increase pruritus, risk of skin breakdown & infection
Pressure ulcers	• Assess risk per Braden Q Scale[48]	• Prevention by repositioning frequently, adaptive mattress, & maximizing skin integrity	• Areas commonly affected in children are scalp, buttocks, & feet.
Pruritus	• Antihistamine • If opioid induced—IV naloxone 0.1 mg IV at a time • 5-HT3 antagonist • If secondary to cholestasis—PO phenobarbital • PO low-dose corticosteroid	• Oatmeal bath • Moisturizing creams • Avoid sources of heat • Ice or cool compresses to areas • Distraction	• May tremendously impact quality of life • The goal is to decrease itching without overly sedating, if possible

28

Appendix 28-A: Pediatric Symptom Management[45-47]—continued

SYMPTOM	PHARMACOLOGICAL/MEDICAL	NONPHARMACOLOGICAL/ MEDICAL	COMMENTS
Integumentary — Tumor necrosis & fistula	• Odor control • Anaerobic organism—topical metronidazole • If bacteria suspected—triple topical antibiotic ointment; apply to wound & cover with dry dressing • Octreotide IV/SC to decrease drainage • Wound care referral	• Cleanse with 3% peroxide or Dakin's solution • Pressure dressing with non-adherent dressing • Collection of copious drainage in ostomy pouch or wound evacuation device	• This rarely occurs in children, but can be devastating when it does • Aggressive support is needed to minimize discomfort; preserve appearance, control odors, & prevent bleeding
Neurologic — Agitation	• Consider & treat underlying cause • Benzodiazepine anxiolytic PO, SC, IV, PR • Lorazepam—0.05 mg/kg every 4-6 hours; max dose 2 mg/dose • Diazepam or haloperidol—0.01 mg/kg every 8-12 hours; max dose 30 mg/day • If tapering opioids, go slowly to prevent withdrawal symptoms	• Gentle touch, soothing • Guided medication, hypnosis. • Decrease environmental stimulation • Encourage constant presence of family member • Support of caregivers	• Goals are to assure causative sources are minimized & reinforce soothing techniques
Delirium/ confusion	• If possible, treat cause (e.g., fever, infection, hypoxia, insomnia, pain, electrolyte imbalance, polypharmacy) • Neuroleptic agent • Haloperidol—PO 0.01 mg/kg/day divided into 2-3 times/day dosing	• Environmental issues • Comfortable & safe • Familiar objects & people • Soothing presence	• Can be very frightening for child & family • Provide support as symptom is usually short duration
Dysphagia	• Glycopyrrolate to reduce secretions if problematic—PO 0.04-0.1 mg/kg every 4-8 hours	• Speech & language pathology consult • Modify consistency of food & fluids to thick honey • Position upright, use chin tuck • Gentle suction as needed	• Caused by loss of coordination of lower cranial nerves, respiratory & gastrointestinal systems
Fatigue	• Treat underlying cause of sleep disturbance (e.g., pain, dyspnea, nausea, anxiety) • Meds to stimulate alertness • Corticosteroids • Modafinil • Methylphenidate	• Conserve energy • Low-intensity exercises • Daily light exposure • Good sleep hygiene • Relaxation & distraction techniques	• Considered by parents to be one most troubling symptoms for children at EOL[24]

28

SYMPTOM	PHARMACOLOGICAL/MEDICAL	NONPHARMACOLOGICAL/ MEDICAL	COMMENTS
Neurologic			
Fever	• Antipyretics • Acetaminophen—PO 10-15 mg/kg/dose every 4-6 hours • Ibuprofen—PO 150 mg/kg/dose every 4-6 hours; treat underlying cause of fever	• Remove clothing & bedding • Tepid-room temperature bath • Fan • Avoid ice-packs & aggressive cooling measures that may lead to shivering & increase temp while decreasing comfort	• Consider whether child is comfortable vs. degree of temperature • Interventions to treat infection may not be beneficial at EOL • Consider family goals of care
Increased intracranial pressure	• Dexamethasone • Analgesic • Mannitol IV, if hospitalized	• Elevate head of bed • Minimal stimulation	• Consider treating symptoms vs. underlying etiology
Insomnia/sleep disturbance	• Antihistamine • Anxiolytic	• Encourage routine • Reduce stimuli • Warm milk, chamomile tea • Minimize stimulation	
Myoclonus/ Tremors	• Change opioid with equianalgesic dosing • Add adjuvant analgesic agent to decrease opioid dose • Hydration as appropriate if reduced renal function	• Reassurance • Decrease stimulation	
Seizures	• Prevention with prophylactic anticonvulsant per neurologist • Acute episode—PO, PR if unable to take PO • Lorazepam—0.05 mg/kg • Neonates—0.1 mg/kg • Infants & children—0.07 mg/kg; max dose 4 mg/dose • Diazepam • Dexamethasone to decrease ICP	• Seizure precautions • Put nothing in their mouth • Turn to side • Protect from falls • Observe where it started, how it progressed, length of time, etc. to assist with planning for prevention	• Seizures can be very disturbing to families & healthcare providers not prepared for them • If the child's condition could lead to seizures, the family must be prepared for them
Spinal cord compression	• Dexamethasone • Analgesics • Adjuvant med for neuropathic pain	• Range of motion exercises • Minimize ADLs • Monitor for urinary retention	• Interventions are dependent on family's goals of care • Emergent surgery or radiation therapy may be indicated if aggressive approaches toward a cure are being considered

28

Appendix 28-A: Pediatric Symptom Management[45-47]—continued

SYMPTOM	PHARMACOLOGICAL/MEDICAL	NONPHARMACOLOGICAL/ MEDICAL	COMMENTS
Agonal respirations	• Oxygen, if indicated	• Position & therapies to assure comfort	• Prepare family for imminent death, which may occur within minutes to days
Cough	• Administer opioid • Nebulized albuterol • Consider postnasal drip; treat with antihistamine • Chest physiotherapy to mobilize secretions	• Humidified air • Avoid respiratory irritants (e.g., smoke, strong odors) • Upright position	• Protective reflex that may weaken at EOL. Goal is to prevent cough from causing pain, loss of sleep or anxiety that may decrease quality of life
Dyspnea	• Oxygen if hypoxic • Opioid analgesic • Anxiolytic	• Humidified air • Avoid respiratory irritants (smoke, strong odors) • Upright position • Calming reassurance • Distraction	• Use of nebulized opioids is controversial without clear indications for use49
Pulmonary edema	• Restrict fluids • Oxygen • Opioid analgesic • Albumin or plasma, if hospitalized • Diuretics	• Position of comfort • Cool mist humidifier • Limit activities that could increase respiratory demands	• Interventions dependent on underlying cause & family's goals of care
Secretions	• Anticholinergic agents • Mucolytic agent • Yankauer oral suction catheter • Consider diuretic • Restrict fluids	• Humidified air • Position to allow drainage	• Noisy respirations, or 'death rattle' can sometimes be alleviated by changing position or gently oral suctioning, if end of life
Wheezing	• Bronchodilator—albuterol • Systemic corticosteroid • Diuretic	• Cool mist humidifier	

Pulmonary

28

	SYMPTOM	PHARMACOLOGICAL/MEDICAL	NONPHARMACOLOGICAL/ MEDICAL	COMMENTS
Renal & Metabolic	Decreased urine output	• Pyridium if pain with urination • Diuretic if fluid retention • Urinary catheter to facilitate emptying of bladder	• Run water to encourage voiding • Inhale peppermint spirits • Ammonia capsule in urinal or bedpan • Increase oral intake	• Prepare family for further system shutdown & EOL
	Urinary frequency/ Incontinence	• Treat underlying cause if indicated	• Facilitate toileting • Restrict fluids • Skin care	• Prepare family of change in consciousness may herald approaching death
	Hematuria	• Treat underlying cause if indicated	• Maximum oral intake	
	Hypercalcemia	• Bisphosphonate—no specific pediatric dosing • Hydration if appropriate	• Maximize activity to level of tolerance	• May cause significant discomfort, lethargy & muscle weakness • Treatment may require short term hospitalization
	Syndrome of inappropriate antidiuretic hormone	• Restrict fluids • If hospitalized, hypertonic saline infusion & diuretic		• Interventions dependent on underlying cause & family's goals of care
	Urinary retention	• Opioid rotation using equianalgesic dose • Low dose naloxone if opioid related • Consider treatment for underlying bladder infection • Consider neurological causes • Urinary catheter as appropriate	• Run water to encourage voiding • Inhale peppermint spirits • Ammonia capsule in urinal or bedpan • Increase oral intake	

KEY:
CPR—cardiopulmonary resuscitation
EOL—end of life
ET—endotracheal tube
IM—intramuscular
IV—intravenous
max—maximum
PO—oral
PR—rectal
SOB—shortness of breath

28

CITED REFERENCES

1. Feudtner C, Hexem K, Rourke MT. Epidemiology and the care of children with complex conditions. In: Wolfe J, Hinds PS, Sourkes BM, eds. *Textbook of Interdisciplinary Pediatric Palliative Care.* Philadelphia, PA: Elsevier/Saunders; 2011:7-17.

2. Friebert S. *NHPCO Facts and Figures: Pediatric Palliative and Hospice Care in America.* Alexandria, VA: National Hospice and Palliative Care Organization; 2009. Available at: www.nhpco.org/files/public/quality/pediatric_facts-figures.pdf. Accessed July 18, 2012.

3. National Hospice and Palliative Care Organization. *ChiPPS White Paper: A Call For Change: Recommendations to Improve the Care of Children Living with Life-Threatening Conditions.* Alexandria, VA: NHPCO; 2001.

4. National Hospice and Palliative Care Organization. *Standards of Practice for Pediatric Palliative Care and Hospice.* Alexandria, VA: NHPCO; 2009.

5. Field MJ, Behran RE. *When Children Die: Improving Palliative and End-of-Life Care for Children and Their Families.* Washington DC: National Academies Press; 2003.

6. Newacheck PW, Houtrow AJ, Romm DL, et al. The future of health insurance for children with special health care needs. *Pediatrics.* 2001;123(5):e940-e947.

7. Berenson S. Management of cancer pain with complementary therapies. *Oncology (Williston Park) Nurse Edition.* 2007;21(4 Suppl):10-22.

8. 11th Congress of United States of America, Title 2, Subtitle D, Section 2302. *Concurrent Care for Children.* 2010. Available at: www.ncsl.org/documents/health/ppaca-consolidated.pdf. Accessed April 30, 2012.

9. World Health Organization. *WHO Definition of Palliative Care.* 2012. Available at www.who.int/cancer/palliative/definition/en/. Accessed April 30, 2012.

10. National Consensus Project for Quality Palliative Care. *Clinical Practice Guidelines for Quality Palliative Care.* 3rd ed. Pittsburgh, PA: NCP; in press.

11. MacDorman MF, Mathews TJ. *Recent trends in infant mortality in the United States.* NCHS Data Brief. No 9. Hyattsville, MD: National Center for Health Statistics. 2008. Available at: www.cdc.gov/nchs/data/databriefs/db09.htm. Accessed March 21, 2011.

12. Widger K, Davies D, Drouin DJ, et al. Pediatric patients receiving palliative care in Canada: results of a multicenter review. *Arch Pediatr Adolesc Med.* 2007;161:597-602.

13. Friebert S, Huff S. NHPCO's Pediatric Standards: A key step in advancing care for America's children. *Newsline.* 2009;February:9-13

14. Friebert S, Osenaga, K. *Pediatric Palliative Care Referral Criteria.* Available at: www.capc.org/tools-for-palliative-care-programs/clinical-tools/consult-triggers/pediatric-palliative-care-referral-criteria.pdf. Accessed March 10, 2011.

15. Feudtner C, Kang TI, Hexem KR, et al. Pediatric palliative care patients: a prospective multicenter cohort study. *Pediatrics.* 2011;127(6):1094-101.

16. Ethier A. Family-centered end of life care. In: Hockenberry MJ, Wilson D, eds. *Wong's Nursing Care of Infants and Children.* 9th ed. St. Louis, MO: Elsevier/Mosby; 2011:876-907.

17. Hinds PS, Oakes LL, Hicks J, et al. "Trying to be a good parent" as defined by interviews with parents who made phase I, terminal care, and resuscitation decisions for their children. *J Clin Oncol.* 2009;27(35):5979-5985.

18. U.S. Department of Education. *Building the legacy: IDEA 2004.* 2004. Available at: idea.ed.gov/. Accessed: March 11, 2011.

19. Cassell E. *The Nature of Suffering and the Goals of Medicine.* 2nd ed. New York, NY: Oxford University Press; 2004.

20. Ferrell BR, Coyle N. *The Nature of Suffering and the Goals of Nursing.* New York, NY: Oxford University Press; 2008.

21. Hesselgrave J, Hockenberry M. Fatigue. In: Wolfe J, Hinds PS, Sourkes BS, eds. *Textbook of Interdisciplinary Pediatric Palliative Care.* Philadelphia, PA: Elsevier/Saunders; 2011:266-271.

22. Lansky LL, List MA, Lansky SB, Cohen ME, Sinks LF. Toward the development of a play performance scale for children (PPSC). *Cancer.* 2006;56(7 Suppl):1837-1840.

23. Hockenberry MH, Wilson D. Chronic illness, disability, or end-of-life care for the child and family. In: Hockenberry MJ, Wildon D, eds. *Wong's Essentials of Pediatric Nursing.* 8th ed. Philadelphia, PA: Elsevier/Mosby; 2008:239-325.

24. Wolfe J, Grier HE, Klar N, et al. Symptoms and suffering at the end of life in children with cancer. *N Engl J Med.* 2000;342(5):326-333.

25. Collins JC, Berde CB, Frost JA. Pain assessment and management. In: Wolfe J, Hinds PS, Sourkes BM, eds. *Textbook of Interdisciplinary Pediatric Palliative Care.* Philadelphia, PA: Elsevier/Saunders; 2011:284-299.

26. Pasero C. Pain assessment in patients who cannot self-report. In: Pasero C, McCaffery M, eds. *Pain Assessment and Pharmacologic Management.* St. Louis, MO: Mosby; 2011:123-131.

28

27. Hummel P, Lawlor-Kloan, Weiss MG. Validity and reliability of the N-PASS assessment tool with acute pain. *J Perinatol.* 2010;30(7):474-478.

28. Suarez A, Knoppert DC, Lee DS, Pletsch D, Seabrook JA. Opioid infusions in neonatal intensive care units. *J Pediatr Pharm Ther.* 2010;15(2):142-146.

29. Herr K, Coyne PJ, Key T, et al. Pain assessment in the nonverbal patient: position statement with clinical practice recommendations. *Pain Manag Nurs.* 20067(2):44-52.

30. City of Hope; American Association of Colleges of Nursing, Inc. ELNEC: *End-of-Life Nursing Curriculum-Pediatric Palliative Care.* Duarte, CA; Washington, DC: City of Hope; American Association of Colleges of Nursing, Inc. 2012. For further information: www.aacn.nche.edu/ELNEC.

31. Anand K. Consensus statement for the prevention and management of pain in the newborn. *Arch Pediatr Adolesc Med.* 2001;155(2)173-180. Available at: archpedi.jamanetwork.com/article.aspx?articleid=190335. Accessed May 17, 2012.

32. Slater R, Fabrizi L, Worley A, Meek J, Boyd S, Fitzgerald M. Premature infants display increased noxious-evoked neuronal activity in the brain compared to healthy age-matched term-born infants. *Neuroimage.* 2010;52(2):583-589.

33. Abdulkader HM, Freer Y, Garry EM, Fleetwood-Walker SM, McIntosh N. Prematurity and neonatal noxious events exert lasting effects on infant pain behavior. *Early Hum Dev.* 2008;84(6):351-355.

34. Catlin A, Carter B. Creation of a neonatal end-of-life and palliative care protocol. *J Perinatol.* 2002;22(3):184-195.

35. Carter B, Levetown M. *Palliative Care for Infants, Children and Adolescents: A Practical Handbook.* Baltimore, MD: John Hopkins University Press; 2004.

36. Goldstein ML, Sakae M. Pediatric pain: knowing the child before you. In: Ferrell BR, Coyle N, eds. *Oxford Textbook of Palliative Nursing.* 3rd ed. New York, NY: Oxford University Press; 2010:1099-1118.

37. Jacobs HH. Ethics in pediatric end-of-life care: a nursing perspective. *J Pediatr Nurs.* 2005;20(5):360-369.

38. Lautrette A, Ciroldi M, Ksibi H, Azoulay E. End-of-life family conferences: rooted in the evidence. *Crit Care Med.* 2006;34:364-372.

39. Jones BL, Gilmer MJ, Parker-Raley J, Dokken DL, Freyer DR, Sydnor-Greenberg N. Parent and sibling relationships and the family experience. In: Wolfe J, Hinds PS, Sourkes BM, eds. *Textbook of Interdisciplinary Pediatric Palliative Care.* Philadelphia, PA: Elsevier Saunders; 2011:135-147.

40. Rushton CH. Ethical decision making at the end of life. In: Armstrong-Daily A, Zarbock A, eds. *Hospice Care for Children.* Boston, MA: Oxford University Press; 2009:457-489.

41. Lindley LC. Healthcare reform and concurrent curative care for terminally ill children. *J Hosp Palliat Nurs.* 2011;13(2):81-88.

42. Kreicbergs U, Validimarsdottier U, Onelov E, Henter JI, Steneck G. Talking about death with children who have severe malignant disease. *N Engl J Med.* 2011;351(12):1175-1186.

43. Pirie A. Pediatric palliative care communication: resources for the clinical nurse specialist. *Clin Nurse Spec.* 2012;26(4):212-215.

44. American Academy of Pediatrics Committee on Bioethics: Guidelines on foregoing medical treatment. *Pediatrics.* 1994;93(3):532-536.

45. Ethier AM, Rollins J, Stewart J, eds. *Pediatric Oncology Palliative and End-of-Life Care Resource 2010.* Glenview, IL: CureSearch, Children's Oncology Group, Association of Pediatric Hematology/Oncology Nurses; 2010.

46. Wolfe J, Hinds PS, Sourkes BM. *Textbook of Interdisciplinary Pediatric Palliative Care.* Philadelphia, PA: Elsevier/Saunders; 2011.

47. Epocrates RX; Version 9.0, 2009.

48. Curley MA, Razmus IS, Roberts KE, Wypij D. Predicting pressure ulcer risk in pediatric patients: the Braden Q Scale. *Nurs Res.* 2003;52(1):22-33.

49. Dudgeon D. Dyspnea, death rattle, and cough. In: Ferrell BR, Coyle N, eds. *Oxford Textbook of Palliative Nursing.* 3rd ed. New York, NY: Oxford University Press; 2010:303-319.

28

ADDITIONAL RESOURCES

Allen PJ, Vessey JA, eds. *Primary Care of the Child with a Chronic Condition.* 4th ed. St. Louis, MO: Elsevier/Mosby; 2004.

Armstrong-Dailey A, Zarbock S, eds. *Hospice Care for Children.* 3rd ed. New York, NY: Oxford University Press; 2009.

Bearison DJ. *When Treatment Fails: How Medicine Cares for Dying Children.* New York, NY: Oxford University Press; 2006.

Carter B, Levetown M, eds. *Palliative Care for Infants, Children and Adolescents.* Baltimore, MD: Johns Hopkins University Press; 2011.

Charastek J, Eull D. *Just in Time Guide: A Primer for Pediatric Palliative Care at Home.* Pittsburgh, PA: Hospice and Palliative Nurses Association; 2010.

Hilden J, Tobin DR. *Shelter from the Storm: Caring for a Child with a Life-Threatening Condition.* Cambridge, MA; Perseus Publishing; 2003.

Pirie A. Pediatric palliative care communication: resources for the clinical nurse specialist. *Clin Nurs Spec.* 2012;26(4):212-215.

Wrede-Seaman L. *Pediatric Pain and Symptom Management Algorithms for Palliative Care.* Intellicard, Inc; 2005.

28

CHAPTER 29

THE OLDER ADULT POPULATION

Susan Derby MA. GNP-BC, ACHPN®

I. INTRODUCTION

- By 2030, one in five people will be age 65 and older.[1]

- The majority of people who suffer from chronic diseases and conditions are older adults, with comorbid chronic illnesses and symptoms increasing during the last years of life.

- Evidence suggests that end-of-life care for many older people is characterized by poor symptom control, inadequate advance care planning, and increased dependence on family and caregivers.

- The older patient may develop symptoms related to various conditions and diseases, treatment related therapies such as those related to cancer, or interaction with a pre-existing comorbid illness.

- APRNs who have clinical expertise in palliative care, are in an ideal position to provide palliative care and end-of-life care.

II. DEMOGRAPHICS

The silver tsunami started in the last decade. The fastest growing population is people over the age of 85. Within the next 20 years, 1 in 5 people will be over the age of 65. This chapter will outline some of the most important palliative care needs of the older population, and highlight how the APRN, in a variety of settings, can impact significantly on symptom management and care at the end of life for this population.

During the last years of life, many people will develop a chronic illness; often these illnesses will be potentially life-limiting. The typical course will be progressive loss of function, decline, and dependence on others and/or placement in institutions for care. From 2002-2006, the median age at diagnosis for cancer of all sites was 66 years of age.[2] Over the past decade, the prevalence rates for arthritis, hypertension, and obesity have increased in persons over age 65; while the reported prevalence of heart problems decreased slightly. In 2005, the percentage of adults with three or more chronic conditions increased with age; from 7% of adults 45–54 years-of-age to 37% of adults 75 years-of-age and over.[3]

One population of individuals that can be expected to achieve greater longevity in increasing numbers is older adults with severe disabilities in need of long-term care. In one retrospective cohort study of 229,543 Medicare beneficiaries with heart failure who died between January 2000 and December 2007, approximately 80% of patients were hospitalized in the last 6 months of life; days in intensive care units increased from 3.5 to 4.6;[4] use of hospice increased from 19% to nearly 40% of patients.[4] This represents a dramatic shift in care at the end of life for older Americans. While cancer remains the most common hospice diagnosis, it is encouraging to see more patients

29

with advanced heart disease using hospice services. One barrier to timely hospice referrals for patients with heart failure is the difficulty in predicting prognosis.

The course of illness for many older people is often accompanied by multiple, frequent, and unpredictable exacerbations of disease, hospitalization and the need for nursing and medical care. Three general stages of progression of chronic illness have been identified

1. Early stage—diagnosis and initial management

2. Middle stage—disease modification and adjustment to functional decline

3. Late stage—preparation for dying

   a) This model applies to many chronic illnesses common in the older adult, but other conditions such as advanced cancer may show a more gradual and steady course over months followed by a rapid decline.

Many older people suffer from multiple chronic illnesses—advanced cardiac disease, diabetes, and advanced cancer. All of these factors can threaten the independence of the older adult, increase symptom burden, and add to the complexity of prognostication.

III. GERIATRIC SYNDROMES AND THE FRAIL ELDERLY

In order to provide comprehensive palliative care and end-of-life care to the older patient, it is important for the advanced practice palliative care nurse to understand and identify the presence of geriatric syndromes in the older patient.

A. The term "geriatric syndromes" is used to describe clinical conditions in older persons that do not fit into discrete disease categories. The use of this term denotes multiple causes for a constellation of signs and symptoms. Geriatric syndromes are multi-factorial, with shared risk factors.

   1. There is no one single mechanism of aging; multiple changes occur over time. Advancing age is associated with both structural and physiological changes in most body systems and changes in physical, emotional, and cognitive function.

   2. The physiological stress response is compromised as is the patient's ability to tolerate medication dosing typically used in younger patients.

   3. These changes, along with the presence of multiple comorbid conditions and the use of multiple prescription drugs place the older adult at greater risk for development of geriatric syndromes.

B. These conditions include functional decline, delirium, dementia, falls, frailty, dizziness, syncope, pressure ulcers, and urinary incontinence.

C. The presence of "geriatric syndromes" indicates both decreased life expectancy and reduced functional reserve.

D. Elderly cancer patients have a higher prevalence of geriatric syndromes than those without cancer.

E. Frailty is a process of physiologic decline that reduces physiologic reserve and predisposes to organ failure. Balducci and Stanta[5] have identified several criteria of frailty that include

29

1. Age of 85 years or more

   a) Comorbidities can include 3 or more conditions with at least 1 of the following—cardiovascular, respiratory, or cerebrovascular

2. Comorbidity index

   a) Presence of one or more geriatric syndromes

      i. Moderate to severe dementia

      ii. 3 or more falls during one month

      iii. Delirium in the presence of upper respiratory infection, urinary tract infection, diuretics, as side effect of medications, or benign prostatic hypertrophy

      iv. Fecal incontinence unrelated to diarrhea or laxatives

3. History of osteoporotic fracture or vertebral compression fracture

4. Failure to thrive

5. Neglect and abuse

6. Other criteria for frailty include

   a) Dependence in activities of daily living (ADLs)

   b) Depression

   c) Malnutrition

   d) Polypharmacy

   e) Prolonged bedrest

   f) Restraints

   g) Sensory impairment

   h) Socioeconomic/family problems including substance abuse, physical or psychological abuse

7. The frail elderly person is generally not a candidate for aggressive life-prolonging treatment but requires management of chronic and acute illnesses and symptom management based on the goals of care as established by patient, family, and caregivers. Goals of maximizing quality of life and preventing further decline in function are often primary and will influence the use and dosing of medications and interventions used to treat common symptoms and conditions, and end-of-life care.

8. One way of assessing the older patient for the presence of geriatric syndromes and frailty is through the use of a comprehensive geriatric assessment in all practice settings. The APRN, through skilled assessment, can identify baseline function including the presence of geriatric syndromes, and plan interventions that may prevent significant morbidity and mortality.

IV. COMPREHENSIVE GERIATRIC ASSESSMENT

Comprehensive Geriatric Assessment (CGA) is a multidisciplinary evaluation directed at uncovering, describing, and explaining problems of the older person. The resources and strengths of the person are cataloged, and a coordinated care plan is developed to focus interventions on the person's problems.[6]

A. The purpose of performing a CGA is to design multidisciplinary and therapeutic interventions aimed at reducing functional impairments, psychological and psychosocial distress, managing symptoms, and reducing caregiver burden and distress. CGA can be part of any initial nursing assessment of the older adult in any setting (e.g., medical, surgical, oncologic).

B. A CGA should include

1. Sensory function (e.g., hearing, vision)

2. Mobility and gait

3. Activities of daily living (ADL) such as toileting, bathing, dressing, and eating

4. Instrumental activities of daily living (IADLs) such as meal preparation, housekeeping, and bill paying

5. Nutritional status

6. Cognitive function

7. Socialization

8. Affect

9. Economic concerns

10. Home environment

11. Symptom assessment

12. Medication use and management.

C. The CGA should also include patient preferences for life-prolonging therapies and the presence of a healthcare agent who is aware of the patient's end-of-life wishes.

D. In settings where a CGA is not a routine part of assessment, the APRN can include many of the components in the initial assessment. The initial physical examination and assessment should include areas listed in the GCA. Ideally it should be performed prior to onset frailty to allow for early identification of those conditions that predispose or trigger frailty.

E. Assessment of physical function begins with an evaluation of the patient's ability to perform ADLs and IADLs, gait, physical strength, and function. Questioning the patient and caregiver about the patient's abilities is a helpful part of this evaluation. If further evaluation is needed, the patient should be referred to a physical and/or occupational therapist for ongoing evaluation and intervention. Establishing baseline function will determine the patient's level of independence, and will assist in the ongoing monitoring and assessment.

1. Gait and mobility can be tested with a simple Get Up and Go evaluation where the patient gets up from a chair and walks 10 feet and turns around, walks back to the chair and sits down. The time required is normally 10 seconds or less. A patient with impaired gait, balance, muscle weakness, or cognitive function will take longer to complete this task.

2. The Minimum Data Set (MDS) is a comprehensive interdisciplinary assessment required by the Centers for Medicare and Medicaid Services (CMS) for all long-term care residents. The assessment sections include identification information; hearing, speech, and vision; cognitive patterns; mood; behavior; preferences for customary routine and activities; functional

29

status; bladder and bowel function; active disease diagnoses; health conditions; swallowing/nutritional status; oral/dental status; skin conditions; medications; special treatments and procedures; restraints; and participation in assessment and goal setting. The final section is an area of care assessment summary to document areas of concern (triggered care areas) brought to light by combined assessment sections and develop a care plan for each triggered areas. The care assessment areas are delirium, cognitive loss/dementia, visual function, communication, activities of daily living functional/rehabilitation potential, urinary incontinence and indwelling catheter, psychosocial wellbeing, mood state, behavioral symptoms, activities, falls, nutritional status, feeding tubes, dehydration/fluid maintenance, dental care, pressure ulcer, psychotropic medication use, physical restraints, pain, and return to community referral.[7,8]

F. An event, such as a fall can lead to a hospitalization and prolonged bedrest. Risk factors for falls are outlined in Table 1.

   1. The frail older adult, with decreased muscle mass and strength, coupled with the physiological effects of bedrest, increases the risk of disability during or after hospitalization.

   2. Medical complications of bedrest and immobility include deep vein thrombosis, pressure ulcers, cardiac and muscle deconditioning, falls, and in some patients, confusion.

G. Ongoing evaluation of mental status can detect early cognitive changes such as dementia, and/or delirium, assessment for depression in relation to functional change is essential.

Table 1: Common Risk Factors for Falls in Older Adults

• Cognitive dysfunction • Environmental hazards—improper fitting shoes, stairs, slippery floors, loose scatter rugs • History of falls • Impaired balance • Improper lighting • Incontinence of bowel and/or bladder • Lymphedema	• Medication use—sedatives, hypnotics, opioids, antihypertensives, diuretics, laxatives • Muscle weakness • Peripheral neuropathy • Pets • Sensory loss—vision and hearing • Small children

V. UNDERSTANDING SYMPTOM CLUSTERS

A syndrome has been defined as "a group of signs and symptoms that occur together and characterize a particular abnormality or condition.[9] A symptom cluster may be defined as "2 or more concurrent symptoms that occur together with a high degree of predictability."[10] Both syndromes and symptom clusters impact clinical interventions and survival.

In the older adult who may present with multiple comorbid illnesses and geriatric syndromes, the impact of symptom clusters further adds to distress and the complexity of symptom management. The presence of symptom clusters often requires multidisciplinary intervention.

A. Symptoms within a cluster should have a stronger association with each other than with symptoms in different clusters. Symptom clusters may or may not have a common etiology. Patients with specific symptom clusters may also have different clinical outcomes and disease course than those with individual

29

symptoms. The cluster phenomenon represents inter-relationships between symptoms occurring in 1 type of cancer or disease, and with other symptom clusters. For example, a patient with depression, pain, and fatigue may share a direct association with a common mediator, such as chemotherapy or radiation therapy. Individuals with pain seem more prone to depression, because of its effect on psychological state. Depression might contribute to the symptoms of pain and fatigue.

1. In one study, evaluating 1366 older cancer patients with gastrointestinal, lung, and breast cancer, symptoms in the years 2005-2007 were assessed using the Edmonton Symptom Assessment Scale (ESAS). Two major symptom clusters were identified—Cluster 1—fatigue, drowsiness, decreased appetite, and dyspnea; and Cluster 2—anxiety and depression.[11] Their findings of psychological distress further support the finding that anxiety and depression are a major source of distress to patients with advanced cancer, and indicate the necessity to use pharmacological management targeted at these symptoms.

B. At the end of life, when it becomes necessary to eliminate all nonessential medications, using multipurpose drugs to manage symptom clusters eases the pill burden. For example, when treating an older adult at the end of life for fatigue, drowsiness, and decreased appetite, it may be prudent to use one multipurpose drug such as a steroid to manage all three symptoms. However, the initiation of these medications should begin at much lower doses such as 0.5-1 mg to account for possibly decreased kidney function.

C. Presently, although there is an incomplete understanding of the causes and mechanisms of clusters, certain clusters have been found to be statistically valid. Ongoing assessment of symptoms using validated tools such as the Edmonton Symptom Assessment System[12] and the Condensed Memorial Symptom Assessment Scale[13] in the older population will further identify symptom clusters in different cancer sites. Understanding the pathophysiology and mechanisms of action can allow clinicians to provide treatment with specific symptom-targeted interventions.

D. Pharmacological intervention is the mainstay of treatment for symptom management in palliative care of the older adult. Knowledge of the physiology of aging will help the clinician prevent significant morbidity and mortality when prescribing drugs used to treat single or multiple symptoms. Aging is characterized by a gradual decline in organ function reserves. This becomes apparent under stress and plays an important role at the end of life when the goal of care is symptom management and comfort. In many organs, function loss begins in the 3rd or 4th decade and proceeds at approximately 1% annually.[14] Aging without disease is normal. Table 2 outlines some common physiological changes of aging.

29

VI. CHALLENGES OF SYMPTOM MANAGEMENT IN THE OLDER ADULT—PAIN, DEPRESSION, AND DELIRIUM

Whether the older patient is in the home, an acute-care setting, or in a long-term care facility, the challenges of providing end-of-life care are similar. All ARPNs have a critical role in contributing to the ongoing management of symptoms in the older adult. Through their collaborative efforts, and working within the context of an interdisciplinary team, they can provide care for these complex patients. Whether

Table 2: Common Physiological Changes of Aging

Organ System	Age-Related Change
Cardiovascular	• Left ventricular (LV) early-diastolic filling rate progressively decreases • Atrial hypertrophy → 4th heart sound • Left ventricular ejection fraction during exercise decreases • Decrease in maximal cardiac output • Diminished cardiac reserve • Diminished LV elasticity • Decreased myocardial perfusion • Increased risk for cardiac events, increased risk for atrial fibrillation
Respiratory system	• Increased chest wall rigidity • Reduced respiratory muscle strength • Decrease in hypoxic and hypercapnic ventilatory drive • Loss of diffusing capacity & elastic recoil • Weakening of intercostal muscles, decreased strength of the diaphragm • Decreased forced expiratory volume in the 1st second of expiration (FEV1) & forced vital capacity (FVC)
Renal system	• Progressive loss of baseline kidney function between the ages of 30 & 85 years—20-25% loss of renal mass, fewer glomeruli • Loss of nephrons due to atherosclerosis & ischemia • Decreased capacity to reabsorb sodium & secrete potassium & hydrogen ions • Impaired concentrating capacity • 10% decline in renal blood flow per decade after age 25 • Decreased glomerular filtration rate (GFR), serum creatinine levels remain normal because of the decreased production of creatinine in the older adult • Decreased ability to tolerate water deprivation & water boluses • The concentration of atrial natriuretic peptide (ANP) is increased → suppression of renin
Endocrine	• Reduced estrogen & testosterone • Increased insulin resistance • Less lean body mass & increase in fat
Reaction time	• Slower mental & physical responses to specific stimuli
Brain	• Gradual loss of brain tissue • Deterioration in memory, insomnia
Immune system	• Functional impairment of T lymphocyte-mediated immunity & increased susceptibility to infections • Increased serum inflammatory mediators • Increase in stress-related natural killer cell activity

29

death is expected within days, weeks, or months, the palliative APRN can provide leadership and skill in maximizing quality of life for the older adult with chronic illness.

A. Pain—as many as 55% of nursing home residents have pain that contributes significantly to impaired quality of life.[15] Most mild pain in nursing homes is related to degenerative arthritis, low-back disorders, and diabetic and post-herpetic neuropathy. Cancer pain accounts for the majority of severe pain. Data from nursing homes suggest that as many as 30-80% of nursing home residents receive inadequate pain management.[16] One of the most troublesome issues in the nursing home population is the difficulty in assessing pain in the cognitively impaired older resident.

1. Self-report is the standard for pain assessment. However, in the older adult with cognitive impairment, the ability of the patient to verbally report their level of pain is diminished and may be in the form of a story. This necessitates that the observer, often unlicensed staff, assess for pain. Identifying pain in a

cognitively impaired patient involves sophisticated clinical skills. Behaviors exhibited by patients with advanced dementia may be indicative of a variety of conditions, including pain. Table 3 outlines common pain behaviors in cognitively impaired older adults. Incorporating a pain assessment tool into the management of cognitively impaired older adults is part of a comprehensive plan of care.

Pain assessment in the older adult is based on observation by the nurse and patient's self-report. A thorough assessment of pain will help the advanced practice registered nurse determine the etiology of pain and establish a pain diagnosis. The basic principles of a pain assessment in the older adult are outlined in Table 4.

A variety of pain assessment tools are available for use by the older adult. For those with mild cognitive impairment, standard scales can be used. For those with severe cognitive impairment, a tool that uses behavioral observations should be used (see Table 5). A 2011 position statement of the

Table 3: Common Pain Behaviors in Patients with Moderate to Severe Dementia

Indication	Example
Facial expression	Frown, sad, grimacing, blank look, wincing
Verbalizations	Moaning, groaning, noisy breathing, calling out, telling an implausible story
Body movements	Guarding, fidgeting, rocking, rigid, massaging affected area, bracing, wandering
Behavioral changes	Aggressive, combative, withdrawn
Changes in activity	Refusing food, decreased interaction, sleeping more than usual, rest pattern changes, changes in ability to wash or dress
Mental status changes	Crying, increased confusion, irritability or distress

Table 4: Principles of Pain Management in the Older Adult[18,19]

- Provide for routine screening of pain
- Identify goals of care—what is the diagnosis and the prognosis, & is the patient and caregiver in agreement with the goals of care
- Perform a thorough pain assessment
- Determine comorbid conditions which may contribute or be the underlying cause of the pain
- Assess functional, cognitive, psychological status including memory loss, depression, anxiety
- Identify level of caregiver support
- Ask about substance abuse—present, recent, or remote
- Perform a physical examination with careful attention to the painful site(s)
- Review past radiology history & imaging studies to determine the etiology of the pain
- Determine barriers to assessment, administration, & compliance with drug treatment plans (e.g., cultural issues, financial, physiological, psychological)
- Determine renal clearance, which may limit analgesic selection. Do not use morphine if impaired renal function
- Review other physiological parameters (e.g., liver function, respiratory status), which may affect analgesic selection
- If indicated, provide for around the clock dosing with long-acting opioids & as needed rescue dosing with short-acting opioids for breakthrough pain
- Avoid drug combinations that may potentiate side effects such as sedation
- Avoid drugs that may potentiate pre-existing comorbidities such as peripheral edema with certain anticonvulsants
- Consider cost & compliance with scheduling when prescribing
- Provide for ongoing education for the patient and caregiver in issues related to addiction and side effects
- Start low and titrate slowly with frequent assessments for side effects and analgesic effect

29

American Society for Pain Management Nursing (ASPMN), *Pain Assessment in Patients Unable to Self-Report* provides additional information about assessment and validated tools.[17]

2. The principles of pain management in the older adult are similar to those in the younger patient with some exceptions. The reader is referred to Chapter 6, Pain, for further details, and to the American Geriatrics Society Panel on the *Pharmacological Management of Persistent Pain in Older Patients* for recommended drugs for the management of persistent cancer pain in older adults.[19]

Pharmacological Management of Persistent Pain in Older Adults

The palliative APRN should be aware of the physiological changes of aging that impact on the effectiveness and toxicity of medications used to treat pain in the older adult (see Table 6).

Pharmacotherapy is the primary treatment of pain; it should not be the only approach in the management of pain in the older patient. A multimodal approach is usually required, and nonpharmacological interventions should be employed, if appropriate. Table 7 outlines some of the most common nonpharmacological interventions. Nonpharmacological intervention, often easy to implement, may benefit the older adult who may be reluctant to take medications. Theses interventions may serve as complementary interventions to pharmacological interventions and provide for an interdisciplinary approach.

B. End-of-Life Depression

Older patients at the end of life are faced with challenges to their sense of control, autonomy, their relationships to family and friends, and issues surrounding progressive symptom burden and dependence on others. As with other patient populations, the older adult may be fearful about uncontrolled pain, loss of cognitive function, and separation from their loved ones. Depression in the older adult is often under-diagnosed, and therefore inadequately treated. Based on the Diagnostic and Statistical Manual of Mental Disorders (DSM1V)[27] at least 5 of the following symptoms must be present for a 2-week period

- Significant change in appetite and weight

- Disrupted sleep or hypersomnia

Table 5: Common Pain Assessment Tools in Cognitively Impaired Older Adults

Pain Assessment Tool	QR Code to Access Tool
Pain Assessment in Advanced Dementia Scale (PAINAD)—for use in acute care and long-term care[20,21]	
Checklist of Nonverbal Pain Indicators (CNPI)—for use with acute and chronic pain in acute care & long-term care.[22,23]	
Non-Communicative Patient's Pain Assessment Instrument (NOPPAIN)—nursing assistant-administered tool for assessing pain behaviors patients with dementia[24-26]	

29

Table 6: Common Pharmacological Changes with Aging Influencing Pain Management[19]

Pharmacological Concern	Change with Normal Aging
Gatrointestinal absorption	• Slowing of transit time may prolong effects of continuous-release enteral drugs • Opioid-related bowel dysmotility may be enhanced in older patients
Transdermal absorption	• Less subcutaneous fat may decrease absorption
Distribution	• Increased fat to lean body weight may increase volume of distribution for fat soluble drugs • May result in long drug half-life
Liver metabolism	• Oxidation is variable and may result in prolonged half-life. May occur in patient with cirrhosis, hepatitis, & extensive tumor infiltration
Renal excretion	• Glomerular filtration rate decreases with aging, resulting in decreased excretion and toxicity
Active metabolites	• Reduced renal clearance will prolong effects of metabolites, resulting in toxicity

Table 7: Nonpharmacological Interventions for Pain Management

• Progressive relaxation • Music therapy • Cognitive-behavioral therapy • Biofeedback • Acupuncture/acupressure • Transcutaneous nerve stimulation (TENs) • Reflexology	• Physical exercise and physical therapy if consistent with goals of care • Reiki • Spiritual activities (e.g., prayer, services, reading holy books, hymns) • Distraction (e.g., participating in an activity, visiting with family & friends)

- Psychomotor agitation or retardation

- Fatigue or loss of energy

- Feelings of worthlessness

- Excessive guilt

- Reduced concentration

- Recurrent thoughts of death or suicidal ideation

Determining a diagnosis of depression in the setting of profound illness and symptoms becomes especially challenging. Estimates of depression may be as high as 25% in the cancer population.[28] Aging, even for the healthiest, includes profound changes and losses—of friends and family, social roles, function and independence. At the end of life, many older, highly symptomatic, patients exhibit many of these symptoms, which are often attributed to medical illnesses.[29] Many older patients who easily acknowledge depression accept it as a normal part of being ill and dying. Focusing assessment on feelings of hopelessness, helplessness, worthlessness, and guilt may help differentiate depression from physical frailty.[30]

Assessing for and treating depression in the older adult should be part of all symptom management endeavors. Psychotherapy as well as pharmacological interventions should be employed to strengthen coping skills. Cognitive-behavioral approaches such as relaxation, deep breathing, and guided imagery may help in reducing anxiety and panic. Pharmacological interventions should include use of antidepressants and psychostimulants. The use of selective serotonin reuptake

29

inhibitors (SSRIs) is recommended, when life expectancy is greater than 2 months. At the end of life when there is limited time to respond to antidepressants, the use of psychostimulants can help enormously in improving mood.[30] (See Chapter 15, *Psychosocial Aspects*)

C. Delirium

Delirium is a common and serious condition in the older adult. Delirium in the older adult is associated with a significant amount of morbidity and mortality, increased hospital stay, increased risk of cognitive decline, functional decline, decreased quality of life, and increased nursing home placement.[31] It can also interfere with symptom assessment and treatment as it limits communication of a patients' distress. Delirious patients experience more falls, develop a greater incidence of pressure ulcers, and are unable to care for themselves.

Delirium is more common in certain patient populations including patients with AIDS or cancer, the critically ill, postoperative patients, and those who are terminally ill. It is more frequent in elderly patients and in patients with a baseline brain dysfunction such as dementia. In cancer patients, delirium is an independent factor of poor prognosis for short–term survival. At the end of life, most older patients experience some degree of diffuse brain abnormalities, often with agitation. Some of these patients may require palliative sedation to control this symptom.

Increasing age, dementia, sensory losses, advanced illness, complex cancer treatments and polypharmacy increases the risk of delirium in the older adult.[31,32] Predisposing factors are the older person's vulnerabilities such as pre-existing dementia, and precipitating factors are the acute and noxious stimuli/insults experienced by the older person, such as surgery, and prolonged hospitalization (see Table 8). Polypharmacy is a major contributing factor to the development of delirium in older patients. Table 9 outlines the most common drugs causing delirium in older patients.

Delirium in older patients is often overlooked or misdiagnosed. It is usually precipitated by an underlying acute medical condition, which in most cases can be identified. The diagnostic criteria for delirium are identified by the DSM IV. See Chapter 12, *Delirium* for further discussion. The APRN who assesses the cognitive status of older patients can be instrumental in the early detection of pathophysiologic states including delirium, dementia, and depression. Knowledge of the course and clinical features of each of these states will allow for further evaluation by the clinician so that an appropriate diagnosis can be made (see Table 10). Evaluation of the older patient should always be based on the goals of care, the extent of disease, and the possible reversibility of the condition or symptom.

29

VII. CAREGIVER ISSUES

In palliative care, the patient and family/caregiver are seen as one unit. In older patients with advanced disease, the caregiver in the home is the primary source of assistance. Patients with advanced disease require assistance with almost all activities of life including dressing, feeding, meal preparation, bill paying, medication administration, and toileting. In some patients, care may be very complicated involving care of ostomies, wounds, tracheostomies, and feeding or drainage tubes. The majority of caregivers are spouses, most of them wives, many older themselves. The family is more vulnerable by being at risk of fatigue and emotional and physical burnout.

Table 8: Factors Contributing to Delirium in Older Adults with Cancer[32]

	Predisposing	Precipitating
General	• Age • Severity of illness	• Prolonged hospitalization, immobility
Central nervous system factors	• Cognitive impairment • Depression • Sensory loss—hearing, seeing • Metastatic cancer to the brain • Previous stroke • Dementia • Atrophy of gray and white matter • Senile plaques in the brain	
Metabolic	• Fever • Electrolyte disturbance—uremia, hypo/hyperglycemia, hypo/hypernatremia • Dehydration • Malnutrition • Vitamin deficiency • Hypoxemia, anemia • Hypo/hyperthyroidism • Disseminated intravascular coagulation • Congestive heart failure • Cardiac arrhythmia	
Infection	• Chemotherapy • Low white blood counts	• Urinary catheters • Intravenous catheters • Prolonged immobility
Substance abuse	• Recent or remote alcoholism • Recent or remote history of drug abuse	• Hospitalization & alcohol or drug withdrawal syndrome • Use of opioids, bensodiazepines
Environmental	• Sleep deprivation	• Hospitalization, room changes, Intensive care unit
Pharmacological	• Polypharmacy • Drug-drug interactions • Chemotherapy	• Use of sedatives, hypnotics, antidepressants, tranquilizers, opioids, steroids, antineoplastics

29

     Over time, all aspects of the caregivers' quality of life often suffer. The burden of caregiving includes a greater number of depressive symptoms, diminished health, and financial problems. If the patient is incontinent, confused, or agitated, the strain is even greater, with greater requirements for monitoring on a 24-hour basis. In the palliative care setting, where the treatment goals are supportive and management includes complex symptoms in addition to daily caregiving, the home caregiver may feel additionally burdened. The palliative ARPN can be of tremendous benefit to the caregiver in establishing priorities, obtaining assistance with home care, financial assistance, transportation, and being a "therapeutic ear" to listen and counsel and promoting interdisciplinary care particularly in the hospice setting. Family grief therapy during this palliative phase of illness has the potential to improve the psychosocial function of caregivers. Kissane and colleagues have used a screening tool to identify dysfunctional family coping, and relieve stress through a model of family grief therapy.[35]

Table 9: Drugs Commonly Causing Delirium in the Older Adult with Cancer[33,34]

Classification	Examples
Antidepressants	Amitriptyline, doxepin
Antihistamines	Chlorpheniramine, diphenhydramine
Diabetic agents	Chlorpropamide
Cardiac	Digoxin, dipyridamole
Antihypertensives	Propanolol, clonidine
Sedatives, barbiturates	Diazepam, flurazepam
Opioids	Meperidine, pentazocine,
Nonsteroidal anti-inflammatory agents and Cox-2 inhibitors	Indomethacin, celecoxib
Antibiotics	Quinolones
Anticonvulsants	Phenobarbital, phenytoin, carbamazepine
Anticholinergics	Atropine, scopolamine
Antiemetics	Phenothiazine, metoclopramide, prochlorperazine, dronabinol,
Antispasmodics	Hyoscyamine, belladonna alkaloids
Chemotherapy	Methotrexate, mitomycin, procarbazine, Ara-C, carmustine, fluorouracil, interferon, interleukin, l-asparaginase, prednisone, ifosfamide, vincristine, vinblastine, cisplatin, bleomycin
Antiparkinson	Amantadine, levodopa
Acetaminophen	
Salicylates	
Alcohol	
H2 receptor antagonists	Cimetidine, ranitidine

VIII. ADVANCE CARE PLANNING AND THE OLDER ADULT

A. Advance care planning (ACP) is a process whereby a patient, in consultation with healthcare providers, family members, and important others make decisions about his or her future healthcare. Grounded in the ethical principle of autonomy and the legal doctrine of consent, advance care planning helps to ensure that the patient's wishes are respected and carried out, if the patient becomes unable to participate in decision-making. This becomes extremely important when the older adult begins to lose capacity to make healthcare decisions due to advanced illness, effects of medications, impact of symptoms clusters, and geriatric syndromes. These conversations should begin when the older person is independent and should continue along the trajectory of illness, recognizing the changing goals of care as death approaches. At the end of life, patients and families should participate in goals of care discussion, and understand the role of comfort care and symptom management. This will lay the framework for decisions about specific clinical interventions such as resuscitation, artificial hydration, transfusions, antibiotics, as well as preferred settings of death. Advance care planning also documents treatment and care preferences in the form of living wills, healthcare proxy forms, do not resuscitate orders. Some states have approved the use of Physician/Provider Orders for Life-Sustaining Treatment

29

Table 10: Clinical Features of Delirium, Dementia, and Depression[31]

Clinical Feature	Delirium	Dementia	Depression
Onset	• Acute	• Insidious	• Variable • Can be abrupt with major life change
Course	• Quick & fluctuating • Often at night	• Slow & progressive • May worsen when stressed	• Variation during the day • May worsen in the morning
Reversibility	• Sometimes	• Not reversible	• Variable
Level of consciousness and orientation	• Disoriented	• Lucid until the late stages	• Intact but may be selective
Attention & memory	• Poor short-term memory • Constant inattention	• Good attention • Poor short-term memory	• Poor attention • Intact memory
Alertness	• Fluctuates, lethargic to hypervigilant	• Generally normal	• Normal
Cognition	• Focal cognitive failure	• Global cognitive failure	• Cognition intact
Thinking	• Disorganized, incoherent at times	• Thoughts impoverished • Judgment impaired • Word-finding difficulty	• Intact • Themes of hopelessness & helplessness
Perception	• Distorted • Illusions & delusions often present	• Misperceptions usually absent	• Intact except in severe cases
Psychomotor behavior	• Variable Hypo/hyperkinetic • Mixed	• Normal	• Variable
Sleep/wake cycle	• Disturbed • Often reversed	• Fragmented	• Disturbed
Psychotic symptoms	• Frequent • Often paranoid	• Less frequent	• Rare
Evaluation & treatment	• Emergent evaluation is needed	• Needs chronic monitoring	• Needs urgent attention and therapy

29

(POLST) or the Medical Orders for Life-Sustaining Treatment (MOLST). These forms document treatment orders at the end of life, and are honored in different practice settings including nursing homes, adult homes, hospices, and hospitals, as well as the emergency medical services (EMS) when the patient is at home and 911 is called.

Advance care planning increases older patient's empowerment, and encourages planning for death. The APRN is in an ideal position to help the older adult address concerns about end-of-life care. The process of addressing end-of-life issues allows the nurse to elicit patient goals and values relevant to medical care, and address any misconceptions the patient or caregiver may have about end-of-life care or life-sustaining interventions. This process can allow the nurse to establish a trusting, therapeutic relationship, face cultural diversity and face his/her own biases.

B. Many studies have found that African-Americans are less likely to complete advance directives and are less likely to have discussed end-of-life preferences with their physician or their family. In addition, members of many minority groups have rates of morbidity and mortality that are higher than nonminority groups. This includes higher incidences of diabetes, lung cancers, and cervical cancers in some minority groups. Older Asian-Americans, Hispanic and African-American residents of nursing homes are also less likely than whites to have sensory and communication aids, such as glasses and hearing aids.[36] It is also known that older minority adults are more likely to live in poverty, and this correlates with limited access to health services. This data suggests that uninformed cultural attitudes and ineffective healthcare professional-patient interactions often contribute to these problems; further suggesting that healthcare clinicians need to become culturally competent in order to address these issues in the older population. Cultural issues are addressed elsewhere in this book, and the core competencies identified in that section pertain to the older adult. (See Chapter 16, *Cultural Considerations*)

C. A strong component of the role of the APRN is to provide for ongoing education throughout the trajectory of illness. This becomes especially important at the end of life when symptoms can rapidly escalate in intensity. Pain, delirium, and dyspnea are frequently managed in the home setting and families and caregivers are often the singular most important person managing these symptoms. Understanding culturally related health beliefs about end-of-life care, use of medications to manage symptoms can make the difference between what one might consider "a good death," where symptoms are managed well and "a bad death" where symptoms are poorly managed.

D. On February 9, 2011, under Chapter 331 of the Laws of 2010 of New York State (commonly known as the Palliative Care Information Act)[37] was enacted and it is hoped that it is a model for other states. Under this statute, physicians and nurse practitioners are required to offer to terminally ill patients information and counseling concerning palliative care and end-of-life options. Under the law, a patient with a terminal illness or condition "reasonably expected to cause death within six months, whether or not treatment is provided." Palliative care as defined by law is "healthcare treatment, including interdisciplinary end-of-life care, and consultation with patients

New York State Department of Health: Palliative Care

and family members to prevent or relieve pain and suffering and to enhance the patient's quality of life, including hospice care." The law is intended to ensure that patients are fully informed of the options available to them when they are faced with a terminal illness. Patients should be given information verbally or in writing about

- Prognosis

- Range of options appropriate to the patient

- Risks and benefits of various options

- Patient's legal rights to comprehensive pain and symptom management at the end of life

IX. CONCLUSION

Older people and their caregivers have a right to expect compassionate and skilled palliative care. For those patients who are coming to the end of their lives, the advanced palliative care nurse can be instrumental in the assessment and management of symptoms, and in providing instruction and teaching about advanced directives and goals of care. It is rare that the older patient has a clear-cut etiology of symptoms; most are often multi-factorial, compounded by the presence of advanced disease, cancer, comorbid conditions, and geriatric syndromes. Nursing care of these patients requires compassion, patience, skill, and knowledge.

CITED REFERENCES

1. Population Resource Center. *The Aging of America.* 2012. Available at: www.prcdc.org/300million/The_Aging_of_America/. Accessed September 13, 2012.
2. National Cancer Institute. Surveillance Epidemiology and End Results. *Table 1.11: Median Age of Cancer Patients at Diagnosis, 2002-2006.* Available at: seer.cancer.gov/csr/1975_2006/results_single/sect_01_table.11_2pgs.pdf. Accessed September 13, 2012.
3. U.S. Department of Health and Human Services, Centers for Disease Control and Prevention, National Center for Health Statistics. *Health, United States, 2007: With Chartbook on Trends in the Health of Americans.* Available at: www.cdc.gov/nchs/data/hus/hus07.pdf. Accessed March 26, 2012.
4. Unroe KT, Greiner MA, Hernandez AF, et al. Resource use in the last 6 months of life among Medicare beneficiaries with heart failure, 2000-2007. *Arch Intern Med.* 2011;171(3):196-203.
5. Balducci L, Stanta G. Cancer in the frail patient: a coming epidemic. *Hematol Oncol Clin N Am.* 2000;14(1):235-250.
6. Ellis G, Whitehead MA, O'Neill D, Langhorne P, Robinson D. Comprehensive geriatric assessment for older adults admitted to hospital. *Cochrane Database of Systematic Reviews.* 2011;Issue 7: Art No;CD006211.DOI:10.1002/14651858.CD00621.pub2. Available at: summaries.cochrane.org/CD006211/comprehensive-geriatric-assessment-for-older-adults-admitted-to-hospital. Accessed March 26, 2012.
7. Centers for Medicare and Medicaid (CMS). *Resident Assessment Instrument (RAI).* CMS's RAI Version 3.0 Manual. Washington, DC: CMS; 2011. Available at: www.cms.gov/NursingHomeQualityInits/25_NHQIMDS30.asp. Accessed March 23, 2012.
8. Centers for Medicare and Medicaid (CMS). Overview to the item-by-item guide to the MDS 3.0. Centers for Medicare and Medicaid. *CMS RAI MDS 3.0 Manual.* Washington, DC: CMS; 2011.
9. Merriam-Webster Online. *Syndrome.* Available at: www.merriam-webster.com/dictionary/syndrome?show=0&t=1310926599. Accessed July 17, 2011.
10. Aktas A, Walsh D, Rybicki L. Symptom clusters: myth or reality? *Palliat Med.* 2010;24(4):373-385.
11. Cheung WY, Le LW, Zimmermann C. Symptom cluster in patients with advanced cancers. *Support Care Cancer.* 2009;17:1223-1230.
12. Bruera E, Kuehn N, Miller MJ, Selmser P, Macmillan K. The Edmonton Symptom Assessment System (ESAS): a simple method for the assessment of palliative care patients. *J Palliat Care.* 1991;7(2):6-9.
13. Chang VT, Hwang SS, Kasimis B, Thaler HT. Shorter symptom assessment instruments: the Condensed Memorial Symptom Assessment Scale (CMSAS). *Cancer Invest.* 2004;22(4):526-536.
14. Knapowski J, Wieczorowska-Tobis K, Witowski J. Pathophysiology of ageing. *J Physiol Pharmacol.* 2002;53:135-146.
15. Jones GT, Macfarlane GA. Epidemiology of pain in older persons. In: Gibson S, Weiner D, eds. *Pain in Older Persons.* Vol 35. Seattle, WA: IASP Press; 2005:3-22.
16. Scherder E, Oosterman J, Swaab D, et al. Recent developments in pain in dementia. *BMJ.* 2005;26:330(7489):461-464.
17. American Society for Pain Management Nursing. *Position Statement: Pain Assessment in the Patient Unable to Self-Report.* Available at: www.aspmn.org/Organization/documents/UPDATED_NonverbalRevisionFinalWEB.pdf. Accessed September 13, 2012.
18. Miaskowski C, Bair M, Chou R, et al. *Principles of Analgesic Use in the Treatment of Acute Pain and Cancer Pain.* 6th ed. Glenview, IL: American Pain Society; 2008:1-101.

29

19. American Geriatrics Society Panel on the Pharmacological Management of Persistent Pain in Older Person. Pharmacological management of persistent pain in older persons. *JAGS.* 2009;57:1331-1346.
20. Warden V, Hurley AV, Volicer L. Development and psychometric evaluation of the Pain Assessment in Advanced Dementia (PAINAD) scale. *J Am Med Dir Assoc.* 2003;4:9-15.
21. Hogas AL. *Assessing Pain in Older Adults with Dementia.* 2012. Available at: consultgerirn.org/uploads/File/trythis/try_this_d2.pdf. Accessed September 13, 2012.
22. Feldt KS. The check list of non-verbal pain indicators (CNPI). *Pain Manage Nurs.* 2000;1(1):13-21.
23. Pain Assessment Tool Guidelines for use: Checklist of Non-Verbal Pain Indicators (CNPI) Available at: www2.massgeneral.org/painrelief/pcs_pain_files/cnvpi_scales.pdf. Accessed September 13, 2012.
24. Zwakhalen SM, Hamers JP, Berger MP. Improving the clinical usefulness of a behavioral pain scale for older people with dementia. *J Adv Nurs.* 2009;58(5):493-502.
25. Snow AL, Weber JB, O'Malley KJ, et al. NOPPAIN: a nursing assistant-administered pain assessment instrument for use in dementia. *Dement Geriatr Cogn Disord.* 2004;17(3):240-246.
26. Snow AL, O'Malley K, Kunik M, et al. *NOPPAIN (Non-Communicative Patient's Pain Assessment Instrument) Activity Chart Check List.* Available at: www.nmmra.org/resources/Nursing_Homes/156_1538.pdf. Accessed September 13, 2012.
27. American Psychiatric Association. *Diagnostic and Statistical Manual of Mental Disorders, IV.* 4th ed. Text Revision. Washington, DC: American Psychiatric Association; 2000.
28. Thompson GN, Chochinov HM. Reducing the potential for suffering in older adults with advanced cancer. *Palliat Support Care.* 2010;8(1):83-93.
29. Goy E, Ganzini L. End-of-life care in geriatric psychiatry. *Clin Geriatr Med.* 2003;19(4):841-856.
30. Block S. Psychological issues in end-of-life care. *J Palliat Med.* 2006;9(3):751-772
31. Fong TG, Tulebaev SR, Inouye SK (2009). Delirium in elderly adults: diagnosis, prevention and treatment. *Nat Rev Neurol.* 2009;5(4):210-220.
32. Holroyd-Leduc MJ, Khandwala F, Sink KM. How can delirium best be prevented and managed in older patients in hospital? *CMAJ.* 2010;182(5):465-470.
33. Cancelli I, Beltrame M, Gigli GL, Valente M. Drugs with anticholinergic properties: cognitive and neuropsychiatric side-effects in elderly patients. *Neurol Sci.* 2009; 30:87-92.
34. Centeno C. Delirium in advanced cancer patients. *Palliat Med.* 2004;18:184-194.
35. Kissane DW, Block S, eds. *Family Focused Grief Therapy. A Model of Family-Centered Care During Palliative Care and Bereavement.* Buckingham UK: Open University Press; 2002.
36. Schneider EC, Zaslavsky AM , Epstein AM. Racial disparities in the quality of care for enrollees in Medicare managed care. *JAMA.* 2002;287:1288-1294.
37. Laws of New York. *An ACT to amend the Public Heath Law in relation to a Patient's Right to Palliative Care Information.* August 13, 2010. Available at: www.health.state.ny.us/professionals/patients/patient_rights/palliative_care/. Accessed September 13, 2012.

ADDITIONAL RESOURCES

Administration on Aging (www.aoa.gov)
American Association of Retired Persons (www.aarp.gov)
Brown University Center for Gerontology and Health Research (www.cher.brown.edu)
City of Hope Pain/Palliative Care Resource Center (www.cityofhope.org)
End of Life/Palliative Education Resource Center (www.eperc.org)
GeroNurse Online (www.geronurse.org)
Indian Health Service-Elder Care Initiative (www.ihs.gov.medicalprograms/eldercare)
International Association for Hospice and Palliative Care (www.hospicecare.com)
John A. Hartford Foundation Institute for Geriatric Nursing (www.hartfordign.org)

29

CHAPTER 30

MEETING THE PALLIATIVE CARE NEEDS
OF THE UNDERSERVED

Anne Hughes, RN, PhD, ACHPN®, FAAN

I. INTRODUCTION

A. Despite the proliferation of hospital-based palliative care programs and increased numbers of hospice and palliative care outpatient and home programs, many Americans lack access to hospice and palliative care services. Disparities in equal access to hospice in the United States have been well documented.[1] More recently, in a report card on access to palliative care services, Morrison and colleagues noted that only 54% of public hospitals had palliative care teams, which amounted to a C grade.[2] The lack of hospital palliative care services available in public hospitals suggests that persons dependent on safety net care providers (i.e., the uninsured and underinsured) may lack access to palliative care.[2] There is also a gap in follow up once patients are discharged due to a lack of outpatient clinics in these programs

B. A recent systematic review of barriers to accessing quality palliative care among the economically disadvantaged concluded that, as of result of economic deprivation, home visits were fewer; hospice services were limited in high crime areas; institutional deaths were more likely with no available caregiver in the home setting; transportation to access specialty care services was problematic; and limited health literacy resulted in more aggressive medical interventions, little clarification of goals of care, and an inability to negotiate complex medical care delivery systems.[3]

C. This chapter will define underserved populations, identify barriers and challenges to providing palliative services to such communities, evaluate the evidence base for providing care for one at-risk group, and recommend clinical interventions and community/policy approaches.

II. DEFINING UNDERSERVED POPULATIONS

Groups or communities that are not well served by the healthcare system, (i.e., the so called underserved) are numerous. A Kellogg Foundation report identified several underserved populations—low-income individuals, uninsured persons, immigrants, racial and ethnic minorities, and the elderly.[4] However, many have argued that even those with healthcare insurance and presumably access to care, are not always well served by the current healthcare system. Terms or concepts used to characterize those lacking access to quality care include health disparities, health inequities, vulnerable populations, and marginalized communities.

A. Describing Underserved Populations for Palliative and Hospice Services

The underserved are at risk for a poor dying process as well as challenged living.[1,5] The underserved in palliative care include persons living in the inner city, in rural or remote areas, the homeless; members of ethnic and racial minorities; undocumented immigrants and persons with limited English language proficiency; persons with mental illness, dementia, or developmental delay; nursing home residents; persons with limited health literacy; and those who are uninsured and underinsured.[1,3,6-11] Factors that contribute to the risk of being underserved shape the challenges and barriers faced in accessing palliative and hospice services. Frequently an individual is a member of more than one underserved group as the case below illustrates.

1. Martin is a middle aged African-American man with chronic kidney disease, and diabetic neuropathy related to poorly controlled diabetes (Hgb A1C = 14.3). He was admitted to a nursing home for long-term care after Adult Protective Services received a referral from a single-room occupancy hotel (SRO) manager who reported Martin's self-neglect and threatened eviction, in spite of the support services he received in the community. He is estranged from his family, homeless, with a history of mental illness, substance abuse, and traumatic brain injury. Martin was determined to lack decision-making capacity and the court appointed a conservator (legal guardian) to make medical and financial decisions.

2. Catherine is an 89-year-old Caucasian nursing home resident with dementia. She has no family in the area. She has poorly controlled diabetes. Her care is covered by Medicaid and she has no assets. Catherine has an attorney as legal guardian who also is responsible for her medical and financial decisions.

Needless to say, addressing the palliative care needs of Martin will be different than those of Catherine. Both individuals are receiving care in an urban nursing home, neither has the capacity to engage in discussions about care, nor have ready or available support systems. Martin and Catharine have multiple interactions with medical and social services, both are vulnerable adults, and both have progressive illnesses. Both are impoverished urban dwellers. That designation, as with any group affiliation, does not account for individual differences nor does it define individual experiences. Understandably, in acute care settings, care is directed toward correcting, stabilizing, or palliating physiological disruptions and toward discharge to the community, rather than to the often complex and convoluted narrative of the person presenting for care. Failure to recognize individual differences results in stereotyping and eliminates the possibility of person-centered care.

B. Subpopulation Focus of this Chapter

The urban poor serve as a prototype for evaluating the palliative care needs of other groups who are underserved. This chapter, therefore, focuses on the urban poor with advanced disease, as representative of some of the issues encountered by underserved populations requiring palliative care. For this group, serious or life-threatening injuries and illness as well as death may be isolating experiences occurring in hospitals, emergency rooms, or in nursing homes.[12] Many persons who are economically disadvantaged live everyday with environmental hazards, such as pollution, crime-ridden and blighted neighborhoods in marginal or substandard housing. Lifestyle-related illnesses linked to tobacco, drug, and alcohol use are common.[13] Poverty, race, and urbanization present particular challenges to providing palliative care.[7] In the United States, persons of color are disproportionately represented among the almost 46.2 million (15.1%) of all Americans who meet the federal criteria for poverty.[14] Consequently, deciphering the contributions of race as opposed to socioeconomic class to health disparities is for all intents and purposes impossible.[15] The average number of deaths annually in the United States is about 2.4 million. The poor (urban and rural) will account for at least 362,400 of those deaths.[16] Hundreds of thousands of urban dwellers who live in poverty will need palliative care services before the terminal phase of illness.

III. BARRIERS AND CHALLENGES PROVIDING PALLIATIVE SERVICES

There are many barriers (structural or community factors) that limit access to quality palliative care for the urban poor and an equal number of challenges (individual and/illness-related factors) that are common among the urban poor with advanced disease.[12]

Barriers that influence the health status of anyone living in an inner city are listed in Table 1 and include factors such as high rates of violence, marginal housing, and limited public transportation to healthcare appointments or pharmacies. Challenges to providing palliative care to the urban poor with advanced disease are both person-specific and illness-related factors. (see Table 2)

Table 1: Barriers Impacting the Health of Persons Living in the Inner City[17-19]

- High rates of violent crime & drug use
- Marginal or substandard housing
- Limited public transportation
- Convenience stores, which sell more tobacco, processed foods, & alcohol than fresh fruits & vegetables
- Environmental pollution
- Oversubscribed & often charity-dependent community health services, if even available
- Lack of pharmacies &/or restricted drug formularies
- Lack of insurance or a reliable income source to meet basic needs

Table 2: Challenges to Providing Palliative Care to the Urban Poor[3,8,12,13,20-23]

Illness-related	• Prevalence of concurrent mental illness and substance abuse • Decisional incapacity • Presentation with advanced disease • Multiple comorbidities • End-organ diseases altering pharmacodynamics
Resource challenges	• Health literacy • Family or friend caregiver availability • Need for designated surrogate in the event of decisional incapacity • Chaotic lives that have little space for day-to-day illness demands • Limited ongoing therapeutic relationships with health or social service providers • Survival or addiction that overshadows illness management • Competing role responsibilities • Functional impairments, geographic distances, & transportation limitation compromise appointment keeping
Relationships with healthcare system or providers	• Cultural history of racism, discrimination, or rejection in healthcare system • As a result of disrespectful, rude, or dismissive interactions in past, may present as angry, avoidant, suspicious, or non-adherent with care recommendations • Healthcare providers often have different cultural & ethnic backgrounds/world views
End-of-life preferences	• Reluctance to relinquish aggressive medical management • Different assumptions about optimal EOL care, particularly in communities of color • Lack of advance care planning, as life is experienced moment to moment • Tendency to equate goals of care modification with abandonment or continued poor care • Spirituality may be a hidden resource for comfort & in guiding decision-making

30

Illness-related challenges include the prevalence of serious mental illness, addiction, and the diagnosis of posttraumatic stress disorder (PTSD); and multiple comorbidities (e.g., end-organ and other chronic diseases). Many seek initial care when disease is in advanced stages and may be less responsive to disease-modifying interventions, even if such therapies were available. Social resource challenges include fragile support systems, limited health literacy, need for a healthcare proxy or agent if a family member or friend is not available, and chaotic lives in which survival frequently overshadows illness management. Relationships with healthcare providers and systems may be frayed if existent. Providers may experience quite different world views and cultural backgrounds than the person in the exam room or the hospital bed presenting for care.

In general, barriers to providing quality palliative care to this population require community level or policy interventions, while individual challenges require person-centered interventions, such as how to engage persons whose lives may be very different than the APRNs caring for them. Both levels of approaches will be discussed following a review of the evidence base for providing palliative care to the urban poor.

IV. EVIDENCE-BASED PALLIATIVE CARE FOR THE URBAN POOR

The evidence base to guide palliative care for the urban poor includes reviews, program evaluations, and research that used both descriptive and clinical trial designs. The reviews were found in textbooks and journal articles.[5,7,24] The program evaluations described shelter-based[25] and home care[20] palliative care programs. Research used in-depth individual and group interviews, survey, and clinical trial approaches. Researchers explored attitudes and beliefs about end-of-life care,[26-28] and barriers to palliative care among low income cancer patients.[17] They tested methods for promoting advance directive completion among this population, using a low literacy version[29] or other methods.[30] Researchers described the experiences of the urban poor with advanced disease who were community dwelling or in a dedicated AIDS nursing home unit.[13,21] and also the hopes and concerns about care at the end of life for inpatients at public hospitals with serious illness.[31]

Appendix 30-A summarizes and evaluates the quality of research evidence to guide care for this underserved population. Only one aspect of palliative care practice has strong evidence for its use in the urban poor (i.e., advance care planning, using a 5th grade reading level version, or other methods including one-to-one coaching or self-completion).[26,29,30]

30

V. CLINICAL INTERVENTIONS AND COMMUNITY/POLICY LEVEL APPROACHES

A. Clinical Interventions—Importance of Relationships

Developing trusting therapeutic relationships is at the very heart of all clinical interventions regardless of whether the person is impoverished and marginally housed, or has social and financial resources. Therapeutic relationships take on a particular salience with those facing serious illness and death. However developing trusting relationships with persons who have experienced rejection, abandonment, or felt unwelcomed in healthcare settings requires patience and time; scarce resources for clinicians in busy clinical settings. Moreover, relationships may be even more highly valued and trusted when clinicians focus on patient-centered, culturally sensitive care more than data driven guidelines.[8]

Multiple qualitative studies of the urban poor with serious or life-limiting illness have demonstrated a desire for therapeutic relationships with healthcare professionals characterized by respect and 'sitting down and listening' with honesty and consistency.[13,21,26,31] When patients and providers come from different life experiences, the most basic principles of therapeutic communication are crucial. For the palliative APRN, these communication tenets include addressing the person formally, unless given permission to use the familiarity of first names; sitting at eye level when interacting; and appreciating that the palliative care philosophy and principles guiding care approach may be quite foreign or even suspect as a means of denying care (again) or as an 'ethically charged' clinical intervention.[5,8] Consequently, the APRN will need patience and appreciation that the establishment of relationship is a process that likely will take time.

B. Assessment Considerations

1. A comprehensive assessment includes—history of illness, treatment, comorbidities, medication, self-care abilities, symptom management, and a physical examination appropriate to the presenting complaint and history. Additionally, the APRN collects psychosocial information that further shapes end-of-life care options. Obtaining information over time, rather than in a single session, is more likely to promote a therapeutic connection and to uncover a richer narrative. Admittedly, a lack of reliable phone numbers for appointment reminders or home visits justify trying to get as much information as possible during an initial encounter, but a focus on completing data collection rather than the person's more pressing need for seeking care on this day, is likely to be perceived as off-putting. While various screening or assessment tools for specific aspects of care are available and recommended in many practice guidelines, the timing of when, or if, to use such standardized instruments need to be evaluated on a case-by-case basis in a population who may be more hesitant to engage in care and suspicious of how this information may be used. In addition to illness, treatment, comorbidities, medication, self-care, and symptom-related assessment, psychosocial areas to assess include but are not limited to—safety, housing, food, transportation, income/entitlements, contact methods, support system, literacy, and substance use.[24] (see Table 3)

2. Besides collecting individual patient data, the APRN needs resource information about the community/neighborhood where the patient lives. This is important for outpatient care or care provided in the community where they live. Are pharmacies available for the patient? Where they are located? What are their hours? Are local pharmacies willing to accept fax or telephone orders? What medications are kept on hand? Are they willing to work with populations that live in rooming houses, boarding houses etc? What supportive services are available, such as food/meal programs, case management services, representative payee programs, supportive housing, and crisis mental health and substance abuse programs? Are there homeless medical or health teams that make visits to where persons are in the community rather than expecting them to come to clinic during "business hours?" What home health or hospice programs service the community, including any restrictions on services because of concerns related to staff safety? Is the hospice or home care flexible in providing care in alternative living situations? Would the hospice or home care admit them into service

30

Table 3: Psychosocial Assessment Domains[24]

Domain	Possible Assessment Questions
Housing	Where do you usually stay at night?
Food	How often are you are hungry from not having enough to eat?
Transportation	How do you get to appointments or to the hospital?
Safety	Do you feel safe where you're staying?
Caregiver availability	Is there a friend or family member or someone else you can count on when you need help?
Other resources accessed	Do you have a case manager, peer advocate, patient navigator, or clinic you go to when you need help?
Literacy	Are you much of a reader?
Spirituality	What role does faith or religion play in your life?
Cultural identity	What beliefs or practices about health and healing are important for us to incorporate into your care?
Income/benefits	Are you receiving any income or benefits?
Preferred contact methods	How can we get in touch with you?
Coping resources	How have you coped in the past when dealing with challenges?
Substance use	Have you used alcohol or drugs to cope? If so, what difficulties has their use presented in your life?

without a primary care giver? How would they deliver interdisciplinary care or have medicines or equipment available?

3. Most often, community-level information can be obtained from social workers or case managers working with a particular client, or from an agency serving this population. Additional community information can be gained from, what is commonly known in community health, as a "windshield community assessment." In other words, the APRN drives in the neighborhoods where her clients are living to observe living conditions, such as the upkeep or decay of buildings and streets, availability of public transportation, access to grocery stores, pharmacies, churches or places of worship, the ethnicity, ages and even language spoken of inhabitants (noted on signage), community centers, and police and fire stations, etc. Appreciating the environments in which patients live allows the APRN to develop plans of care that take into account what is possible for an individual patient, given the environment he/she calls home.

C. Substance Abuse and Mental Illness—Challenges in Clinical Management

1. Substance abuse and mental illness, common comorbidities in this population, present special challenges in providing palliative care in at least two key areas—pain management[32] and capacity determination for advance care planning.

2. The management of pain in persons with a history of opioid dependence whether in recovery or actively using, requires thoughtful consideration and informed consent regarding its attendant risks. Various types of agreements or pain medication contracts developed between patient and provider have sought to establish mutual pain management goals, stipulate how opioid

30

dosages will be adjusted, dispensed, or refilled, and outline monitoring strategies for potential aberrant behaviors. No evidence was located that identifies a pain contract that has been tested for this purpose in this population. However even without empirical support, many providers have incorporated the use of agreements to protect the patient and themselves as prescribers, because of Risk Evaluation and Mitigation Strategies (REMS). (See Chapter 33, *Substance Abuse*)

3. Furthermore, most clinical pain management guidelines include assessment of substance use history, realistic goal setting, consultation with pain and addiction specialists, use of a multidisciplinary approach, frequent re-evaluations, possible referrals to interventional pain services, evaluation and treatment of comorbid psychiatric illness, incorporation of cognitive behavioral and complementary approaches, evaluation of opioid dosing escalation, home and social environment evaluation, and frequent documentation of patient monitoring efforts.[32,33] The evidence base for the use of screening tools to predict risk of aberrant drug-related behaviors however, is sparse.[34]

4. The end-of-life care needs of the mentally ill, and those who have abused substances, many of whom are poor and without connection to care, have not been well studied.[9,32] Grounded in the ethical principle of respect for autonomy, the basis for informed consent, capacity is critical to advance care planning. Decision-making capacity may be compromised by self-medicating mental illness symptoms with drugs and alcohol. An additional assessment consideration, related to decision-making, is determining if the patient has a court appointed conservator or decision-maker. If so, what are the domains of the agent's decision-making authority? For example, some mentally ill persons may have a court appointed conservator whose authority is restricted to authorizing the use of psychiatric treatment and not end-of-life care decisions. Furthermore, a patient's inability to make decisions about psychiatric treatment does not exclude her/his right to participate in decision-making regarding palliative care. Capacity determinations are always situational and require review with each care transition decision point. Capacity changes and may decline over time as illness progresses.[35]

5. A patient who presents for care who is incapacitated or lacks decision-making capacity presents a dilemma. Often the person is without an available family decision-maker, without court appointed proxy, and no documentation of prior wishes or known preferences to guide care goals. In such cases, the APRN investigates past medical records for (1) past primary care provider who may have information about patient's wishes, (2) any previously discussed advance directives found in available medical records, and/or (3) for any emergency contacts or next of kin who may be able to articulate the patient's values. This investigator role of the APRN may or may not be effective, in which case—ideally, access to ethical and legal consultation may be available.

D. Program, Community or Policy Level Approaches

1. While there are no clinical practice guidelines developed specifically to define palliative care of the underserved, *Clinical Practice Guidelines for Quality Palliative Care* does serve as useful framework for developing and evaluating services to meet the unique needs of this population.[36] In particular, the preferred practices addressing social aspects of care (Domain 4), spiritual,

30

religious, and existential aspects of care (Domain 5) and cultural aspects of care (Domain 6) can be used to shape program development and service evaluation.

2. Two programs designed to meet the palliative care of the poor, one home care-based program in Hawaii[20] and a shelter-based program in Canada[25] documented cost savings and favorable results for other quality indicators. The home-based program for older, ethnically diverse, rural homebound Hawaiians with chronic progressive illnesses used a palliative care team approach. The team included a physician, nurse, psychologist/chaplain, case manager, interpreters, and volunteers. The goals of the service were to assess and manage symptoms, provide support to patients and caregivers, facilitate advance directive completion and linkage to hospice, with a secondary goal of decreasing emergency and acute care service utilization. Health service utilization patterns were compared to pre-service utilization. Outcomes from this program included 25% hospice enrollment, fewer acute hospitalizations, and greater caregiver satisfaction.

    The Canadian shelter-based palliative care pilot program used harm-reduction principles to engage homeless individuals with liver disease, HIV/AIDS, malignancies, and other diseases. The program offered nursing support 7 days a week, case management and physician services on site. The pilot demonstrated over 1 million dollars cost savings, as clinically important, and reunited many persons who had been estranged from their families.[25]

3. Another study, the Kellogg Foundation's report, *Patient-Centered Care for Underserved Populations: Definition and Best Practices,*[4] noted the commitment to patient-centered care for vulnerable populations must occur simultaneously on multiple levels of the organization, the patient, the provider, and the community, in order to be successful. Moreover, the Kellogg report identified barriers to patient-centered care for the underserved, core components of patient-centered care along with organizational or institutional supports necessary to develop programs grounded in patient-centered beliefs for underserved populations. These recommendations and findings are printed in Appendix 30-B with the permission of the Kellogg Foundation.

4. Finally, it should be emphasized that the U.S. Department of Veterans Affairs (VA) does provide healthcare services and assistance for Veterans who may be homeless or have limited incomes, substance abuse issues, and other diagnoses. All homeless people should be queried about military service. They may have access to benefits even if they do not want to stay overnight in VA facilities.[37]

VA Homeless
Veterans

VI. CONCLUDING OBSERVATIONS

Providing palliative care for persons who are members of underserved communities, who have lived at the margins of society, is eminently rewarding and often simultaneously overwhelming. Witnessing the ravages of deprivation can leave an APRN wondering what she/he can achieve.

Expect that relationship building will likely take longer than you would expect. Once relationships are established, transitions in care may be difficult. So if an

30

underserved person establishes a relationship with a home care or palliative team, the transition to other venues of care may not occur.

Attempt to get as much collateral information about how to reach the person should housing be lost or phone service disconnected without seeming intrusive or unnecessarily inquisitive.

Using professional and community networks, obtain information about the neighborhoods where your patients live, including what resources are available.

Assess for factors impacting decisional-capacity, such as substance abuse or serious mental illness, and link with mental health professionals or law enforcement when a patient's or others' safety is compromised.

Given chaotic lives, in which survival frequently trumps self-care, anticipate challenges with adherence, follow up, and hesitancy to discuss goals of care or consider placement options as illness progresses. Focus on what's most important to the person at that moment.

Finally, keep in mind that the person sitting in front of you most often will remember being heard, being recognized as a human being deserving of care whose illness concerns were taken seriously. The APRN can serve as to advocate and to provide continuity across the system as he or she may be the only provider the person trusts. It is important for the APRN to assure communication and to provide a holistic picture of care.

30

Appendix 30-A: Evidence Table for Palliative Care of the Urban Poor

Year/Author	Study Question Purpose/Aim or Hypothesis	Design/Sample/Setting	Measurement/Data Collection/Analysis	Findings/Implications	Level of Evidence*
2011 Lewis et al[3]	Evaluate literature in the developed world regarding barriers to palliative care access	Systematic review of published literature n = 67 articles included; 49% (33) articles from U.S.	Results were summarized & themes identified using 4 dimensions of access—availability, affordability, acceptability, & geographic accessibility	Availability of services influenced uptake; likelihood of home death while preferred was unlikely; geographic location & distance of health services influenced access. Acceptability was affected by absence of caregivers, stigma & mistrust, communication, & health literacy	V
2010 Dzul-Church et al[31]	Describe experiences, concerns, preferences on improving EOL care in underserved inpatients	Qualitative interviews of 20 ethnically diverse & seriously ill inpatients at a university-affiliated public hospital	Semi-structured interview conducted by single interviewer; audio taped; transcribed; thematic analysis completed by 2 researchers	Difficult life histories influenced end-of-life experiences & patient-provider interactions. Recommendations included—improved provider relationships, increased access to chaplaincy services, & home based services	VI
2010 Lyckholm et al[17]	Pilot study to identify barriers to EOL care	Cross sectional survey design. Surveys were distributed to terminally ill cancer patients in hematology-oncology clinic [29], 15 unmatched caregivers, & 34 healthcare providers in urban medical center. Patients were older & more racially & ethnically diverse than healthcare providers (HCP)	Investigator developed survey instrument based on clinical experience & consistent with literature (face validity); convenience sampling	Barriers reported by patients & families differed from HCP. Caregivers & HCPs believed hospice was discussed more often than patients reported. 48% of patients reported having an advance directive & 72% enjoyed life most of the time. HCP endorsed barriers such as, transportation, hospice home visits access & insurance, which were not reported by patients	VI
2010 Fernandes et al[20]	Measure symptom, quality of life, health services use, & advance care planning	Prospective program evaluation of home-based palliative care (HBPC) team to 46 adult ethnically diverse homebound patients (median age 71 years) & 45 matching caregivers in a medically underserved area near Honolulu. 67% were living below the federal poverty line. Pre-program health services utilization data were used as historical controls	Instruments used at admission & with each follow up visit included—Palliative Care Performance Scale, Edmonton Symptom Assessment Scale, Missoula Quality of Life Index, Adapted Caregiver Satisfaction survey, advance care documentation & health services utilization	Median LOS = 7 months Median visits = 3.5. More than 50% had neurodegenerative diseases (stroke, cerebral palsy or dementia); 70% were dependent in ADLs & IADLs. No statistically improvement in symptom management. Significant improvement in overall wellbeing using Missoula Vitas QOL Index. Significant differences were noted in advance directive completion, clarification of code status, & fewer hospitalizations. Caregiver satisfaction rated after death of patient was extremely high. Case management service was most utilized	IV

30

Year/Author	Study Question Purpose/Aim or Hypothesis	Design/Sample/Setting	Measurement/Data Collection/Analysis	Findings/Implications	Level of Evidence*
2008 Song et al[30]	Explore (1) advance directive (AD) completion among homeless persons & (2) if completion of an AD improved knowledge, & change attitudes & beliefs regarding EOL care	Prospective, randomized pilot trial to improve EOL decision-making process for homeless persons by facilitating advance care planning (ACP). Convenience sample of 59 English speaking adult homeless persons receiving services at drop in center. Average age was 42 years, 89% had completed at least high school education, 51% were African-American; 24% Veterans, & 53% reported chronic illness or disability	Participants randomized to self completed (SG) or counselor assisted (CG) group to complete advance directive. Follow up in 3 months was conducted to determine who had completed AD. Repeated measurement of knowledge, attitude, & behaviors were completed at study entry & at follow up	Overall AD completion for all samples was 44%; CG was statistically more likely to complete AD than SG; 50% of African-Americans completed AD versus 33% of Caucasians. 41% returned at 3 month follow up. There were no changes in EOL knowledge for those who returned; those who completed AD were more likely to report decreased worry, & had plan to write to their surrogate decision-maker about their wishes	II
2008 Hughes et al[21]	Describe the meaning & experiences of dignity for those receiving care in an urban AIDS dedicated nursing home unit	Ten ethnically diverse adults with advanced HIV disease participated in semi-structured group interviews, which occurred in a large urban publicly owned skilled nursing facility in western U.S. Average age 45 years (range 35-58), 7 African-Americans & three mixed racial participants were in the sample of 5 males, 3 females, & 2 transgendered persons	Part of a larger mixed methods study. Interpretive phenomenology guided analysis of transcribed interviews. Researchers read transcripts & reviewed drafts of interpretive memos by primary author until a credible account was achieved	Most believed that dignity was important. Dignity was usually defined as respect, respect received from & given to others, & respect for self. At least one participated reported not understanding the word & its meaning. Meeting care needs such as call lights & toileting assistance in a timely manner; being listened to & addressed to in a respectful manner, & not put down were ways nurses' actions demonstrated respectful care. Dedicated unit may have helped diminish stigma of HIV/AIDS & the social isolation, affronts to dignity	VI

*KEY38

II = Evidence obtained from well –designed randomized controlled trials (RCTs)
IV = Evidence from well-designed case-control and cohort studies
V = Evidence from systematic reviews of descriptive and qualitative studies
VI = Evidence from single descriptive or qualitative studies

30

Appendix 30-A—*continued on next page.*

Appendix 30-A: Evidence Table for Palliative Care of the Urban Poor—*continued*

Year/Author	Study Question Purpose/Aim or Hypothesis	Design/Sample/Setting	Measurement/Data Collection/Analysis	Findings/Implications	Level of Evidence*
2007 Sudore et al[29]	To determine whether an AD redesigned to meet most adults literacy needs (5th reading level with graphics) was more useful for advance care planning than a standard form (> 12th grade reading level)	205 adults from urban medical clinic were randomized to redesigned or standard AD groups & followed up at 6 months to assess form completion & interview. Sample was English & Spanish speaking. Average age of groups was 59.4 years to 61.9 years respectively; more than 70% of subjects were persons of color; approximately 50% had high school or less education; Mean literacy levels for all subjects was 9-10th grade	After assignment to different AD versions, subjects were asked acceptability of both versions & knowledge. Six months later phone interviews were completed to determine whether subjects had completed AD or had an advance care planning discussion. Group differences were computed using standard statistical analyses	Redesigned AD group reported significantly greater ease & personal usefulness in treatment decision discussions. There was no difference in time to complete. 84% of entire sample was available for follow up, of those 173 participants, 146 did not complete AD regardless of group assignment. Of 81 in the redesign group, 15 completed the form; & in 91 of the standard form group, 7 completed the AD. There were no differences between groups in advance care planning discussions	II
2007 Hughes et al[13]	Understand the meaning of dignity to urban poor & describe experiences living with advanced cancer	14 adult persons with stage III or IV solid tumor, ranging in age from 45-69 (mean 56 years), 50% persons of color, 8 females & 6 males, 50% had histories of homelessness; 7 participants died during the data collection period	Interpretive phenomenology guided analysis of audio taped & transcribed 32 interviews. Participants were interviewed up to three times	Many participants could not relate to the concept of dignity & were unable to articulate its meaning. Three themes emerged—difficult backgrounds, living not dying of cancer, & struggling with healthcare systems & providers. Exposure to violence, family abandonment or estrangement, drug & alcohol use were common. Few spoke about death as a possibility, even those very near the end of their lives. Most vividly described were problems with accessing care—rude or insensitive treatment from staff, delays in call lights being answered, long waits for appointments & prescriptions, inpatient nursing care delays, & perceived racial discrimination in the care provided	VI

30

Year/Author	Study Question Purpose/Aim or Hypothesis	Design/Sample/Setting	Measurement/Data Collection/Analysis	Findings/Implications	Level of Evidence*
2006 Podymow et al[25]	Evaluate the effectiveness of a 15-bed shelter based palliative care pilot program in Ottawa	Retrospective analysis of cohort & cost comparisons were calculated if care had been obtained in another setting. Twenty eight persons (25 men, 2 females & 1 transgendered person), average age 49 years, 89% Caucasian, 50% were shelter house prior to shelter hospice unit admission	Demographic, medical & psychiatric histories, symptom management, self care, religious services, family contacts & place of death, & alternative care site cost estimations computed	Length of stay (LOS) of persons ranged from 3-523 days, with median LOS 31-90 days. 86% had Karnofsky Scores < 59/100. Causes of death—alcohol cirrhosis, cancer, & HIV. 43% diagnosis of depression, 50% alcohol abuse, & 21% injection drug use. 82% (n = 23) died in the shelter hospice unit. Most common symptom—pain (89%), nausea (68%), confusion (61%), & SOB (50%). Cost estimates concluded that the program may have saved $1.39 million for the 28 patients	IV
2005 Tarzian et al[26]	Give voice to homeless or similarly marginalized individuals' EOL experiences & treatment preferences	Focus groups were conducted using semi-structured interview guide at a free urban health clinic. 20 participated in one of 5 focus groups. 16 were African-American & 4 Caucasian; age range was 19 -63 years; 12 males & 8 females. None were actively psychotic during the interviews. Minimal demographic information was collected to encourage trusting atmosphere. Some information was voluntarily disclosed during interviews	Part of a larger study evaluating the effectiveness of team on palliative care for persons with HIV	All had experienced multiple losses & drug addiction. Five main themes were uncovered—valuing an individual's wishes (who is dying); acknowledging emotions; the primacy of religious beliefs & spiritual experience; seeking relationship-centered care; & reframing advance care planning to prime directives	VI

*KEY38

II = Evidence obtained from well –designed randomized controlled trials (RCTs)
IV = Evidence from well-designed case-control and cohort studies
V = Evidence from systematic reviews of descriptive and qualitative studies
VI = Evidence from single descriptive or qualitative studies

30

Appendix 30-B: Components of Patient-Centered Care (PCC) For Underserved Populations, Institutional Supports, and Barriers to Implementation[4]

Core Components of Patient-Centered Care for Underserved Populations	<ul><li>Welcoming environment—provide a physical space & an initial personal interaction that is "welcoming," familiar, rather than intimidating</li><li>Respect for patients' values & expressed needs—obtain information about patient's care preferences & priorities; inform & involve patient & family/caregivers in decision-making; tailor care to the individual; promote a mutually-respectful, consistent patient-provider relationship</li><li>Patient empowerment or "activation"—educate & encourage patient to expand their role in decision-making, health-related behaviors, & self-management</li><li>Socio-cultural competence—understand & consider culture (ethnic traditions as well as culture of homelessness, addiction, etc.), economic & educational status, health literacy level, family patterns/situation, & traditions (including alternative/folk remedies); communicate in a language & at a level that the patient understands</li><li>Coordination & integration of care—assess need for formal & informal services that will have an impact on health or treatment, provide team-based care & care management, advocate for the patient & family, make appropriate referrals & ensure smooth transitions between different providers & phases of care</li><li>Comfort & support—emphasize physical comfort, privacy, emotional support, & involvement of family & friends</li><li>Access & navigation skills—provide what patient can consider a "medical home," keep waiting times to a minimum, provide convenient service hours, promote access & patient flow; help patient attain skills to better navigate the healthcare system</li><li>Community outreach—make demonstrable, proactive efforts to understand & reach out to the local community</li></ul>
Institutional Supports for Patient-centered Care	<ul><li>Feedback & measurement—seek & respond to suggestions & complaints from patients & families; develop, collect, & evaluate data on measures of patient-centered care, & feed back the results into further improvements; incorporate accountability for addressing deficiencies & continually improving indicators</li><li>Patient/family involvement—include patients & family members in the planning, design, & ongoing functioning of the organization; consider the patient a member of his/her care team</li><li>Workforce development—employ, train, & support a workforce that reflects, appreciates, & celebrates the diversity of the communities & cultures that the organization serves; reward & recognize staff exhibiting patient centeredness principles; develop communication skills among all levels of staff; empower staff to be part of patient-centered teams</li><li>Leadership—top management, board, & department heads make a clear, explicit commitment to patient centeredness & act as role models</li><li>Involvement in collaboratives, pilot projects—seek out & pilot research projects & collaborative relationships with other organizations that attempt to "push the envelope" in developing new methods to operationalize patient-centered principles</li><li>Technology & structural support—use electronic systems/user-friendly software programs that promote patient/family education & compliance, & minimize medical errors; structure the physical environment to optimize patient flow & safety</li><li>Integration into institution—tie patient-centered care to other priorities such as patient safety, quality improvement, etc., & incorporate patient-centered practices into daily operations & culture</li></ul>
Barriers to Implementing Patient-centered care (PCC) for Underserved Populations	<ul><li>Difficulty recruiting & retaining underrepresented minority physicians</li><li>Lack of defined "boundaries" for outreach staff who may be overwhelmed dealing with interrelated health, social, cultural, & economic issues of patients</li><li>Strict hiring requirements that pose obstacles to hiring neighborhood residents</li><li>Lack of tools to gauge & reward PCC performance</li><li>Financial constraints</li><li>Traditional attitudes among staff unwilling to change the "old school" provider/patient relationship or acknowledge & address cultural & socio-economic issues</li><li>Fatigue & competing priorities</li></ul>

30

CITED REFERENCES

1. Jennings B, Ryndes T, D'Onofrio C, Baily MA. Access to hospice care: expanding boundaries, overcoming barriers. *Hastings Cent Rep.* 2003;33(2 Suppl):S3-S7, S9-S13, S15-S21.
2. Morrison RS, Augustin R, Souvanna P, Meier DE. America's care of serious illness: a state-by-state report card on access to palliative care in our nation's hospitals. *J Palliat Med.* 2011;14(10):1094-1096.
3. Lewis JM, DiGiacomo M, Currow DC, Davidson PM. Dying in the margins: understanding palliative care and socioeconomic deprivation in the developed world. *J Pain Symptom Manage.* 2011;42(1):105-118.
4. Silow-Carroll S, Alteras T, Stepnick L. *Patient-Centered Care for Underserved Populations: Definition and Best Practices.* Washington, DC: The W. K. Kellogg Foundation; 2006,1-43. Available at: www.esresearch.org/documents_06/Overview.pdf. Accessed September 6, 2012.
5. Hughes A. Poor, Homeless and underserved populations. In: Ferrell BR, Coyle N, eds. *Oxford Textbook of Palliative Nursing.* 3rd ed. New York, NY: Oxford University Press; 2010:745-755.
6. Jennings B, Kaebnick GE, Murray TH. Improving end of life care: why has it been so difficult? *Hastings Cent Rep.* 2005;Spec No:S1-S60.
7. Hughes A. Poverty and palliative care in the U.S.: issues facing the urban poor. International *J Palliat Nurs.* 2005;11:6-13.
8. Dula A, Williams S. When race matters. *Clin Geriatr Med.* 2005;21:239-253.
9. Foti ME. "Do It Your Way": a demonstration project on end-of-life care for persons with serious mental illness. *J Palliat Med.* 2003;6(4):661-669.
10. Payne R. Palliative Care for African Americans and other vulnerable populations: access and quality issues. In: Foley KM, Gelband H, eds. *Improving Palliative Care for Cancer.* Washington, DC: National Academy Press; 2001:153-160.
11. Volandes AE, Paasche-Orlow M, Gillick MR, et al., Health literacy not race predicts end-of-life care preferences. *J Palliat Med.* 2008;11(5):754-762.
12. Moller DW. *Dancing with Broken Bones: Portraits of Death and Dying Among Inner-City Poor.* New York, NY: Oxford University Press; 2004.
13. Hughes A, Gudmundsdottir M, Davies B. Everyday struggling to survive: experiences of the urban poor living with advanced cancer. *Oncol Nurs Forum.* 2007;34(6):1113-1118.
14. DeNavas-Walt C, Proctor BD, Smith JC. Income, Poverty, and Health Insurance Coverage in the United States: 2010. *U.S. Census Bureau, Current Population Reports.* Washington, DC: U.S. Government Printing Office; 2011:P60-239. Available at: www.census.gov/prod/2011pubs/p60-239.pdf. Accessed September 6, 2012.
15. Koenig BA, Gates-Williams J. Understanding cultural difference in caring for dying patients. *West J Med.* 1995;163(3):244-249.
16. National Center for Health Statistics. Deaths/Mortality FastStats. Washington, DC: Centers for Disease Control and Preventions, U.S. Department of Health and Human Services; 2007.
17. Lyckholm LJ, Coyne PJ, Kreutzer KO, Ramakrishnan V, Smith TJ. Barriers to effective palliative care for low-income patients in late stages of cancer: report of a study and strategies for defining and conquering the barriers. *Nurs Clin North Am.* 2010;45(3):399-409.
18. Morrison RS, Wallenstein S, Natale DK, Senzel RS, Huang LL. "We don't carry that"—failure of pharmacies in predominantly nonwhite neighborhoods to stock opioid analgesics. *N Engl J Med.* 2000;342(14):1023-1026.
19. United Way of the Bay Area. University of Washington – Center for Woman's Welfare, National Economic Development and Law Center (U.S.), Wider Opportunities for Women. *The Bottom Line: Setting the Real Standard for Bay Area Working Families.* San Francisco, CA: United Way of the Bay Area; 2004:28.
20. Fernandes R, Braun KL, Ozawa J, Compton M, Guzman C, Somoqyi-Zalud E. Home-based palliative care services for underserved populations. *J Palliat Med.* 2010;13(4):413-419.
21. Hughes A, Davies B, Gudmundsdottir M. "Can you give me respect?" Experiences of the urban poor on a dedicated AIDS nursing home unit. *J Assoc Nurses in AIDS Care.* 2008;19(5):342-356.
22. Hughes A, Gudmundsdottir M, Davies B. Exploring spirituality in the urban poor with advanced cancer (poster abstract). *Oncol Nurs Forum.* 2008;35(3):535.
23. Williams BR. Dying young, dying poor: a sociological examination of existential suffering among low socio-economic status patients. *J Palliat Med.* 2004;7(1):27-37.
24. Kushel MB, Miaskowski C. End-of-life care for homeless patients: "She says she is there to help me in any situation." *JAMA.* 2006;296(24):2959-2966.
25. Podymow T, Turnbull J, Coyle D. Shelter-based palliative care for the homeless terminally ill. *Palliat Med.* 2006. 20(2):81-86.
26. Tarzian AJ, Neal MT, O'Neil JA. Attitudes, experiences, and beliefs affecting end-of-life decision-making among homeless individuals. *J Palliat Med.* 2005;8(1):36-48.
27. Song J, Ratner ER, Bartels DM, Alderton L, Hudson B, Ahluwalia JS. Experiences with and attitudes toward death and dying among homeless persons. *J Gen Intern Med.* 2007;22(4):427-434.

30

28. Song J, Ratner ER, Bartels DM, Alderton L, Hudson B, Ahluwalia JS. Dying on the streets: homeless persons' concerns and desires about end of life care. *J Gen Intern Med.* 2007;22(4):435-441.
29. Sudore RL, Landfeld CS, Barnes DE, et al., An advance directive redesigned to meet the literacy level of most adults: a randomized trial. *Patient Educ Couns.* 2007;69(1-3):165-195.
30. Song J, Wall MM, Ratner ER, Bartels DM, Ulvestad N, Gelberg L. Engaging homeless persons in end of life preparations. *J Gen Intern Med.* 2008;23(12):2031-2036; quiz 2037-2045.
31. Dzul-Church V, Cimino JW, Adler SR, Wong P, Anderson WG. "I'm sitting here by myself ...": experiences of patients with serious illness at an Urban Public Hospital. *J Palliat Med.* 2010;13(6):695-701.
32. Kirsh KL, Passik SD, Palliative care of the terminally ill drug addict. *Cancer Invest.* 2006;24(4):425-31.
33. Passik SD, Kirsh KL. The interface between pain and drug abuse and the evolution of strategies to optimize pain management while minimizing drug abuse. *Exp Clin Psychopharmacol.* 2008;16(5):400-404.
34. Chou R, Fanciullo GJ, Fine PG, Miaskowski C, Passik SD, Portenoy RK. Opioids for chronic noncancer pain: prediction and identification of aberrant drug-related behaviors: a review of the evidence for an American Pain Society and American Academy of Pain Medicine Clinical Practice Guideline. *J Pain.* 2009;10(2):131-146.
35. Lyness JM. End-of-life care: issues relevant to the geriatric psychiatrist. *Am J Geriatr Psychiatry.* 2004;12(5):457-72.
36. National Consensus Project for Quality Palliative Care. *Clinical Practice Guidelines for Quality Palliative Care.* 2nd ed. Pittsburgh, PA: HPNA; 2009. Available at: www.nationalconsensusproject.org. Accessed September 6, 2012.
37. U.S. Department of Veterans Affairs. *Homeless Veterans: About the Initiative.* 2012. Available at: www.va.gov/HOMELESS/about_the_initiative.asp. Accessed July 25, 2012.
38. Melnyk BM, Fineout-Overholt E. Making the case for evidence-based practice and cultivating a spirit of inquiry. In: Melnyk BM, Fineout-Overholt E, eds. *Evidence-based Practice in Nursing & Healthcare.* Philadelphia, PA: Wolters Kluwer Health/Lippincott Williams & Wilkins; 2011:e-book.

ADDITIONAL RESOURCES

Center on Budget and Policy Priorities—a nonpartisan research organization and policy institute that conducts research and analysis on a range of government policies and programs with an emphasis on those affecting low- and moderate-income people. Available at: www.cbpp.org/.

Center for Community Change—a grassroots building organization that helps low-income people build powerful, effective organization through which they can change their communities and public policies for the better. Available at: www.communitychange.org/.

Center for Law and Social Policy (CLASP)—a nonprofit organization that seeks to improve the economic security of low-income families with children and secure access for low-income persons to our civil justice system. Available at: www.clasp.org/. Accessed June 8, 2012.

Coalition on Human Needs—an alliance of national organizations working together to promote public policies that address the needs of low-income and other vulnerable populations. Available at: www.chn.org/.

Community Action Partnership—national association representing the interests of the 1,000 Community Action Agencies (CAAs) organized to change people's lives, embody the spirit of hope, improve communities, and make America a better place to live. www.communityactionpartnership.com/.

National Alliance to End Homelessness—nonprofit, non-partisan, organization committed to preventing and ending homelessness in the United States. By improving policy, building capacity, and educating opinion leaders, the Alliance has become a leading voice on this issue. Available at: www.endhomelessness.org/.

U.S. Census Bureau—Poverty Reports. Available at: www.census.gov/hhes/www/poverty/.

Spotlight on Poverty and Opportunity: Focus on Health—a non-partisan initiative that brings together diverse perspectives from the political, policy, advocacy and foundation communities to find genuine solutions to the economic hardship confronting millions of Americans. Through the ongoing exchange of ideas, research and data, Spotlight seeks to inform the policy debate about reducing poverty and increasing opportunity in the United States. Available at: www.spotlightonpoverty.org/health_and_poverty.aspx.

30

CHAPTER 31

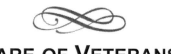

CARE OF VETERANS

Carma Erickson-Hurt, APRN, ACHPN®, LCDR, USN, RET

I. DEMOGRAPHICS

A. One out of every four dying Americans is a Veteran.[1]

B. More than 1,800 Veterans die every day in the United States or about 54,000 per month.[1]

C. Although significant numbers of the dying population are Veterans; approximately 4% of Veterans die in a Veteran's Health Administration inpatient facility, which is a division of the U.S. Department of Veterans Affairs (VA).[1]

D. Only 10-15% of all Veterans in the United States receive healthcare through the VA system.

E. Because the majority of dying Veterans are not served by the VA, it is essential that palliative APRNs understand their unique needs.

II. DEFINING THE VETERAN POPULATION

A. A Veteran is anyone who served any length of active duty, reserve, or guard service in the United States Navy, Marines, Army, Air Force, Coast Guard, Public Health Service, or National Oceanographic and Atmospheric Administration. Identifying a Veteran in the community is the initial step in providing Veteran centric care.

B. Different Types of Veteran Service

1. Active duty is determined by the amount of full time service a Veteran fulfilled in the military. This can vary from a few years to thirty years.

2. The Reserves are military personnel who chose to combine a civilian career with a military career. During drills (one weekend a month and approximately 2 weeks or more a year with a military unit on active duty), reservist perform mock military operations, . Always on call, Reserves personnel could be ordered to enter active duty based upon the needs of their military branch. The current global war on terror utilizes the Reserves to support operations.

3. The Army and Air National Guard (National Guard) are similar to the Reserves. Again, these are military personnel who combine a civilian and military career. Historically the National Guards provide support to individual states to protect the life and property of the citizens of that state during times of emergencies such as natural disasters, riots, etc. However, The National Guards have also deployed troops in support of past and current wars and conflicts.

31

4. Retired military indicates that a person served at least 20 years of active duty service, but has retired from further service. Upon retirement, he/she is entiled to receive a pension and medical insurance benefits.

C. A Veteran's discharge from military service form is known as a DD214 or "Certificate of Release or Discharge from Active Duty." The DD214 is issued upon a military member's retirement, separation, or discharge from Active Duty military and serves as proof of military service. It is an essential element in the VA enrollment process and most Veterans will know what a DD214 is, but the family may not be aware of the need for this document. It is important to make sure the family is aware of the location of the DD214 or how to retrieve it.

III. THE MILITARY HISTORY CHECKLIST

A. It is impossible to treat a Veteran's needs if his/her military status is unknown. All patients should be asked, "Did you ever serve in the military?" or "Are you a Veteran?"

1. If the answer to both questions is "yes," then a military history checklist, relating to branch, period of service, perception of service experience, and military benefits, can serve as a guide to identify how military service has affected their life.

2. If the answer is yes to service in the military but no to a Veteran, it may be an indication the person had a dishonorable discharge from the military. They will not have access to care but will have the same experiences from service and the same healthcare issues.

B. Those men and women who have served in the military are part of a distinct culture with its own language, rituals and norms, and experiences. This culture can define the functioning of entire families; especially when there is a strong familial history of military service. Within this culture, there are significant subcultures based on—the era of service; combat versus noncombat service; voluntary entry into service or drafted into service; and whether the Veteran served as an officer or enlisted serviceman.

C. Once a Veteran has been identified, he/she should be asked "Which branch of service were you in?" Each branch of service is distinct in its methods of training, instruction, and socialization. The focus of each branch also partially determines the likelihood of combat related trauma. For example, a Marine or Army Veteran is more likely to have seen combat than a Coast Guard Veteran.

D. The Veteran should then be asked "Which war era or period of service did you serve?" Each era of service and war has its own unique history and influences upon the Veteran. This can dramatically influence the outcome of the Veteran's experience. Medical issues seen in the various eras and locations of service may be associated with presumptive disabilities.

E. Once the background information is gathered on the Veteran's military service, the service man or woman can be asked, "Overall, how do you view your military service?" Understanding how the Veteran views his/her service, positively or negatively, may help the clinician gain insight into how the Veteran may perceive his/her serious or life-threatening condition, especially if the condition is related to his/her military service.

31

1. Many Veterans often take great pride in their service, considering it as a meaningful period of time when he/she made a difference in the world. This positive perspective may be in spite of being subjected to imprisonment, torture, wounding, exposure to atrocities, or other traumatic experiences.

2. However, other Veterans view their service negatively. They feel they did sacrifice their time, but may not feel they made any difference. This perception may have subsequent implications and may warrant further exploration of potential existential questions and concerns. The palliative APRN can provide opportunities during follow up visits for discussion and exploration to promote healing and build trust.

F. If hospice is involved in the care of the Veteran, they may ask, "If available, would you like a hospice staff member or volunteer with military experience?" The military Veteran culture, which is often able to span eras and theaters of service despite the previously mentioned differences, can be a powerful force even at the end of life. A volunteer or staff member who is part of the military culture can provide support in a unique way, helping to bridge the patient-provider relationship. It may also provide an outlet for the stories and experiences never previously communicated to family or others in the Veteran's life.

1. Volunteer opportunities are often a path to healing war related trauma for the volunteer.

2. Veteran volunteers may benefit from education, training, and additional support when caring for fellow Veterans at the end of life, as their own trauma may also be re-triggered.

G. Finally the Veteran should be asked, "Are you enrolled in the VA?" All Veterans who were honorably discharged may be eligible for VA benefits. These vary from healthcare coverage to disability compensation. Eligibility for most VA benefits is based on honorable discharge from active military service.

1. Veterans must be enrolled in the VA in order to be considered for these benefits. If a Veteran is enrolled in the VA, it may be helpful to ask if they receive any benefits or if they have a service-connected condition.

2. Many Veterans may receive their medications through the VA. A Veteran enrolled in the VA for healthcare benefits may receive their medication from their VA primary care provider at a reduced rate. The name and contact information of the VA facility and provider should be obtained to promote collaboration, communication, and continuity of care.

3. If the Veteran is enrolled in hospice, they would receive their medications related to their terminal diagnosis from the hospice and the medications not related to the terminal diagnosis from the VA.

H. Those who were dishonorably discharged are not eligible for VA benefits.

I. Only 10-15% of Veterans receive their healthcare at the VA.[3] One cannot assume that because they are a Veteran they can use the VA. The majority of Veterans are not enrolled in the VA system, but instead may carry private insurance. Therefore, they are unfamiliar with the VA system and its healthcare facilities, because they receive their care elsewhere. Therefore identification of Veterans in non-military healthcare settings is vital to helping the Veteran access benefits they may be missing.

31

IV. HONORING VETERANS

A. Once the military status is known, it is important to respect the Veteran's service, feelings, and any suggestions they might offer. It may take longer for Veterans to build trusting relationships than other patients.

   1. Patience and listening will build trust and rapport with the Veteran. Most Veterans will not share their entire story on the initial visit. Rather, pieces of the story may be revealed with time. The expectation and willingness to allow the sharing of information to occur over a period of time will help the APRN.

   2. Veterans may have strong political feelings and/or positive or negative feelings about their military service. Allow them to express their feelings without being judgmental. Be supportive and validate their feelings and concerns.

   3. Similar to any palliative care, it is best that the APRN avoid statements such as, "I understand how you feel," as usually the clinician has not shared the same experience. Statements such as, "That must have been very hard for you," validate the feelings the Veteran is expressing.

B. Simple acts of gratitude, particularly at the end of life, can make up for a lifetime of pain because some Veterans were never welcomed or thanked for their service. A general statement such as, "Thank you for your service," may be appreciated. A specific statement such as, "Thank you for your service in Vietnam," may be more authentic. Hospice and palliative care staff may provide the last opportunity for Veterans to feel that their service was not in vain, and they are appreciated. Additionally, showing appreciation to the family of the Veteran for their sacrifice is also important.

C. The National Hospice and Palliative Care Association (NHPCO) and the Department of Veterans Affairs have developed the *We Honor Veterans* program to assist hospice and palliative care providers in caring for the unique needs of Veterans.[2]

D. The Hospice and Palliative Nurses Association (HPNA—www.HPNA.org) and the End-of-Life Nursing Education Consortium (ELNEC—www.aacn.nche.edu/elnec) have developed education aimed at all levels of nursing about palliative care for Veterans.

V. CHARACTERISTICS OF PARTICULAR WAR ERAS

A. World War II (WW II) lasted from 1939-1945. There are over 2 million WWII Veterans living, all of whom are over 80 years old.[3] WWII had a clear mission and these Veterans came home to a hero's welcome. For the most part the country was supportive of the war efforts.

   1. Many service personnel have a positive view about their military experience and felt they had a duty to serve their country. Veterans fought in several countries in extreme climates and conditions.

   2. Those who served aboard ships may been exposed to asbestos. WWII Veterans may have also been exposed to infectious diseases, extreme temperatures, nuclear weapons, and chemical agents.

   3. Although WWII ended triumphantly with soldiers viewed as heroes, some providers may not realize that these Veterans are still at risk for posttraumatic

31

stress disorder (PTSD). However, PTSD had not yet been identified or accepted as a specific diagnosis. Thus, the term "shell shock" was applied to soldiers experiencing the traumatizing effects of war. These Veterans experienced disturbing events, such as multiple deaths of dying comrades in the field, and mangled injuries from various bombs. They relive these deaths once back in the United States. Those soldiers at highest risk for PTSD in this population included those engaged in high levels of combat, detained as prisoners of war, or were wounded in action.

B. The Korean conflict lasted from 1950 to 1953. Currently there are around 2.4 million living Korean Veterans.[3] Because of the short duration and lack of media attention, the Korean conflict is sometimes termed "The Forgotten War."

1. Because the war was overshadowed by WWII and Vietnam, soldiers' efforts were minimized and traumas ignored.

2. Soldiers served in harsh weather conditions, with inadequate equipment exposing them to cold temperatures. Battlefield conditions, themselves, made treatment for cold injuries difficult.[4] Injuries related to cold exposure often caused long-term sequelae, though delayed and worsen with age. The long-term effects of cold exposure included peripheral neuropathy, skin cancer in frostbitten areas such as the heels and earlobes, arthritis in injured areas, chronic tinea pedis, fallen arches, and stiff toes. Moreover, with aging, these soldiers developed conditions such as diabetes and peripheral vascular disease, placing them at risk for late amputations.[4]

3. Soldiers who experienced the traumatizing effects of war were diagnosed as having "combat fatigue."

C. The Cold War lasted from 1945 until the fall of the former Soviet Union in the early 1990s. This period of tension between the United States and its allies and the Soviet bloc began after WWII.

1. Veterans of this era are often referred to as "Atomic Veterans" because of exposure to atomic weapons and radiation.[4]

2. A major fear of the Cold War era was nuclear war with associated health concerns about exposure to ionizing radiation. Service members during this time may have participated in nuclear weapons testing and cleanup. Exposure to radiation has been associated with leukemias and other cancers and cataracts.[4]

3. Atomic Veterans are eligible to participate in the VA's Ionizing Radiation Program. This includes access to an Ionizing Radiation Registry Examination performed within the VA. In addition, there is special eligibility for treatment of conditions recognized by VA as potentially radiogenic, whether or not they have had a radiation compensation claim approved.[4] See Appendix 31-A for the list of Presumptive Disability Benefits for Certain Groups of Veterans.

D. The Vietnam conflict began in 1962 and lasted until 1975. There are over 7.9 million Vietnam Veterans, comprising the largest number of combat Veterans.[4] The proportion of Vietnam-era Veterans over the age of 65 continue to increase through 2014, when Vietnam Veterans will account for nearly 60% of all Veterans in that age group.[5] Many soldiers who served in Vietnam were drafted—not serving in the military willingly. Because of the stigma associated with this unpopular war, many of these Veterans were personally attacked upon return home by their fellow citizens who opposed the war.

31

1.   Many Veterans may have negative or hidden feelings and attitudes toward their service. This situation magnified the trauma associated with their combat experiences.[2] Contributing to the stress experienced by many Veterans was the lack of unit cohesiveness. Many soldiers were sent to Vietnam as individuals, not as units, and left upon completion of a year's tour.[2] Because they did not leave Vietnam with their fellow soldiers, many Vietnam Veterans did not have the opportunity to begin the closure process or sharing experiences.

2.   Vietnam Veterans may have been exposed to an herbicide and defoliant chemical spray, called by the military code name Agent Orange. Extensive research identified the long-term health effects of exposure to Agent Orange. The government took many years to recognize the side effects of contact with this chemical. The VA assumes that all Vietnam Veterans who served in the Republic of Vietnam, from January 9, 1962 to May 7, 1975, were exposed to Agent Orange and now offers Veteran's benefits related to Agent Orange exposure. (see Appendix 31-A)

   a)   Under VA Code of Federal Regulations, Veterans who served in Vietnam between 1962 and 1975 (including those who even briefly visited Vietnam), and have a disease the VA recognizes as being associated with Agent Orange, are presumed to have been exposed to Agent Orange.[6]

   b)   Updates are now published every 2 years in reports issued by the Institutes of Medicine. Unfortunately, there is no concrete data to determine how much exposure to Agent Orange herbicide Vietnam Veterans experienced. Additionally, it has yet to be determined the amount of Agent Orange exposure resulted in various conditions or increased the risk of developing such conditions. Presumptive diseases related to Agent Orange exposure include

      i.   Malignant diseases—non-Hodgkin's lymphoma, Hodgkin's, multiple myeloma, sarcoma, prostate and respiratory cancers, chronic lymphocytic leukemia, and hairy cell leukemia.

      ii. Nonmalignant diseases—birth defects in children of Vietnam Veterans, spinal bifida, type II diabetes, peripheral neuropathy, ischemic heart disease, and Parkinson's disease.

3.   Education is important as many Vietnam Veterans are unaware that their disease is related to military service that would qualify them for benefits. Or they may have been denied claims in the past by the VA, but now would be eligible. It is important to encourage Veterans to seek a VA evaluation.

31

E.   The Gulf War lasted from 1990 to 1991. Currently approximately 5.7 million Gulf War era Veterans are living.[3] The Gulf War was considered a brief and successful military operation with fewer injuries and deaths of American troops in comparison to other conflicts. Most Gulf War Veterans resumed their normal activities after returning from the war.

1.   Troops were exposed to smoke from burning oil fields, various unknown chemical and biological agents, depleted uranium from weapons, and infections such as leishmaniasis. The effects of these exposures are still unknown.

2. Many soldiers soon began reporting a variety of unexplained health problems they attributed to their participation in the Gulf War recognized by the VA as "Gulf War Syndrome." The problems included chronic fatigue, muscle and joint pain, loss of concentration, forgetfulness, headache, rash, fibromyalgia, and irritable bowel syndrome. A registry was established for all Veterans for evaluation of complaints and symptoms. "Gulf War Syndrome" was later changed to "Gulf War Illness." (see Appendix 31-A)

F. Operation Iraqi Freedom (OIF) and Operation Enduring Freedom (OEF) began in 2003 with the wars in Iraq and Afghanistan. Most recently, Operation New Dawn (OND) was initiated. Similar to Gulf War Veterans, OIF/OEF/OND Veterans may experience complications from immunizations, chemical and biological agents, and infections. It is important to note that many OIF/OEF/OND Veterans have other health insurance plans after leaving the military and may not seek healthcare through the VA system. OIF/OEF/OND soldiers survived injuries that would have been fatal in previous conflicts. Due to advances in technology

1. Polytrauma is common in this group of Veterans. Polytrauma is defined as 2 or more injuries to physical regions or organ systems, 1 of which may be life-threatening, resulting in physical, cognitive, psychological, or psychosocial impairments and functional disability.[7] One particular polytrauma triad comprised of chronic pain, PTSD, and traumatic brain injury (TBI), presents a diagnostic and treatment challenge.[7,8]

2. TBI is the hallmark injury of OIF/OEF/OND Veterans. TBI is the result of head injuries sustained when the head forcefully hits an object, when an object penetrates the skull, or when brain tissue undergoes sudden acceleration, deceleration or both.[9] There are almost 44,000 Veterans with TBI because military duties increase the risk of TBI.[10] It is estimated that 10-20% of all soldiers returning from Iraq and Afghanistan have sustained some type of TBI.[9]

a) Blasts are a leading cause of TBI for military personnel in combat. Other causes of TBI in the military may include bullets or fragments, motor vehicle accidents, assaults, and falls.

b) TBI symptoms can appear immediately or can be delayed over time. These can include memory loss, decreased cognitive function, behavioral and personality changes, dementia, and PTSD. Neurological symptoms include seizures, headaches, impaired reflexes, nervous ticks, and post-concussive syndrome, which can manifest as dizziness, headaches, vertigo, nausea, insomnia, and depression.

c) A common complication of TBI is chronic pain syndromes. Therefore, an assessment of chronic pain is crucial.[9] Some symptoms resolve within a month of injury while others persist for months or years.[7]

d) Long-term implications of TBI are not known; further research is needed to determine how to care for Veterans with TBI.

3. OIF/OEF/OND combat Veterans can receive cost free medical care for any condition related to their service in the Iraq/Afghanistan Theater for five years after the date of their discharge or release. Other benefits may also be available. In order to take advantage of these benefits, OIF/OEF/OND Veterans need to enroll in the VA's healthcare system.

31

4. Often due to length of conflicts, service personnel participate in multiple tours of duty in which they have come back to the United States in-between being in the war zone. This may be seen as an accomplishment. However, the prolonged timeline of these conflicts has meant that military personnel and their families often endure multiple tours of combat duty.

VI. WOMEN VETERANS

A. The role of women has evolved with each conflict. Thus, women in World War II had a much different role and military experience than today's women Veterans. Identification of women's Veteran status and military occupation can help to identify unique issues.

B. Women comprise approximately 14% of the U.S. Armed Forces.[11] Women Veterans account for nearly 1 in 100 adult female patients in the United States.[12] Most of today's 1.7 million women Veterans obtain all or most of their healthcare outside of the VA system. It is common that a women's Veteran status is unacknowledged when accessing a civilian healthcare system.[8]

C. Exposure to combat environments and harsh duty assignments can affect a woman's health. The top three diagnostic categories for women treated within the VA system are PTSD, hypertension, and depression.[13] Because of their military experiences, women Veterans have unique healthcare needs as compared to their non-Veteran peers.

D. However, the sequelae for women deployed to a combat area are still largely unknown.[8] Many women, like their male counterparts, return from combat traumatized by the events they have experienced. Researchers and healthcare providers are beginning to recognize that gender plays a large role in how Veterans process the psychological trauma of war. The greatest hope for answers lies in the Women Veterans Cohort Study; a longitudinal study to identify gender-associated disparities in healthcare utilization among OIF/OEF/OND Veterans receiving care in the VA system. This may help to determine the healthcare needs of women Veterans.

VII. HOMELESS VETERANS

A. Veterans comprise 23% of the homeless population.[14] A large number of these are displaced and at-risk Veterans. They live with lingering effects of PTSD and substance abuse, compounded by a lack of family and social support networks.[15] Since 1987, the VA has addressed the problems of homelessness among Veterans through the development of specialized programs geared to facilitate access to services and care.

1. The VA has a strategic initiative to end Veteran homelessness by 2015.[16] To accomplish this, the VA has established a range of specialized resources, services, and programs to promote easy access to programs and services for Veterans at risk for homelessness or attempting to exit homelessness. Programs and resources include prevention and early intervention services, a national call center, housing support services, treatment, employment and job training, benefits, and resources, all of which collaborate with community and national programs. The local VA Medical Center or Vet Center will have information on the programs available to homeless Veterans.

31

2. Most homeless Veterans will be able to access medical care through the VA system if they were honorably discharged from active military service. However, because of the complex process of obtaining eligibility for care from the VA, many Veterans may not have accessed care through the VA system. Few homeless Veterans are able to navigate the system assistance. Social workers can help connect the homeless Veteran with the VA system. Veteran Service Organizations (VSOs) such as the Veterans of Foreign Wars (VFW) or Disabled American Veterans (DAV) can provide free assistance navigating the VA system.

B. Many homeless Veterans may have issues with healthcare providers such as the VA, large institutions, or the government.[17] Many Veterans also pride themselves in self-reliance and their ability to survive. This pride may result in a preference for sleeping out in the rough rather than staying in shelters. They may have experienced or heard about "red tape" bureaucracies and the lack of coordination of services. Many may feel resentful about not receiving services and benefits to which they feel entitled to. Efforts to promote outreach, collaboration, and access to services and care are essential to navigate the homeless Veteran to appropriate programs and resources available in the VA and community.

VIII. VETERAN (VET) CENTERS

A. The Veteran Centers or VET Centers are community based and part of the U.S. Department of Veterans Affairs. The VET centers are a VA program designed to provide readjustment counseling to Veterans exposed to the uniquely stressful conditions of military service in a combat theater of operations. The goal of a VET center program is to provide a broad range of counseling, outreach, and referral services to eligible combat Veterans in order to help them make a satisfying post-war readjustment to civilian life. The VET center program encourages early intervention to promote better readjustment and makes every effort to remove the stigma of seeking assistance. They provide services in a non-clinical environment without the stigma sometimes associated with some other mental health or readjustment care. Because many Veterans prefer to confidentially speak with a fellow Veteran regarding readjustment from military to civilian life following active service in a combat zone; the counseling staff at most VET centers are Veterans themselves.

B. The VET Centers are located within the community, with services tailored to the specific needs of the Veteran population within that community. VET center staff members are always available to welcome Veterans and family members, and to provide useful information about available services. Eligible Veterans have access to a wide range of services. These include professional readjustment counseling for war-related social and psychological readjustment problems, family military related readjustment services, substance abuse screening and referral, military sexual trauma counseling referral, bereavement counseling services, employment services, and multiple community-based support services such as preventative education, outreach, case management, and referral services.

C. To accommodate Veteran's work schedules, VET centers maintain flexible schedules. VET centers have no waiting list. Veterans may be seen by a counselor the same day they stop by for an initial assessment. They can schedule subsequent appointments at their convenience.

31

D. VET Center Services include bereavement counseling to surviving parents, spouses, children, and siblings of service members who died while on active duty. Bereavement counseling includes a broad range of transition services including outreach, counseling by volunteers or a chaplain, and referral services for family members. Often counseling is available in the family's home or where the family feels the most comfortable. There is no cost for VA bereavement counseling in the VET centers.

IX. VETERAN SERVICE ORGANIZATIONS (VSO)

A. VSOs differ from VET centers in that VSOs are not part of the VA system. VSOs are located in every community. The larger VSOs have a national office with posts or chapters in communities across the United States. VSOs include, but are not limited to—the Veterans of Foreign Wars (VFW), American Legion, Disabled American Veterans (DAV), American Veterans (Am Vets) and Vietnam Veterans of America (VVA). These service organizations can provide information, support, and volunteers to assist Veterans in accessing benefits. They are non-profit community based organizations devoted to serving the interests of Veterans, usually supported by a Veteran membership base. Some VSOs have a Veteran's advocate service officer who may legally represent and support Veterans on issues related to their Veteran status, including application for benefits, etc.

X. POSTTRAUMATIC STRESS DISORDER (PTSD)

A. PTSD is an anxiety disorder that can occur after a traumatic event, serious or life-threatening situation. Veterans are at higher risk than the general population of developing PTSD by the very nature of military service.[4] Specific military situations that may cause PTSD for Veterans are—combat or military exposure; terrorist attacks; sexual, psychological or physical assault in military service; accidents in vehicles, planes, or boats; and participation in disaster relief or stabilization efforts related to hurricanes, tornadoes, floods, or earthquakes. However, not all Veterans have PTSD. (See Chapter 15, *Psychosocial Aspects*)

B. The Diagnostic and Statistical Manual of the American Psychiatric Association (DSM-IV-R) specifies criteria for the diagnosis of PTSD.[18] Diagnostic criteria for PTSD include a history of exposure to a traumatic event meeting two criteria and symptoms from each of three symptom clusters—intrusive recollections, avoidant/numbing symptoms, and hyper-arousal symptoms. The fifth criterion delineates duration of symptoms and the sixth criterion assesses functioning.

   1. Criterion A—stressor.[18] The person has been exposed to a traumatic event in which both of the following have been present—the person has experienced, witnessed, or been confronted with an event or events that involve actual or threatened death or serious injury, or a threat to the physical integrity of oneself or others; and the person's response involved intense fear, helplessness, or horror.[18]

   2. Criterion B—intrusive recollection.[18] The traumatic event is persistently re-experienced in at least one of the following ways

      a) Recurrent and intrusive distressing recollections of the event, including images, thoughts, or perceptions

      b) Recurrent distressing dreams of the event

31

      c) Acting or feeling as if the traumatic event were recurring (includes a sense of reliving the experience, illusions, hallucinations, and dissociative flashback episodes; including those that occur upon awakening or when intoxicated).

      d) Intense psychological distress at exposure to internal or external cues that symbolize or resemble an aspect of the traumatic event

      e) Physiologic reactivity upon exposure to internal or external cues that symbolize or resemble an aspect of the traumatic event

3. Criterion C—avoidance/numbing.[18] Persistent avoidance of stimuli associated with the trauma and numbing of general responsiveness (not present before the trauma), as indicated by at least 3 of the following

      a) Efforts to avoid thoughts, feelings, or conversations associated with the trauma

      b) Efforts to avoid activities, places, or people that arouse recollections of the trauma

      c) Inability to recall an important aspect of the trauma

      d) Markedly diminished interest or participation in significant activities

      e) Feeling of detachment or estrangement from others

      f) Restricted range of affect (e.g., unable to have loving feelings)

      g) Sense of foreshortened future (e.g., does not expect to have a career, marriage, children, or a normal life span)

4. Criterion D—hyper-arousal.[18] Persistent symptoms of increasing arousal (not present before the trauma), indicated by at least two of the following

      a) Difficulty falling or staying asleep

      b) Irritability or outbursts of anger

      c) Difficulty concentrating

      d) Hyper-vigilance

      e) Exaggerated startle response

5. Criterion E—duration. Duration of the disturbance (symptoms in B, C, and D) is more than 1 month.

6. Criterion F—functional significance. The disturbance causes clinically significant distress or impairment in social, occupational, or other important areas of functioning.[19]

C. Despite its prevalence, PTSD often goes unrecognized and therefore untreated in Veterans. This is common because Veterans find it difficult talking about traumatic experiences. Veterans with PTSD may have experienced a traumatic event in which they witnessed something horrific or caused them to fear for their lives. The result is a feeling of helplessness because they could not change the course of events. It is theorized that strong emotions caused by the event create changes in the brain that may result in PTSD. Many Veterans who experience a traumatic event have some initial anxiety symptoms; yet only some will develop PTSD. The reason for this is not clear. Potential factors affecting whether a Veteran will develop PTSD include

31

1. The intensity or duration of the trauma, as the more severe trauma, the more likely the development of PTSD

2. The death or injury of a close comrade or friend

3. The physical proximity to a traumatic event—PTSD is worse the closer the soldier was to witness the event.

4. The amount of control the Veteran had over the events—suffering may be worse if they felt they could have done more, or if they felt helpless to do anything.

5. The extent of the support the Veteran received after the event—Veterans of recent wars such as OIF/OEF/OND are benefitting from earlier PTSD screening and early interventions. Veterans from WWII, Korea, and Vietnam did not receive the same PTSD routine screening or intervention following their homecoming.

D. When speaking with a Veteran about PTSD, it is important to consider the era under which they served, because they may use terms other than PTSD. As stated before, PTSD known as "shell shock" in WWI and WWII, and "battle fatigue" in The Korean War.

E. Stigma may exist in the Veteran population regarding mental health services.[20] Stoic attitudes are pervasive in the military culture. Many soldiers view seeking help as a sign of weakness. Often, Veterans experiencing PTSD fit the profile of the "difficult" patient; the one who is persistently confused, angry, depressed, abusing alcohol and other drugs, and/or otherwise emotionally dependant and demanding. He/she may have tried to cope alone without seeking treatment. The result is that they have yet to recover from the trauma and are in daily struggle to come to terms with what they witnessed or experienced.

F. PTSD symptoms often start soon after the traumatic event. However just as often, they may be delayed until months or years later. Symptoms may also wax and wane over many years. If the symptoms last longer than 4 weeks, they may cause great distress, or interfere with work or home life, the individual probably has PTSD.[4]

G. Many soldiers who develop PTSD improve. However, 1 out of 3 continue to experience PTSD symptoms. Treatment can help to prevent symptoms from interfering with everyday activities, work, and relationships. Types of PTSD symptoms may include

1. The presence of repetitive, disturbing memories, nightmares, flashbacks, and/or hallucinations is common. The Veteran may feel the same fear and horror as when the event originally took place. The Veteran may experience a flashback, including nightmares or the re-experience of the event itself. Sometimes a trigger, such as a sound or sight, causes the Veteran to relive the event. An example of such triggers may be the sound of a car backfiring reminding the Veteran of gunfire, or the sound and light of fireworks reminding him/her of a bomb dropping.

2. Veterans may avoid thoughts, people, places, and activities that resemble the traumatic event. Additionally, Veterans may keep very busy to distract them from thinking or talking about the event. Or they may avoid seeking help so that they do not have to focus on the details of the trauma.

31

3. Suppressing trauma related memories and emotions can lead to amnesia for aspects of the trauma or a sense of being emotionally "numb."[21] Even if the Veteran remembers aspects of the trauma, he/she may be unable to talk about them or they may find it difficult to express feelings about it. The Veteran may lack loving feelings toward others and have distress in relationships. Previously enjoyed activities may no longer be of interest.

4. Symptoms of hyper-arousal, hyper-vigilance, irritability, heightened startle response, insomnia, attention difficulties or anger may be present.[7] The feeling of always being on edge, constantly looking out for danger, a sense of being anxious or jitteriness, may manifest as sudden anger or irritation. Hyper-vigilance can amplify pain experiences.

5. Psychosocial issues such as depression, general anxiety, and survivor guilt are often present with PTSD.[21] The Veteran may have concomitant substance abuse issues such as alcohol or drug problems. They may express feelings of hopelessness, shame or despair, and may have employment problems.

H. Brief, direct questions about trauma exposure and posttrauma symptoms as part of a routine assessment can quickly identify when traumatic experiences are continuing to have a significant impact on functioning. The following questions can be sure to screen for PTSD

   – Have you ever had any experiences that were frightening, horrible, or upsetting in the past?

   – Have you had nightmares about the event or thought about it when you did not want to?

   – Have you tried hard not to think about it or went out of our way to avoid situations that reminded you of it?

   – Are you constantly on guard, watchful, or easily startled?

   – Do you feel numb or detached from others, activities, or your surroundings?

   If the patient answers "yes" to any two of the above questions, it is a positive screen for PTSD.

I. Survivors of trauma may not complain directly of PTSD symptoms such as re-experiencing the trauma or avoidance of discussing the trauma. Instead, they may complain of sleeping disturbances or insomnia.

J. Questioning the Veteran, as well as his/her family members, co-workers, or friends improves the identification of PTSD. Therefore, the palliative APRN should consider asking specific questions about sleep problems, (e.g., flashbacks, nightmares), hyper-arousal (e.g., an exaggerated startle response or sleep disturbance), agitation, and/or depression and anxiety. In particular, the APRN should assess for signs of suicidal ideation.

K. The hospice/palliative APRN may need assistance in the diagnosis of PTSD. By detecting PTSD, the APRN can refer patients for further evaluation to mental health professional as appropriate. It is assumed that APRNs develop ongoing collaborative relationships with mental health professionals at the local VA clinic or hospital.

31

L. Treatment of PTSD may include both pharmacological and nonpharmacological modalities. Medications prescribed for PTSD symptoms act upon neurotransmitters related to the fear and anxiety circuitry of the brain including serotonin, norepinephrine, GABA, and dopamine to name a few. Most often, medications do not entirely eliminate the symptoms, but rather provide symptom reduction. As with other psychiatric diagnoses, medications are best used in conjunction with an ongoing program of trauma specific psychotherapy.[6]

1. The only FDA approved preferred class of medication for treatment of PTSD is selective serotonin reuptake inhibitors (SSRIs). They have been found to alleviate avoidance and numbing symptoms.[21] SSRIs primarily affect the neurotransmitter serotonin, which is important in regulating mood, anxiety, appetite and sleep and other bodily functions. Specific medication within the class is based upon the individual patient history of comorbidities, as well as previous response to medications and side effect profiles.[6] The strongest evidence supports the use of fluoxetine, paroxetine, or sertraline. The use of serotonin norepinephrine reuptake inhibitors (SNRIs) may also be used. In this class, venlafaxine has the strongest support in the treatment of PTSD. Venlafaxine acts primarily as an SSRI at lower dosages and at higher dosages, it acts as a combined SSRI and SNRI.[22]

2. Antidepressants that work through other routes of neurotransmission in altering serotonin neurotransmission are also helpful in PTSD. Mirtazapine may be particularly helpful for treatment of insomnia in PTSD. Trazodone is also commonly use for insomnia in PTSD, even though there is little empirical evidence available for its use. Nefazodone carries a black box warning regarding liver failure, so liver function tests need to be monitored and precautions taken as recommended in the medication's prescribing information.[22]

3. Atypical antipsychotics may also be used in PTSD treatment. While originally developed for patients with a psychotic disorder, this class of medications is being used for patients with myriad psychiatric disorders including PTSD. These medications primarily act on the dopaminergic and serotonergic systems and relieve hyperarousal and re-experiencing symptoms. The evidence for their use as adjunctive therapy in PTSD for patients who have residual symptoms following the use of the first line agent such as SSRIs and venlafaxine is mixed.[6] These medications must be used with caution and require monitoring for elevation of blood glucose and cholesterol levels. There is also a small risk of developing extrapyramidal side effects as well as tardive dyskinesia. A rarer side effect is neuroleptic malignant syndrome. Dosages vary widely for olanzapine and risperidone.

31

4. There are a number of other medications that can be helpful for specific PTSD symptoms or used as second line agents. One medication is prazosin for decreasing nightmares, although it has not been found to be effective for other PTSD symptoms at this time. Tricyclic antidepressants (TCAs) and monoamine oxidase inhibitors (MAOIs) act on a number of neurotransmitters. Again as second line treatment, TCAs are thought to alleviate intrusive symptoms as well as anxiety and depression.[21] However, both have high side effect profiles. The TCAs have cardiac effects such as ventricular arrhythmias, especially in overdose.[22] The MAOIs can cause potentially fatal reactions due to hypertensive crisis when taken with other medications or with certain foods rich in tyramine (e.g., aged cheeses, smoked fish, cured

meats, some types of beer). MAOIs can also provoke the potentially fatal serotonin syndrome when used concurrently with SSRIs.[6] While evidence supports their use, their use as second line therapy warrants judicious and attentive monitoring of safety and side effects.

5. Benzodiazepines such as clonazepam, alprazolam, and lorazepam act directly on the GABA system, which produces a calming effect on the nervous system. Studies have not shown them to be useful in PTSD treatment because they seem to affect core PTSD symptoms. There is also the concerns of the potential addictive and disinhibition symptom necessitating their cautious use in PTSD.[6]

6. Because of the delayed onset of effects of SSRIs and TCAs, patients with days or weeks to live may require medications with more rapid action. Short acting benzodiazepines or neuroleptics may be the most effective relief for Veterans experiencing intense PTSD symptoms at the end of life.[21]

M. Nonpharmacological treatment of PTSD may include support groups with other Veterans suffering from PTSD, complementary and interventional therapy approaches that facilitate a relaxation response such as mindfulness, yoga, acupuncture, and/or massage, which can be adjunctive treatment of hyperarousal symptoms. Hypnotic techniques can be considered, especially for symptoms such as pain, anxiety, dissociation, and nightmares.[6] Group therapy such as PTSD support groups may be very helpful. Veterans considering group therapy should agree to the underlying rationale of trauma work, and the willingness to participate in self-disclosure within the group work.

N. Spiritual support may be desired by the Veteran. The spiritual provider can explore PTSD as well as grief and loss in the areas of physical being, psychological stamina, and loss of future hopes and aspirations.

O. Maintaining an egalitarian stance with all patients is important, but even more so in the Veteran population who may be distrustful of the medical system. A Veteran may be more open to treatment when he/she feels an equal voice in their care. Emphasis should be placed on the Veteran's control over decisions, allowing options and choices whenever possible.

P. A Veteran's family should be educated about PTSD symptoms, including potential consequences of exposure to traumatic stress, practical ways of coping with symptoms, and potential treatments. When Veterans and their family members begin to understand that much of the distress and associated problems are connected to the war experiences and posttraumatic stress, there is often more willingness to reach to the many kinds of available help.

XI. END-OF-LIFE PAIN AND SYMPTOM MANAGEMENT

A. Veterans experiencing chronic pain, particularly headache disorders and fibromyalgia (FM), associated with psychological traumas need a special management strategy.

1. Obtaining the clinical history of a traumatic event or diagnosing PTSD in chronic pain patients can guide treatment.

2. Stoicism is valued in the military culture. While on active duty, service personnel may be less likely to report pain because of peer pressure, fear of being medically evaluated, and/or potential separation from fellow soldiers.[9] Consequently, it is important to build trust with Veterans. They must be given

31

reassurance that it is not a sign of weakness to report pain or discomfort or take pain medication. Moreover, pain medication can improve activity and function.

B. Factors can influence how the Veteran experiences the dying process.

1. The threat to life from a terminal illness may mimic the threat to life experienced in military service, leading to significant distress.[23] For some Veterans it may seem inconceivable that they survived a war only to die of something else.

2. The process of life review, common at the end of life, can lead to anxiety, guilt, anger, and sadness. Allowing time and space for life review and facilitating the conversation on their military experience are both very important for all Veterans for closure. Encouraging the family to interact with the Veteran and listen to his/her stories may be helpful and healing.

3. Avoidance behaviors, which are common in Veterans with PTSD, can manifest as non-adherence. The Veteran may cope by ignoring problems.

4. Distrust can cause excessive questioning of medical personnel and possible refusal of care. Building trust takes time and dedication.

5. Isolation and avoidance behaviors may lead to broken relationships resulting in a lack of caregivers at the end of life due to the Veteran repeatedly pushing away family and friends.

6. All of these factors can influence how the Veteran experiences the dying process, sometimes with more agitation and restlessness.

XII. CAREGIVERS

A. Caregiver support coordinators at each VA Medical Center are available to assist family caregivers in identifying benefits and series of enrolled Veterans. The Caregiver Support Coordinators are well versed in the VA programs and have information about other local public, private, and non-profit agency support series that are available to support Veterans and their family caregivers at home. There is education and training on the caregiver role including how to best meet the Veteran's care needs, the importance of self-care when in a care-giving role. Caregivers for Veterans of all eras are eligible for respite care.

B. As of May, 2011, wounded Veterans and their caregivers may apply for new benefits under the Caregivers and Veterans Omnibus Health Services Act of 2010.[24] The law directs the Department of Veterans Affairs to assist caregivers of Veterans needing ongoing personal care services because of serious injury (including TBI and psychological trauma) incurred in the line of duty on or after September 11, 2001. These benefits include education and training for caregivers, in-home and community-based care, respite care, counseling, health insurance, and a monthly stipend. For a complete explanation of eligibility criteria and benefits, please refer to the VA Medical Center or VA website (www.va.gov). Additional supports for primary family caregivers of eligible post 9/11 Veterans and service members may include a stipend, mental health series, and access to healthcare insurance, if they are not already entitled to care of services under a healthcare plan.

XIII. VA BENEFITS

A. A Veteran must be enrolled in the VA to receive healthcare benefits and other Veteran services. Eligibility for most VA benefits depends upon departure from active military, naval, or air service under honorable discharge. In addition, current and former members of the Reserves or National Guard, who were called to active duty by a federal order and completed the full period for which they were called or ordered to active duty, may be eligible for VA health benefits. If the Veteran is not enrolled in the VA, it may be possible to expedite enrollment by working with the nearest VA Medical Center, a county Veterans Service Officer, or a Veterans Service Organization.

B. Some benefits and services require that the Veteran have a service-connected disability, such as an injury or a disabling condition sustained during his/her time in the military. The VA will determine if the disability was incurred or aggravated in the line of active duty. The extent of an injury or disabling condition that has incapacitated a Veteran determines his/her level of service-connected disability. Service-connected disability ranges from 0-100%. A VA benefits specialist rates the Veterans' percentage of service connection of the condition and reviews a Veteran's service history to determine eligibility. There are conditions (e.g., amyotrophic lateral sclerosis) that are presumed to be service connected. See Appendix 31-A for the list of Presumptive Disability Benefits for Certain Groups of Veterans. Some, but not all, Veterans that are rated with a service-connected disability may receive a monthly monetary stipend. However, both types of Veterans are eligible for VA healthcare and services. Additionally, the survivors of a service-connected Veteran may be eligible for monetary benefits.

C. To qualify for using the VA system, a Veteran with an honorable discharge from active military, naval, or air under any condition may be eligible for some benefits. Service personnel with a dishonorable or bad conduct discharges issued by a general court martial are disqualified from VA benefits. However, prison inmate or parolee Veterans may be eligible for certain VA benefits. Local VA benefits offices can assist in determining eligibility.

XIV. THE VA HOSPICE AND PALLIATIVE CARE BENEFIT FOR ENROLLED VETERANS

A. Hospice and palliative care are included in the VA healthcare benefits for all enrolled Veterans. Veterans can receive both VA and community services concurrently. Under the Veterans' Healthcare Eligibility Reform Act of 1996, the VA determines need and provides or purchases hospice and palliative care services for an enrolled Veteran.[25] These can occur in either the home or VA inpatient setting.

B. VA provided hospice and palliative care

1. All VAs have interdisciplinary consult palliative care teams headed by a palliative care coordinator. These teams have been established throughout VA facilities serving both acute settings and outpatient clinics.

2. Many VA facilities have inpatient hospice and palliative care beds. Inpatient hospice care is provided directly in VA acute care facilities and nursing homes (Community Living Centers [CLCs]). The latter is the preferred option for many Veterans.

31

C. For Veterans needing skilled care, the VA may purchase hospice care through a VA community contracted nursing home or State Veterans Home under some specific conditions.

D. There is collaboration with community hospices for out-of-VA referrals. The VA purchases hospice care from a community hospice provider.

1. This may be purchased from the community hospice provider if the VA physician and patient/family agree care is appropriate.

2. The VA and the hospice have a written contract agreement

3. Contracted hospice services mirror the Medicare hospice benefit with its comprehensive, per diem coverage, including home visits by professional and paraprofessional staff, medications, supplies, biological, durable medical equipment, and ancillary services as outlined in the plan of care. If a Veteran needs care unrelated to the terminal diagnosis stated in the admission paperwork, the Veteran is admitted to a VA hospital.

E. All Veterans enrolled in the VA are eligible for hospice care. If an individual is not currently enrolled in the VA, evidence of an honorable discharge and income verification will be needed to enroll. The process to enroll in the VA can be time consuming, so early assessment of enrollment status is essential. The DD214 form, which is used by all branches of service as proof of military service, is necessary for enrollment into the VA. The VA itself does not provide home hospice, but they contract and pay for hospice care to be provided by a community hospice.

F. To better serve the needs of Veterans and to ensure access, care coordination, and continuity of care, it is beneficial for community organizations to continue efforts to collaborate with the Veteran's preferred VA Medical Center Palliative Care Consult team, social workers, and community health nurse coordinator.

XV. TRICARE

A. TRICARE is a regionally managed healthcare program for the active duty and retired members of the uniformed services, their families, and survivors.

B. A military retiree or the spouse of a Veteran who was killed in action will always be a TRICARE beneficiary.

C. Veterans eligible for TRICARE can obtain care from military hospitals and clinics. Military hospitals and clinics are not the same as the VA system as military facilities are located on or near military installations.

D. It is important to note that TRICARE is not available to all Veterans—only Veterans who qualify based on service.

E. The TRICARE hospice benefit is very similar to most insurance coverage for hospice care.

31

XVI. BURIAL AND MEMORIAL BENEFITS

A. Veterans discharged from active duty under conditions other than dishonorable and service members who die while on active duty, or active or inactive training duty, as well as spouses and dependent children of Veterans may be eligible for VA burial and memorial benefits. It is recommended Veterans be asked in particular about their preferences regarding military honors at burial.

B. The Burial and Memorial Benefit is a guaranteed right to all Veterans who served honorably. Most funeral directors are aware of Veteran benefits.

C. Burial and Memorial benefits include the following

1. If a burial with full military honors is desired, it can be requested by the Veteran at no charge.

2. A plot internment allowance and a small burial benefit may be available to some Veterans.

3. The VA will provide a headstone marker with the branch of service and rank noted if desired. The spouse's name can also be added to the headstone.

4. Veterans may be buried in a Veteran's cemetery, and if desired the spouse can be buried in the Veteran's plot. There may be rules and regulations about cremated remains of a spouse of a retired service member being buried with the Veteran.

5. Veterans may elect to have a burial at sea. This can be arranged through the United States Navy Mortuary Affairs, the various branches of military, or the Maritime Funeral Directors. The rules vary for each of these organizations.

6. A burial flag is provided along with a presidential memorial certificate signed by the current president of the United States.

XVII. CONCLUSION

A. The unique needs of Veterans and their families can best be met by providing a family and patient centered care approach to health and end-of-life care.

B. The palliative APRN should promote identification of a Veteran patient for military service.

C. With evaluation of the medical history of the Veteran, including the impact of the Veteran's military service on how they view their disease, the APRN may understand how the military service affects the dying process of the Veteran. This can facilitate optimal care, with referral to and access of appropriate VA Services and Benefits.

D. The APRN can relieve suffering and promote healing with treatment of potential PTSD, and support for family.

E. Finally, by their presence and sensitivity to subsequent effects of military service, the APRN can promote respect for Veterans in honoring and acknowledging their service.

31

Appendix 31-A: "Presumptive" Disability Benefits for Certain Groups of Veterans[26]

What is "Presumptive" Service Connection?

VA presumes that specific disabilities diagnosed in certain Veterans were caused by their military service. VA does this because of the unique circumstances of their military service. If one of these conditions is diagnosed in a Veteran in one of these groups, VA presumes that the circumstances of his/her service caused the condition, and disability compensation can be awarded. For more information call 1-800-827-1000 or go to www.VA.gov.

What Conditions are "Presumed" to be caused by Military Service?

Veterans in the groups identified on the next page—Entitlement to disability compensation may be presumed under the circumstances described and for the conditions listed.

Veterans within one year of release from active duty—Veterans diagnosed with chronic diseases (such as arthritis, diabetes, or hypertension) are encouraged to apply for disability compensation.

Veterans with continuous service of 90 days or more—Veterans diagnosed with amyotrophic lateral sclerosis (ALS)/Lou Gehrig's disease at any time after discharge or release from qualifying active service is sufficient to establish service connection for the disease, if the Veteran had active, continuous service of 90 days or more.

Former Prisoners of War	Vietnam Veterans (Exposed to Agent Orange)	Atomic Veterans (Exposed to Ionizing Radiation)	Gulf War Veterans (Undiagnosed Illness)
(1) Imprisoned for any length of time, **and** disability at least 10 percent disabling • Psychosis • Any of the anxiety states • Dysthymic disorder • Organic residuals of frostbite • Posttraumatic osteoarthritis • Heart disease or hypertensive vascular disease and their complications • Stroke and its residuals **(2)** Imprisoned for at least 30 days, and disability at least 10 percent disabling • Avitaminosis • Beriberi • Chronic dysentery • Helminthiasis • Malnutrition (including optic atrophy) • Pellagra • Any other nutritional deficiency • Irritable bowel syndrome • Peptic ulcer disease • Peripheral neuropathy • Cirrhosis of the liver	Served in the Republic of Vietnam between 1/9/62 and 5/7/75 • Acute and subacute peripheral neuropathy* • AL amyloidosis • B-cell leukemias • Chloracne or other acneform disease similar to chloracne* • Chronic lymphocytic leukemia • Diabetes type 2 • Hodgkin's disease • Ischemic heart disease • Multiple myeloma • Non-Hodgkin's lymphoma • Parkinson's disease • Porphyria cutanea tarda* • Prostate cancer • Respiratory cancers (lung, bronchus, larynx, trachea) • Soft-tissue sarcoma (other than osteosarcoma, chondrosarcoma, Kaposi's sarcoma or mesothelioma) *Must become manifest to a degree of 10 percent or more within a year after the last date on which the Veteran was exposed to an herbicide agent during active military, naval, or air service.	Participated in atmospheric nuclear testing; occupied or was a POW in Hiroshima or Nagasaki; service before 2/1/92 at a diffusion plant in Paducah, KY, Portsmouth, OH, or Oak Ridge, TN; or service before 1/1/74 at Amchitka Island, AK • All forms of leukemia (except for chronic lymphocytic leukemia) • Cancer of the thyroid, breast, pharynx, esophagus, stomach, small intestine, pancreas, bile ducts, gall bladder, salivary gland, urinary tract (kidneys, renal pelves, ureters, urinary bladder and urethra), brain, bone, lung, colon, ovary • Bronchiolo-alveolar carcinoma • Multiple myeloma • Lymphomas (other than Hodgkin's disease) • Primary liver cancer (except if cirrhosis or hepatitis b is indicated)	Served in the Southwest Asia Theater of Operations during the Gulf War with condition at least 10 percent disabling by 12/31/11. Included are medically unexplained chronic multi-symptom illnesses defined by a cluster of signs or symptoms that have existed for six months or more, such as • Chronic fatigue syndrome • Fibromyalgia • Irritable bowel syndrome • Any diagnosed or undiagnosed illness that the Secretary of Veterans Affairs determines warrants a presumption of service connection *Signs or symptoms of an undiagnosed illness* include fatigue, skin symptoms, headaches, muscle pain, joint pain, neurological symptoms, respiratory symptoms, sleep disturbance, GI symptoms, cardiovascular symptoms, weight loss, menstrual disorders.

31

CITED REFERENCES

1. National Hospice and Palliative Care Organization (NHPCO). *Military History Checklist Guide.* Available at: www.nhpco.org/files/public/veterans/Veterans_Military_History_Guide.pdf. Accessed March 21, 2011.
2. National Hospice and Palliative Care Organization (NHPCO). We Honor Veterans. 2010. Available at: www.wehonorveterans.org/i4a/pages/index.cfm?pageid=3295. Accessed March 28, 2011.
3. National Center for Veteran Analysis and Statistics. Veteran Population. Washington, DC: U.S. Department of Veterans Affairs. 2011. Available at: va.gov/vetdata/Veteran_Population.asp. Accessed March 26, 2011.
4. National Hospice and Palliative Care Organization (NHPCO). Veterans Hospice Resources. 2009. Available at: www.wehonorveterans.org/i4a/pages/index.cfm?pageid=1. Accessed March 21, 2011.
5. U.S. Department of Veterans Affairs. VA is leader in hospice and palliative care. *Reuters.* January 8, 2008. Available at: www.reuters.com/article/pressRelease/idUS163739+08-Jan-2008+PRN20080108. Accessed March 7, 2011.
6. U.S. Department of Veterans Affairs, U.S. Department of Defense. *Clinical Practice Guideline for Management of Post-Traumatic Stress.* 2010. Available at: www.healthquality.va.gov/ptsd/ptsd-sum_2010a.pdf. Accessed May 10, 2011.
7. Lew HL, Otis JD, Tun C, Kerns RD, Clark ME, Cifu DX. Prevalence of chronic pain, posttraumatic stress disorder, and persistent postconcussive symptoms in OIF/OEF Veterans: polytrauma clinical triad. *J Rehabil Res Dev.* 2009;46(6):697-702.
8. Iraq & Afghanistan Veterans of America. *Women Warriors.* New York, NY: IAVA; 2009. Available at: iava.org/issues-and-campaigns/improve-care-female-veterans. Accessed March 7, 2011.
9. Nampiaparampil DE. Prevalence of chronic pain after traumatic brain injury. *JAMA.* 2008;300(6):711-719.
10. Reinberg S. Report finds gaps in health services for U.S. Veterans. *Health Day.* April 9, 2011. Available at: healthomg.com/2011/04/09/report-finds-gaps-in-health-services-for-u-s-veterans/. Accessed March 7, 2011.
11. The Associated Press. *Healthcare for Female Vets Lags Behind.* June 13, 2008. Available at: www.msnbc.msn.com/id/25147195/ns/health-womens_health/. Accessed March 7, 2011.
12. Murdoch M, Bradley A, Mather S, Klein R, Turner CL, Yano EM. Women and war. What physicians should know. *J Gen Intern Med.* 2006;21(Suppl 3):S5-S10.
13. U. S. Department of Veterans Affairs, Office of Policy and Planning. *Women Veterans: Past, Present and Future.* 2007. Available at: www.va.gov/womenvet/docs/womenvet_history.pdf. Accessed March 2, 2011.
14. National Coalition for Homeless Veterans. 2009. *Background and Statistics.* Available at: nchv.org/index.php/news/media/background_and_statistics/. Accessed March 10, 2011.
15. U. S. Veterans Administration (VA) Advisory Council. *Homeless Veterans at Life's End.* (PowerPoint presentation). 2009. Available at: www.nhpco.org/files/public/veterans/Homeless_Veterans.ppt. Accessed March 25, 2011.
16. U.S. Department of Veterans Affairs. *Homeless Veterans.* Available at: www.va.gov/HOMELESS/index.asp. Accessed February 23, 2012.
17. McMurray-Avila M, National Health Care for the Homeless Council. *Homeless Veterans and Health Care: A Resource Guide for Providers.* 2001. Available at: www.nhchc.org/wp-content/uploads/2011/10/HomelessVetsHealthCare.pdf. Accessed September 4, 2012.
18. American Psychiatric Association. *Diagnostic and Statistical Manual of Mental Disorders (DSM-IV-TR).* Revised 4th ed. Washington, DC: APA; 2000. Available at: www.psychiatry.org/practice/dsm/dsm-iv-tr. Accessed April 11, 2012.
19. U.S. Department of Veterans Affairs. *National Center for PTSD.* Available at: www.ptsd.va.gov/professional/pages/dsm-iv-tr-ptsd.asp. Accessed March 30 2012.
20. Seal K H, Bertenthal D, Maguen S, Gima K, Chu A, Marmar CR. Getting beyond "don't ask; don't tell": an evaluation of U.S. Veteran's administration postdeployment mental health screening of Veterans from Iraq and Afghanistan. *Am J Public Health.* 2008;98(4):714-720.
21. Feldman DB, Periyakoil VS. Posttraumatic stress disorder at the end of life. *J Palliat Med.* 2006;9(1):213-218.
22. U.S. Department of Veterans Affairs, National Center for PTSD. *Clinicians Guide to Medications for PTSD.* Available at: www.ptsd.va.gov/professional/pages/clinicians-guide-to-medications-for-ptsd.asp. Accessed March 30, 2012.
23. Duffy SA, Rosin D, Fowler, K, Schim SM, Jackson FC. Differences in Veterans' and nonveterans' end-of-life preferences: a pilot study. *J Palliat Med.* 2006;9(1):1099-1105.
24. Caregivers and Veterans Omnibus Health Services Act of 2010. Public Law 111-163—May 5, 2010. Available at: www.gpo.gov/fdsys/pkg/PLAW-111publ163/pdf/PLAW-111publ163.pdf. Accessed March 30 2012.
25. Veterans Health Care Eligibility Act Reform Act of 1996. Public Law 104-262 [H.R. 3118]—October 9, 1996. Available at: www.tavausa.org/PL%20104-262.pdf. Accessed March 30, 2012.
26. U.S. Department of Veterans Affairs. "Presumptive Disability Benefits for Certain Groups of Veterans. 2011. Available at: www.vba.va.gov/VBA/benefits/factsheets/. Accessed July 11, 2012.

31

ADDITIONAL RESOURCES

Freeman SL, Berger AM. Nebraska Veteran's preferences for end-of-life care. *Clinical J Oncol Nurs.* 2009;13(4):399-403.

Grassman DL. *Peace at Last: Stories of Hope and Healing for Veterans and their Families.* St. Petersburg, FL: Vandamere Press; 2009.

MacLean A, Edwards R. The pervasive role of rank in the health of U.S. Veterans. *Armed Forces Soc.* 2010;36(5):765-785.

Pols H, Oak S. War and military mental health: the US psychiatric response in the 20th century. *Am J Public Health.* 2007;97(12):2132-2142.

U.S. Department of Veterans Affairs. *PTSD Guidebook for Providers, Independent Study Course.* 2002. (www.publichealth.va.gov/docs/vhi/posttraumatic.pdf)

CHAPTER 32

CARE OF THE ACTIVELY DYING PATIENT

Maureen Lynch, MS, APN, BC, AOCN, ACHPN®, FPCN

I. INTRODUCTION

A. In the United States, most people will die after age 65. In the weeks to months before death, individuals will experience a period of declining health caused by an ultimately terminal illness, a serious though chronic illness, or the frailties of advanced age.[1] The National Academy of Science defines this period as end of life, regardless of age and even if death is not clearly imminent.[2] For others, death will come unexpectedly as the result of accident or sudden catastrophic illness.

B. The time of active dying or imminent death constitutes the final hours to days before death, regardless of cause. During the dying process, a shutting down of normal physiological processes produces a pattern of common signs and symptoms that herald approaching death. The specific cause of dying, and the use of medications and other interventions to treat pathophysiology and/or symptoms will affect the signs and symptoms seen and experienced in the peri-death period. This chapter focuses on care of the imminently dying.

C. Role of APRNs

1. APRNs are well positioned to care for patients at the end of life and into the peri-death period. Their knowledge and skills blend disease management, symptom management, and communication skills to provide patients and families with the bio-psycho-social-spiritual support needed during this transition time. The National Consensus Project for Quality Palliative Care and the National Quality Forum Preferred Practices for Palliative Care's Domain 7 *Care of the Imminently Dying* delineate key aspects of care of the imminently dying.[3,4] Palliative care APRNs provide these essential aspects of care by eliciting the values, goals and concerns of the patient and family, providing education about the dying process, planning for and providing care during the dying process and immediately after death, and providing bereavement support for families. See Chapter 36, *National Guidelines and APRN Practice* for a listing of the Preferred Practices for Domain 7.

II. ADVANCE CARE PLANNING

A. Overview

1. Advance care planning (ACP) is the process of setting goals of healthcare based on patient values and preferences. It may include appointing a proxy decision-maker or surrogate to advocate for one's healthcare preferences, and to make specific decisions about limiting life-sustaining therapies such as cardiopulmonary resuscitation, mechanical ventilation, artificial hydration and nutrition, or other therapeutics if one is unable to communicate these preferences. ACP may also include stating preferences about settings of care, organ donation, or autopsy. Completing a living will, POLST

(physician/provider orders for life sustaining treatment) or MOLST (medical orders for life sustaining treatment) form may be part of the process.

B. APRN Role in Advance Care Planning

1. The American Nurses Association affirms the nurse's role in end-of-life care and counseling surrounding end-of-life choices.[5] APRNs are ideally positioned to initiate this process. Healthcare crises often trigger advance care planning discussions but addressing the issues as part of routine healthcare, or early in the trajectory of illness incorporates patient choices and values throughout healthcare.

2. Patient's preferences for types of care and goals of care may change over time so the process of advance care planning is ongoing. The patient's understanding of the course of illness, current condition, prognosis, functional status, predicted outcomes of treatment, benefits, and burdens of therapeutic options may influence decisions. Familiarity with the healthcare system, previous experiences with death of others, a trusted relationship with the healthcare provider, and a desire to lessen burden for surrogate decision makers may also influence decisions about care.[6] With an understanding of the patient and families illness experience, current concerns and future desired outcomes, the APRN can initiate a plan of care that is consistent with patient's values and wishes, and assist the patient and family to revisit the advance care plan as changes in condition warrant.

C. Prognosis

1. The patient's understanding of their prognosis often influences healthcare decisions. Yet, predicting the timing of death, even in terminal illness, is not a simple process. Clinicians are often hesitant to discuss prognosis, and when they do, are often optimistic in the prognostic estimates communicated to patients and families.[7] The APRN can promote discussion of prognosis and provide information to the patient and family while maintaining hope. Critical to this process is sensitivity to patient's readiness and ability to hear information, and an understanding of their perspective on quality of life.[8]

2. Declining functional status and increasing number of symptoms may indicate shorter survival. The use of tools such as Palliative Prognostic Index or Palliative Prognostic Score may be helpful in estimating survival.[9] In one study, a physician's "no" answer the question, "Would I be surprised if this patient dies in the next year?" correlated with a 7 times greater likelihood of death in the next year.[10]

D. Transition from "Living With" to "Dying Of"

1. What marks the transition from living with a progressive serious or life-threatening condition (e.g., heart, renal, or liver failure; amyotrophic lateral sclerosis; chronic obstructive pulmonary disease; cancer) to dying of that condition? Key indicators include current status of the disease, and the physiological, functional, psychosocial, and cognitive changes associated with disease progression. These may occur acutely and/or develop over time.

2. Increasing number and severity of symptoms that may include asthenia (e.g., weakness, fatigue, loss of strength), anorexia, dyspnea, dry mouth, confusion, and retained respiratory secretions.

32

3. Changes in physical appearance such as temporal wasting (e.g., sunken temples, deepening of eye sockets, hollowing of cheeks) associated with weight loss and dehydration.

4. Decrease socialization/engagement with family and friends.

5. Declining ability to focus on issues beyond day to day living.

6. Increase utilization of healthcare resources.

7. Increased need for informal caregiving.[9,11,12]

8. Clinical observations suggest that psychosocial and cultural factors may also influence timing of death. For example, the patient who seems to wait for a special anniversary or event before dying, or who dies very shortly after being told that further disease directed therapies are not indicated.

E. Communicating Prognosis

1. Communicating to patients and families that death is near is ideally done in the context of advance care planning that has been an ongoing process.[13] Respect for the patient and family's personal and cultural preferences about information handling, and interdisciplinary collaboration assist communication. While information and understanding of an illness allow patients and families to more fully participate in decision-making and prepare them for anticipated events, it is important to ascertain what the patient and family know, what they would like to know or are concerned about, and their preferences for how and to whom information is conveyed.

   a) The strategy of ask-tell-ask is particularly suited to this circumstance.

      i. Ask the patient and family about their sense of how the patient has been doing over last days to weeks and what they think it means in terms of disease state, the future, and directions of care.

      ii. Tell them what you see in terms of changes in function, symptoms, and physiological parameters and what it means.

      iii. Ask (explore) the emotional impact of the information and their understanding of the information. Correct any misunderstandings about facts.

      iv. End by making a plan for next steps including ongoing care, communicating with other family members and significant others, and continued education and support as try confront the dying process.[14]

III. SETTING OF DEATH

A. Although many people voice a theoretical wish to die at home, the trend is tht most death occur out of the home.[15,16] While the desire for death at home may be one means of maintaining dignity and control, the place of death may ultimately be less important than attention to individual's current needs and preferences for physical and psychosocial comfort, safety, and support. Some factors that may influence decisions about place of death include

   1. Patient's medical and psychological condition and requirements of care.

32

2. Possibility of severe respiratory difficulties or airway occlusion, bleeding, seizures, and difficult to manage or intractable pain or other symptoms.

3. Availability of resources including the willingness and ability of home caregivers and support services.

4. Financial, safety, and legal considerations including insurance coverage.

5. Cultural and religious beliefs regarding place of death.

B. Because the dying process may be unpredictable, contingency plans for inpatient or residential care should be in place if home care is chosen.

IV. PATIENT AND FAMILY CONCERNS ABOUT THE DYING PROCESS

A. Dying is a highly individual process affected not only by disease, comorbidities and symptom management, but the beliefs, values, wishes, and culture of the dying person.

B. Common concerns of patients and families around dying adults involve the 5 C's

1. Comfort

2. Control

3. Communication with loved ones and healthcare providers

4. Continuity of care

5. Completion of life tasks

6. Coming to peace[17-19]

C. Completing Life Tasks

1. Byock delineated five tasks of dying well

a) Offer forgiveness

b) Seek forgiveness

c) Offer gratitude

d) Offer sentiments of love

e) Say good-bye[20]

Acknowledging the impending death, allows patient and families to work towards resolution of conflicts and unfinished business. This includes practical planning, advance directives, and finding peace and meaning in one's life. Active listening, encouragement of reminiscences and reflections on meaning, and current emotions and concerns of the patient and family are ways that nurses provide a comforting presence during this time and into the time of death, and facilitate completing life tasks as important to the patient. (See Chapter 14, *Spiritual Concerns*)

D. Death and Children—the cited studies around dying were done in an adult population. None the less, dying children are often aware of their impending deaths and will provide cues about when and how much they would like to talk about what is happening. Talking with children about death, their own or that of a loved one, requires an appreciation of the child's concept of death, based on their own experiences with death and their cognitive and emotional development, and the families wishes in this regard. A 2004 study demonstrated that parents who

32

talked to their dying child about death did not regret it.[21] Siblings of a dying child may experience less loneliness, anxiety, anger, and jealousy if they are kept abreast of the illness trajectory in a supportive manner.[22]

E. Family and Caregiver Education about the Dying Process

    1. General themes of education about dying process include

        a) What to expect as death approaches. (see Table 1)

        b) Possible complications specific to patient's condition such as hemorrhage or seizure and their management.

        c) Recognition that death has occurred. (see Table 2)

        d) Immediate post death events such as care of the body and removal from site of the death.

        e) Information including funeral/burial arrangements, autopsy, and organ transplant.

            i. Patients may want to know less than their caregivers about specific aspects of the dying process but need reassurance about maintaining comfort, dignity, and continuity of care.[23] Home caregivers need practical information about physical and psychological care, expected occurrences given the patients disease and status, how to access help at home via visiting nurse, hospice, or home care agency, including transfer to skilled nursing facility or hospital if care becomes too complicated, and psychosocial support to reduce anxiety and sense of burden. Information will often need to be repeated and focused on current issues.

V. COMFORT CARE AT END OF LIFE

A. Comfort is a major concern of patients and families facing death. Comfort is a broad concept. Providing comfort care requires collaboration with interdisciplinary team. (See Chapter 14, *Spiritual Concerns* and Chapter 15, *Psychosocial Aspects of Palliative Care*)

B. The management of pain and other symptoms in all their dimensions is an essential component of comfort care as are attention to

    1. Basic physical needs such as safety, hygiene, elimination; care of skin, eyes, mouth, and grooming.

    2. Psychosocial needs such as dignity, control, completion of life tasks, coping with loss.

    3. Spiritual needs such as finding meaning in life and death, and proactively planning for religious rituals before, during, and after death.

C. Symptom Distress

    1. Symptom distress has multiple etiologies as death approaches. Assessment to determine the etiology of the symptom allows for development of an individualized care plan for proactive symptom management. Assessment includes the patient's experience and description of the symptom, if possible. If the patient is unable to communicate, caregiver reports may be helpful, as will observation and knowledge of previous symptom issues. The assessment includes how the symptom impacts function and quality of life, the meaning of

32

Table 1: Common Signs and Symptoms of Imminent Death[24-26]

Sign or Symptom	Cause	Common Interventions and Points for Patient and Family Education
Decreasing oral intake	• Disease progression • Weakening of swallowing muscles → dysphagia	• Address burden/benefits artificial hydration & nutrition • Mouth care
Cardiovascular changes • Tachycardia • Hypotension • Decreased urine output • Peripheral coolness • Mottling of skin	• Decreased cardiac output & intravascular volume • Decreased kidney perfusion	• Parenteral fluids will not reverse
Cognitive changes • Diminished interaction • Diminished sensory • perceptions • Sleeping more • Delirium	• Multiple etiologies including disease progression, medication effects, changes in metabolic function • Often irreversible unless a specific etiology identified	• Avoid benzodiazepines as initial treatment • Use of antipsychotics such as haloperidol for delirium • Limited hydration may temporarily reverse • Distinguish from pain, hyperalgesia
Inability to close eyes	• Loss of retro-orbital fat pad	• Artificial tears
Loss of sphincter control	• General muscle weakness & neurological dysfunction	• Use of padding/disposable briefs • Skin care • Benefits/burdens urinary catheters or rectal tubes for diarrhea
Near death awareness		• Distinguish from delirium
Respiratory changes • Cheyne-Stokes • Diminished secretion management	• Neurological dysfunction	• Distinguish from respiratory distress • Use of anticholinergics to dry secretions
Weakness • Decreased stamina	• Disease progression	• Passive range of motion to prevent joint fatigue • Position changes

Table 2: Signs that Death has Occurred[24-26]

1. Non-responsiveness to verbal or tactile stimuli	5. Release of urine &/or stool with loss of sphincter control
2. Absence of breathing	
3. Absence of heartbeat/pulse	6. Pallor
4. Pupils fixed & dilated	7. Lack of muscle tone

the symptom to patient and caregiver, and the response to past and current management strategies.

    D.   Individualizing Symptom Management

        1.   Symptoms may be caused by progression of the underlying disease process, other new or pre-existing conditions, or reversible causes such as constipation, distended bladder, or medication side effects. Even if further diagnostic testing is not appropriate to goals of care, the APRN uses critical thinking to determine the known or presumed cause of the symptom. This allows for a rationale, evidence-based management plan that will include treating reversible causes, if possible, appropriate to goals of care, optimal use of medications, nonpharmacological approaches to symptom relief, and

consideration of procedures such as paracentesis, or nerve blocks for pain control. At end of life, changes in organ perfusion and metabolism may lead to variable therapeutic responses to symptom management medications requiring careful monitoring for symptom relief and side effects. For example, poor renal clearance may lead to prolonged drug effect or accumulation of drug metabolites.

E. Medication Administration in Actively Dying

1. The oral route of medication delivery is preferable but as the patient becomes weaker, swallowing may become difficult. Prioritizing medications and utilizing alternate routes of delivery such as rectal, intravenous, or subcutaneous may be needed. Abrupt discontinuation of certain medications can cause withdrawal, so these should be among the essential medications to continue. Opioids and benzodiazepines are examples of such medications.

2. Some medications are available in forms designed for non-oral administration.

   a) Rectal administration of some medications is possible. Patient's dignity, caregiver burden, availability of rectal dosing forms, and contraindications such as painful rectal lesions are factors that may preclude use.[27]

   b) Oral disintegrating tablets (ODT) bypass the need to swallow medication but rely on gastrointestinal absorption. Many medications commonly used in palliative care are available in such formulations including olanzapine, ondansetron, metoclopramide, and lorazepam.[28]

   c) Fentanyl products for breakthrough pain in opioid tolerant patients are absorbed via transmucosal routes.

   d) Oral solutions of morphine and other products meant for oral administration are minimally absorbed via transmucosal route and depend on gastrointestinal absorption.[27]

   e) Other non-oral formulations include transdermal patches of scopolamine, fentanyl, and diclofenac, which are absorbed systemically, and lidocaine, which provides topical benefit.

   f) Despite clinical reports of efficacy, there is little evidence to support use of compounded transdermal gels to deliver medications such as corticosteroids, opioids, and antiemetics.[27] Access to compounded medications may be limited by cost, availability of a compounding pharmacy, and insurance coverage.

3. Parenteral administration via intravenous and subcutaneous routes may offer more reliable absorption. Availability and feasibility of these routes may be limited by cost, access to medications and technology, and patient/caregiver competency.

F. Palliative Sedation

1. In rare cases at end of life, pain and other distressing symptoms are not manageable despite optimum use of available symptom relieving therapies. In these cases, palliative sedation may be required. Palliative sedation is the monitored use of non-opioid medications to relieve refractory symptoms by inducing varying degrees of unconsciousness in imminently dying patients.[29]

32

Its use in management of refractory physical symptoms is more accepted than its use for existential suffering alone.[30-32]

a) As with opioids, appropriate use of palliative sedation does not, and is not intended to, hasten death.[24,33] Rather it is distinct from euthanasia and related practices such as "hanging a morphine drip" on dying patients in the absence of a target symptom.

b) Guidelines for palliative sedation are well delineated in literature.[34] Organizational policies or guidelines for palliative sedation are recommended.

2. An essential component of a palliative sedation guideline is the need for interdisciplinary assessment and goals.

a) Palliative sedation is directed toward relief of suffering associated with an intractable symptom in imminently dying patients.

b) Consultation with an interdisciplinary team that may include palliative care and other specialists, as necessary, to assure that the conditions of imminent death and refractoriness of the symptom are met. The patient (as appropriate), family, and all members of IDT participate in assessment, establishing goals of care, and the need for, and intention of palliative sedation.

3. Appropriate medication selection (see Table 3)

a) Mediations used for palliative sedation may include benzodiazepines, and barbiturates but other agents such as propofol may be used. Selection of the drug, the doses, and route of administration is based on target symptom, patient's current plan of care, and specific organizational policies and procedures. Selected medications are titrated to symptom relief and acceptable level of altered consciousness. Monitoring for medication effectiveness and side effects is continuous. In addition to the sedative used to induce unconsciousness, opioids may be required for ongoing pain relief.

4. Although palliative sedation may be focused on particular symptoms, total care is not eliminated. Other aspects of care are continued including attention to hygiene, elimination, skin care, and administration of other medications or therapies needed to maintain comfort and dignity are continued.

5. Position statements or guidelines for palliative sedation are available from the Hospice and Palliative Nurses Association (HPNA), American Medical Association (AMA), National Hospice and Palliative Care Organization (NHPCO), and Veterans Administration Committee on Ethics.[29-32] Principles of beneficence, non-maleficence, and the rule of double effect provide ethical support of the practice. Legal support is found in a 1997 Supreme Court decision that denied a constitutional right to assisted dying but upheld the provision of palliative care, including administration of medications to the point unconsciousness if needed for relief of suffering.[25]

Table 3: Medications Commonly Used For Palliative Sedation[34]

• Lorazepam	• Pentobarbital
• Midazolam	• Propofol
• Chlorpromazine	

32

VI. COMMON CHANGES IN ACTIVELY DYING PATIENTS

A. Dying involves the shutting down of normal physiological processes; the signs and symptoms of dying are result of this process.[24,26,35] The process may occur rapidly as a result of a catastrophic health event, or gradually as a result of a prolonged illness. The changes outlined below are commonly seen in the final hours to days of life at the end of a prolonged illness. These changes are more difficult to discern when death comes more suddenly.[24]

1. Increasing weakness, lethargy, variable levels of consciousness due to decrease in cerebral perfusion, and changes in metabolic processes are elements of dying process. As function declines, the patient spends more time in bed and the need for assistance with activities of dally living increases. Although some patients remain alert until time of death, many people experience sleepiness that evolves to a coma state. Social interactions may become limited although response to auditory stimulation and touch may continue, so that talking with the patient, playing music, holding hands may be comforting to both family and patient if culturally appropriate.

2. Incontinence of bladder and bowel may accompany generalized weakness.

3. Low blood pressure, and increasingly weak and irregular pulse, as cardiac contractions weaken are common.

4. Cool, mottled extremities caused by poor tissue perfusion.

5. Increased respiratory effort and abdominal distention as heart contractions weaken and circulatory efficiency declines causing pulmonary and hepatic congestion may occur. The congestion may diminish as dehydration from decreased intake progresses.

6. Cheyne-Stokes respirations are caused by failing neurological controls. Periods of irregular rapid shallow breaths are punctuated by periods of apnea. Expiratory grunting is common. Reassure families that this is not painful, nor indicative of respiratory distress.

7. Noisy respirations of the "death rattle" are caused by weakening of respiratory and swallowing muscles that leads to an inability to clear secretions. It is not clear if this is distressing to patients, but it is distressing to many families. Management includes elevation of head of the bed, turning the patient, use of anticholinergic medications such as scopolamine patch, atropine, hyoscyamine, or glycopyrrolate. Suctioning is discouraged as it is uncomfortable for the patient and can promote further secretion accumulation.

8. Appetite declines with a corresponding decrease in intake of food and fluids. Fat pads that shape the facial contours are lost to dehydration and weight loss causing a hollowed eyed, sunken cheek appearance. Caregivers may worry about starvation and need reassurance that this is not the case. Discussion about limited benefit of artificial hydration and nutrition (ANH) should be based on goals of therapy.[36] ANH will not reverse the dying process. It may increase pulmonary congestion and secretions, peripheral edema, increase the risk for aspiration, and cause abdominal distention with nausea and vomiting. Limited hydration may benefit some patients in select circumstances, such as opioid toxicity. Some patients may intentionally limit oral intake in an attempt to hasten death.[37]

32

9.   Urine output decreases as patients eat and drink less and renal perfusion diminishes in response to failing circulation.

10.   Intestinal peristalsis decreases in response to neuromuscular changes and diminished intake resulting in nausea and constipation.

11.   Up to 80% of dying patients experience delirium. For most, a reversible cause will not be identified. Care focuses on safety and comfort for both the patient and family.[38] (See Chapter 12, *Delirium*)

12.   Near death awareness or end-of-life experiences are common in dying patients and may be difficult to distinguish from delirium. These experiences are thought to be part of the patient's preparation for death. They may take the form of recounting a conversation or visit with deceased loved one, or requests for something needed to achieve closure or peace.[39] Families may be helpful in distinguishing these phenomena from delirium, and be reassured by being prepared for them.

13.   Pain at end of life requires ongoing assessment and treatment.

     a)   As death approaches, pain may change, often worsening. This may reflect new or unaddressed dimensions of suffering, worsening disease, altered analgesic metabolism, or other changes in physiologic function such as constipation, urinary retention, pressure ulcers, or other conditions.

     b)   A declining level of consciousness complicates pain assessment. Consider use of assessment tools for non-verbal patients.[27]

     c)   Difficulty in swallowing may require altered routes of administration as described above.

     d)   Changes in renal, circulatory, and hepatic function and dehydration may require changes in doses or pain management medications to maintain analgesia, and avoid over sedation and drug toxicities.[27] (See Chapter 6, *Pain*)

VII. DEATH PRONOUNCEMENT

Death pronouncement and death certificate requirements are regulated by state and local government. These often must be met to allow for disposition of the body. The requirements generally include identifying the patient, certifying that death has occurred (see Table 3), ascertaining time, date, and manner of death. Completing legal and institutional procedures, including documentation in medical record, notification of family, the attending/collaborating physician, other providers, and regulatory agencies are part of the process of pronouncement. State regulations and institutional/organizational policies govern ability of APRNs and hospice nurses to pronounce death and complete death certificates.

32

For families, this marks the transition from caregiving to bereavement. If they are present at the time of death, the APRN should offer condolences.[24] The APRN should explain the formal pronouncement process to family who are present. This may be especially helpful if there is a delay in the formal pronouncement, although it is clear that death has occurred. Whether or not to witness the formal pronouncement is the family's choice.

VIII. CARE AFTER DEATH

After death has occurred, care of the body continues with the same respect and compassion shown to the living person. In most cases, this involves

A. Care of the Body

1. This includes removal of tubes (as allowed by law), bathing, dressing, positioning, and transporting the body away from the setting of care. Family members may want to provide or assist with this care. Specific cultural, religious, and personal beliefs of the patient and family may dictate if, when, and who will care for the body. Notification of clergy or pastoral care workers may be appropriate. If possible, inquiry about special care and rituals should be made prior to death so any needed arrangements can be made. If the death occurred in the home and 911 was called, movement of the body or providing after death care may not be permitted until the paramedics receive word of official pronouncement of death.

B. Disposition of Body

Families may have concerns about where the body goes after death. Setting of death may dictate disposition of the body.

1. In institutional settings, the body may be placed in bag or other wrapping before transport to a morgue or holding area. For some families this process can be upsetting. Some locations have progressive statutes that allow transport of the body from hospital room to a funeral home without going to a morgue. Some families find this more comforting.

2. In a home death, families may need added support at the time the body is transported from the home—a final journey. This may mean having them go to another room when the body is being placed into the body bag and moved to the hearse.

C. Autopsy

1. Some patients authorize an autopsy to promote science. An autopsy may also be requested by families or healthcare providers to understand the cause of patient's illness and death. Since the authority of the healthcare proxy ends at time of patient's death, authorization, if not patient initiated, must be sought from next of kin. Though rare, an autopsy may be required by law or at least inquired about with the coroner if the death was unexpected or following a traumatic event such as a fall. As with death pronouncements, state and local statues may dictate the APRNs legal responsibilities in autopsy requests and authorizations. None the less, educating the family about the reason for the request and helping them access information needed to make the decision is part of the APRN role.

D. Discussion of Organ Donation

1. Federal law and Medicare regulations require hospitals to inform surviving family about the possibility of organ donation.[40] APRNs may initiate the topic of possible organ donation but healthcare providers with specialized training in organ donation procurement have the specific discussions. State law and institutional regulations may further dictate the requirements for these discussions and associated documentation. Cultural and religious mores and personal values influence organ donation decisions. While some families may

32

find it comforting to make such a donation even if donation is limited by the patient's disease process, others may find the concept distressing.

IX. GRIEVING—PATIENTS AND FAMILIES

Grief is a normal response to loss for patients and families.

A. Anticipatory Grief

1. In cases of death from progressive illness, grieving may begin before the actual time of death. This anticipatory grief is a response not only to knowledge of future loss through death, but of the losses inherent in living with serious or life-threatening illness, such as loss of independence, mobility, self image.[41] Although anticipatory grieving does not seem to lessen the grief of family members at time of death, preparation for death is associated with better adjustment to the loss.[42]

B. Grief and Bereavement Immediately Following Death

1. After the death, family members may initially feel numb, and have difficulty deciding what to do next. The practical tasks of burial rituals and other duties, such as notifying government agencies and bringing closure to financial matters may help bereaved family members focus their energies. Over months, feelings of yearning, anger, and sadness eventually yield to adaptation to the loss. The effectiveness of routine interventions for normal grief has not been established.[42] However, individuals who seek such support may derive the most benefit; therefore providing information about resources for support is useful.[42]

C. Complicated Grief

1. While grief is normal, complicated grief may require specialized psychosocial care. Grief that is prolonged, delayed, or exaggerated is complicated and represents denial or avoidance of accepting the loss. Criteria for complicated grief include intrusive thoughts, distressing yearning, avoiding reminders of the deceased, sleep disturbances occurring more than one year after the loss.[41] (See Chapter 15, *Psychosocial Aspects of Palliative Care*)

X. CONCLUSION

Cicely Saunders wrote "how people die remains in the minds of those who live on."[43] Attention to physical, emotional, social, and spiritual needs of dying patient and their families requires active listening, communication, and collaboration with the interdisciplinary team, knowledge of symptom assessment and management including pharmacological and nonpharmacological interventions. The APRN in palliative care is well positioned to provide this care, and to provide education and support for interdisciplinary colleagues involved in care of the dying patient. By being, and role modeling, an informed and compassionate presence the APRN can make it better than it would have been if she/he were not there.[44]

32

CITED REFERENCES

1. National Academy of Science. *Describing Death in America: What We Need to Know.* 2003. Available at: www.nap.edu/openbook.php?isbn=0309087252. Accessed September 2, 2012.
2. Miniño AM, Xu J, Kochanek KD, Tejada-Vera B. Death in the United States. 2007. *NCHS Data Brief.* 2009;26. Available at: www.cdc.gov/nchs/data/databriefs/db26.pdf. Accessed September 2, 2012.
3. National Consensus Project for Quality Palliative Care. *Clinical Practice Guidelines for Quality Palliative Care.* 3rd ed. 2013.
4. National Quality Forum. *A National Framework and Preferred Practices fro Palliative and Hospice Care Quality.* Washington, DC: National Quality Forum; 2006.
5. American Nurses Association. *Position Statement: Registered Nurses Role and Responsibilities in Providing Expert Care and Counseling at End of Life.* 2010. Available at: www.nursingworld.org/MainMenuCategories/EthicsStandards/Ethics-Position-Statements/etpain14426.aspx. Accessed April 4, 2011.
6. Wendler D, Rid A. Systematic review: the effect on surrogates of making treatment decisions for others. *Ann Intern Med.* 2011;154(5):336-346
7. Christakis NA, Iwashyna TJ. Attitude and self reported practices regarding prognostication in a national sample of internists, *Arch Intern Med.* 1998;158(21):2389-2395.
8. Reinke LF, Shannon SE, Engleberg RA, Oung JP, Curtis JR. Supporting hope and prognostic information: nurses perspective on their role when patients have life limiting prognoses. *J Pain Symptom Manage.* 2010;39(6),982-992.
9. Glare PA, Sincliar CT. Palliative medicine review: prognostication. *J Palliat Med.* 2008;11(1):84-103.
10. Moss AH, Lunney JR, Auber M, et al. Prognostic significance of the "surprise" question in cancer patients. *J Palliat Med.* 2010;13(7):837-840.
11. Lunney JR, Lynn J, Foley DJ, Lipson S, Guralnik JM. Patterns of functional decline at end of life. *JAMA.* 2003;289(18):2387-2392.
12. Georges JJ, Onwuteaka-Phillipsen BD, van der Heide A, van der Wal G, van der Maas P. Symptoms, treatment, and dying peacefully in terminally ill cancer patients: a prospective study. *Support Care Cancer.* 2005;13:160-168.
13. Dahlin CM. Communication in palliative care: an essential competency for nurses. In: Ferrell BR, Coyle N, eds. *Oxford Textbook of Palliative Nursing.* 3rd ed. New York, NY: Oxford University Press. 2010:107-136.
14. Back AL, Arnold RM, Baile WF, Yulsky JA, Fryer-Edwards K. Approaching difficult communication tasks in oncology. *CA Cancer J Clin.* 2005;55(3):164-177.
15. Tang ST. When death is imminent: where terminally ill patients prefer to die and why. *Cancer Nurs.* 2003;26:245-251.
16. Gomes B, Higginson IJ. Where people die (1974-2030): past trends, future projections, implications for care. *Palliat Med.* 2008;22(1):32-41.
17. Steinhauser KE, Chirstakis NA, Clipp EC, et al. Factors considered important at end of life by patients, families, physicians and other care providers. *JAMA.* 2000;284(19):2476-2482.
18. Singer PA, Martin DK, Kelner M. Quality end of life care: patients' perspective. *JAMA.* 1999;281(2):163-168.
19. Emanuel L, Bennett K, Richardson VE. The dying role. *J Palliat Med.* 2007;10(1):159-168.
20. Byock I. *The Four Things that Matter Most: A Book about Living.* New York, NY: Free Press, 2004.
21. Kreicbergs U, Valdimirasdottir U, Henter JI, Steineck G. Talking about death with children who have severe malignant disease. *NEJM.* 2004;351(12):1175-1186.
22. Nolbris M, Hellström AL. Siblings' needs and issues when a brother or sister dies of cancer. *J Pediatr Oncol Nurs.* 2005;22(4):227-233.
23. Clayton JM, Butow PN, Arnold RM, Tattersall MHN. Discussing end of life issues with terminally ill cancer patients and their carers: a qualitative study. *Cancer.* 2005;13:589-599.
24. Hallenback J. Palliative care in the final days of life: "They were expecting it any time." *JAMA.* 2005;293(18):2265-2271.
25. Vacco v. Quill, 521 U.S. 793, 1997.
26. Heidrick DE. The dying process. In: Kuebler KK, Heidrich DE, Esper P, eds. *Palliative & End of Life Care: Clinical Practice Guidelines.* 2nd ed. St Louis, MO: Sanders; 2007:33-45.
27. Paice JA. Pain at end of life. In: Ferrell BR, Coyle N, eds. *Oxford Textbook of Palliative Nursing.* 3rd ed. New York, NY: Oxford University Press; 2010:161-186.
28. Hirani JJ, Rathod DA, Vadalia KR. Oral disintegrating tablets: a review. *Trop J Pharm Res.* 2009;8(2):161-172.
29. Hospice and Palliative Nurses Association. *Position Statement: Palliative Sedation.* Pittsburgh, PA: HPNA; 2011. Available at: www.hpna.org/DisplayPage.aspx?Title=Position%20Statements. Accessed September 2, 2012.

32

30. American Medical Association Report of the Council of Ethical and Judicial Affairs. *Sedation to Unconsciousness at End of Life*. CEJA Report 5-A-08. Available at: www.ama-assn.org/resources/doc/code-medical- ethics/2201A.pdf. Accessed April 16, 2011.

31. National Ethics Committee of the Veterans Health Administration. *The Ethics of Palliative Sedation.* Washington, DC: Department of Veterans Affairs: National Center of Ethics in Health Care, 2008.

32. Kirk TW, Mahon MM. National Hospice and Palliative Care Organization (NHPCO) position statement and commentary on the use of palliative sedation in imminently dying terminally ill patients. *J Pain Symptom Manage.* 2010;39(5):914-923.

33. Maltoni M, Pittureri C, Scarpi E, et al. Palliative sedation therapy does not hasten death: results from a prospective multicenter study. *Ann Oncol.* 2009;20(7):1163-1169.

34. Knight P, Espinosa L A. Sedation for refractory symptoms and terminal weaning. In: Ferrell BR, Coyle N, eds. *Oxford Textbook of Palliative Nursing.* 3rd ed. New York, NY: Oxford University Press; 2010:525-543.

35. Berry P, Griffe J. Planning for actual death. In: Ferrell BR, Coyle N, eds. *Oxford Textbook of Palliative Nursing.* 3rd ed. New York, NY: Oxford University Press; 2010:629-644.

36. Ersek M. Artificial hydration and nutrition. In: Nelson P, ed. *Withdrawal of Life Sustaining Therapies.* Pittsburgh: PA: Hospice and Palliative Nurses Association; 2010:59-66.

37. Schwarz JK. Stopping eating and drinking. *AJN.* 2009;109(9):53-61.

38. Heidrich DE, English N. Delirium, confusion, agitation, and restlessness. In: Ferrell BR, Coyle N, eds. *Oxford Textbook of Palliative Nursing.* 3rd ed. New York, NY: Oxford University Press; 2010:449-467.

39. Fenwick P, Lovelace H, Brayne S. Comfort for the dying: five year retrospective and one year prospective studies of end of life experiences. *Arch Gerontol Geriatr.* 2010;51(2):173-179

40. Centers for Medicare and Medicaid Services. *482.45 Electronic Code of Federal Regulations.* Available at: ecfr.gpoaccess.gov/cgi/t/text/text-idx?c=ecfr&tpl=/ecfrbrowse/Title42/42cfr482_main_02.tpl. Accessed October 20, 2011.

41. Corless IB. Bereavement. In: Ferrell BR, Coyle N, eds. *Oxford Textbook of Palliative Nursing.* 3rd ed. New York, NY: Oxford University Press; 2010:597-611.

42. Maciejewski PK, Zhang B, Block SD, Prigerson HG. An empirical examination of the stage theory of grief. *JAMA.* 2007;297(7):716-723.

43. Saunders C. Pain and impending death. In: Wall PD, Melzak R, eds. *Textbook of Pain.* 2nd ed. Edinburgh, UK: Churchill Livingstone; 1989:624-631.

44. Rando TA. Grief, Dying, and Death. Champaign, IL: Research Press Company; 1984:272.

CHAPTER 33

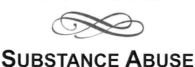

SUBSTANCE ABUSE

Carol R. Matthews, APRN, ACHPN®

I.   GUIDELINES FOR ASSESSMENT AND MANAGEMENT

Substance abuse is a growing problem in our society that impacts both physical and psychological health. Healthcare providers are witnesses to the medical complications of alcoholism, tobacco abuse, illicit drug use, and increasingly, the misuse of prescription drugs. Clinicians who encounter substance abuse in patients need to be aware of the unique treatment concerns for these patients, which include comprehensive assessment, risk management, and frequent visits and evaluations. Substance abuse treatment is multi-modal and often includes management of co-existing conditions, such as mental illness, posttraumatic stress, history of physical or psychological abuse, and other psychosocial factors.

II.   SUBSTANCE ABUSE WITHIN PALLIATIVE CARE

Palliative care practitioners excel in providing pain and symptom management to patients with potential and actual life-limiting illnesses. This care includes the evaluation of the symptoms, the probable cause, the patient's experience, and meaning of the symptoms and their effect on the patient's role in society and functional status. In writing about cancer-related pain and risk management, Miaskowski points out that a balanced perspective is needed to deliver pain management, while recognizing the concerns that patients, families, caregivers, and clinicians have about the development of tolerance, physical dependence, and addiction to opioids.[1] Patient and family related barriers to pain management include a strong conviction to not utilize medication, fear of stigmatizing interactions with clinicians and family members, and intractable side effects of opioid use is also essential.[1] While managing these concerns, palliative care practitioners must be aware of substance abuse/misuse issues.

Approximately 6-15% of the U.S. population suffers from substance abuse disorder.[2] Although studies suggest that the prevalence of addiction and misuse may be lower in the medically ill population, the problem is growing.[3] Among patients with cancer, there are a growing number of survivors with chronic pain syndromes and an increasing percentage of cancer patients with non-cancer pain. In non-cancer diagnosis, such as HIV/AIDS, hepatitis C, there may already be prior issues with substance abuse. This requires the identification of patients at risk and treatment approaches to mitigate risk in this population even as they deal with serious or life-threatening diseases. Although many palliative APRNs have had little experience in caring for patients with substance abuse, a basic knowledge of how to assess and approach substance abuse/misuse is essential.

A.   Prevalence and Substance Abuse

According to the 2009 National Survey on Drug Use and Health, an estimated 6.8% of Americans report heavy alcohol consumption, 22.7% tobacco use and

8.7% of those 12 and older report illicit drug use, which includes nonmedical use of prescription medications. The economic effect of substance abuse is significant. In 2006, the cost of nonmedical use of prescription drugs was $53.4 billion, of which $42 billion (79.9%) was attributed to lost productivity, $8.2 billion (15%) to criminal justice costs, $2.2 billion (4%) to substance abuse treatment, and $0.9 billion to medical complications (2%).[4] The Centers for Disease Control and Prevention reported the cost of smoking was estimated at $193 billion[5] and The Department of Health and Human Services estimated the total cost of alcohol abuse at $184.6 billion.[6]

The increased use of opioids for pain management has mirrored an increase in reported abuse, misuse, and diversion of these medications. In 2009, there were 1,224,679 emergency department visits involving the use or misuse of prescription medications, increased substantially from 627,291 in 2004.[7] Added consequences of substance abuse include hospital admissions, deaths, worsening of emotional and mental health problems, and increased criminal behavior.

B. Terminology

Substance abuse is defined by the DSM-IV as a psychiatric disorder. This definition does not accurately describe the use or misuse of medications in the medically ill population, nor does the DSM-IV define tolerance and physical dependence as it applies to medical practice for symptom management. A consensus document of the American Academy of Pain Medicine, American Pain Society, and the Academy of Addiction Medicine provided definitions of the terms misuse, tolerance, physical dependence and pseudoaddiction that are more applicable to pain and symptom management in the medically ill.[8] (see Table 1)

Table 1: Definitions

Tolerance	A state of adaptation in which exposure to a drug induces changes that result in a diminution of one or more of the drug's effects over time.[9, p. 2]
Physical dependence	A state of adaptation that is manifested by a drug class specific withdrawal syndrome that can be produced by abrupt cessation, rapid dose reduction, decreasing blood level of the drug, and/or administration of an antagonist.[9, p. 2]
Addiction	A primary, chronic, neurobiologic disease, with genetic, psychosocial, and environmental factors influencing its development and manifestations. It is characterized by behaviors that include one or more of the following—impaired control over drug use, compulsive use, continued use despite harm, and craving.[9, p. 2]
Pseudo-addiction	Behaviors that appear to be addictive; however the motivation directing the misuse of medications is influenced by a desire to achieve symptom management and usually subsides when the symptom management plan is adjusted to achieve acceptable symptom control.[9]
Substance misuse	The use of medications for other than the purpose for which it was intended. When describing the use of prescription medications, it may include increases in amount and frequency of the medication, use for other purposes than prescribed (i.e., pain medication for anxiety), and to obtain effects other than treating a target symptom (euphoria vs. analgesia). In a legal sense, this may also mean underage use of a substance or diversion of medication.[10]
Diversion	The removal of medications from legitimate distribution and dispensing channels therefore diverting drugs to persons other than those to whom it is prescribed.[8]

33

C. Substance Abuse Impact and Considerations

1. Substance abuse/addiction produces suffering and impacts all aspects of a person's life as their craving overpowers their choices and actions. Important points for the palliative APRN to remember are

a) It is not the drug or substance that causes the addictive behaviors. Importantly not all persons who use a drug or substances have addiction.[11]

b) The prevalence of co-existing psychosocial conditions further complicates care of the patients with substance abuse. These include anxiety, depression, posttraumatic stress, previous personal abuse, and other psychological disorders.

2. Addiction or substance abuse treatment is not specifically within the scope of practice of the palliative APRN. None the less, collaboration with experts in the field of addiction is consistent with the advanced practice role, for comprehensive care.

3. An important principle for palliative APRNs is that these patients should not be cared for alone.

a) Comanagement with pain specialists, psychiatry, and addiction programs is essential.

b) Referral to community resources for addictions counseling including 12-step programs, psychosocial counseling, support groups, and detoxification centers as needed should also be part of the management plan.[11]

4. Concurrent treatment of all conditions is recommended and ideally should be include open communication between the specialties to assure continuity of care.[11] Access to mental health specialties may be limited by health insurance coverage, lack of local services, patient's compromised medical condition, and even transportation difficulties. These barriers emphasize the need for a team approach to care of these individuals utilizing the full complement of services to reduce suffering.

III. PALLIATIVE CARE AND SUBSTANCE ABUSE

A. The goal of palliative care is to prevent and relieve suffering and promote the best quality of life for patients and their families, regardless of past medical history and comorbid conditions. The relief of suffering and symptom management may include the use of substances with abuse potential. One of the most challenging substance abuse disorders is the misuse of prescription medications. Although opioid mediations are probably the most widely abused medications, other classes of medications such as benzodiazepines are also subject to abuse.[12]

B. APRNs perform comprehensive assessments of their patients that should include previous substance abuse details, risk assessment for potential misuse, physical exam pertinent to pain and symptom complaints, and close monitoring and reassessment of the safety and effectiveness of interventions for symptom management. Screening tools facilitate assessment and will be discussed in detail later in this chapter. However, clinical judgments need to be individualized to each patient and the interdisciplinary team helps support all domains of care.

33

IV. ASSESSMENT OF SUBSTANCE ABUSE AND RISK

A. "First do no harm…"

Ideally, a complete screening and assessment for drug abuse should occur prior to prescribing opioids and benzodiazepines. However, patients may present to us with a history of previous use or misuse of opioids, benzodiazepines, or other illict drugs, and may have a variety of mediations prescribed by other providers. The comprehensive history and physical will include specific details targeting contributing and risk factors for substance abuse. The history and physical should include screening tools and questions eliciting information that promotes the development of an individualized plan of care. A caring approach and nonjudgmental demeanor in eliciting this information helps to develop a therapeutic relationship focused on goals of care. Risk assessments such as opioid risk tool are designed to identify which patient will be at risk for developing substance abuse but other tools are more appropriate to identify active misuse in patients already taking opioids.[11]

B. Suggested components of the assessment may include

1. Detailed description of current diagnosis and comorbid conditions.

2. Past medical history including diagnosis of mental health problems, physical and/or psychological abuse, anxiety, depression, and other psychiatric conditions.

3. Past surgical history and influences on current symptoms.

4. Family history including substance abuse indicators. Note any substance abuse history in the family or anxiety or depression in other family members.

5. Social history including work history, marital or significant relationship status.

6. Review of systems—ask detailed information of all symptoms including severity, duration, alleviating and precipitating factors, as well as nonpharmacological interventions.

7. Substance history[2,11,13]

   a) The use of self reporting documentation completed prior to the visit maybe helpful but underreporting of issues may occur especially if the patient is threatened by the content.

   b) Interview questions are delivered in a nonjudgmental manner to elicit honest report and initiate a trusting relationship between the patient and the practitioner. It is important to frame this discussion by indicating the clinician needs to know everything a patient is using to make safe choices for medical interventions for future symptom management.[2]

      i.   Allergies to medications

      ii. What medications were not effective in treating your symptoms now and in the past? Note type and dosage used.

      iii. What medications have been effective for you now and in the past? Especially note the use of narcotics and medications for insomnia, anxiety, and depression.

      iv. Current medications—doses frequency, indication, effectiveness, side effects, and current prescriber.

33

        v.   Detailed smoking history and/or current use; 75-95% of patients being treated for substance abuse disorder smoke.

      vi.   Current and past alcohol use including duration, quantity, and type of alcohol consumed.

     vii.   How much alcohol are you currently drinking?

   viii.   How much did you drink in the past?

      ix.   Have you ever had a problem with or resulting from alcohol use?

       x.   If currently abstinent, when was your last drink?

  c) Detailed evaluation of previous substance use or misuse including illicit and prescription medications.

       i.   Are you currently using marijuana, cocaine, heroin, or other street drugs? If yes, time of last use?

      ii.   Have you used them in the past?

     iii.   Have you or are you using someone else's prescription medication?

C. Screening Tools

  1. Screening tools can be useful in identifying patients who may be at risk for substance abuse/misuse.

    a) The purpose of screening for substance abuse is not to exclude the patient from opioid therapy but to highlight the need for additional monitoring to facilitate safe medical management.[2,11]

    b) Patients who demonstrate a positive score should be further evaluated to manage a substance abuse condition if present.

  2. When choosing tools keep in mind that they should demonstrate ease of use, be specific to the information you wish to elicit, be brief to meet time constraints, and effective in their outcomes.[11]

  3. While many tools are designed to screen for specific substances (e.g., alcohol), most researched tools are related to alcohol abuse. Some of the tools developed for alcohol abuse screening have been adapted to screen for drug misuse but have not been validated for that purpose.

  4. Tools designed to detect current and life-long substance abuse particularly alcohol abuse

    a) The widely known CAGE (cut, annoyed, guilty, eye) tool asks questions regarding a patient's alcohol consumption and its impact on their interactions with others.

    b) Other tools for alcoholism include the TICS (Two Item Conjoint Screen), MAST (Michigan Alcohol Screening Test) and the AUDIT (Alcohol Use Disorders Identification Test).[11]

  5. Some of these tools have been adapted for use with other drugs.

    a) CAGE-AID—although it is not specific to opioid use it may be useful to screen conjointly for alcohol and drug abuse. Dr. L. Webster[11] suggests that this tool may be more beneficial in screening opioid-treated patients when the questions are asked in an open ended fashion rather than a yes/no fashion (i.e., how often have you tried to cut down…?). (see Table 2)

33

Table 2: The CAGE-Adapted to Include Drugs Questionnaire[11]

In the past have you ever
- Tried to **cut** down or change your pattern of drinking or drug abuse?
- Been **annoyed** or **angry** by others' concern about your drinking or drug use?
- Felt **guilty** about the consequences of your drinking or drug use?
- Had a drink or used a drug in the morning (an "**eye**-opener") to decrease a hangover or withdrawal symptoms?

Implications for prescribing
- One positive response to any questions suggests caution.
- Two or more positive responses may have sensitivity of 60-95% and a specificity of 40-95% for diagnosing alcohol or drug problems. Strongly suggest assessment by an addiction specialist before opioids are prescribed.
- A CAGE test result may have less predictive value in certain populations (e.g., older adults, college students, women, and certain ethnic groups).

Reprinted with permission from Sunrise Press

Table 3: TICS: A Two-Item Conjoint Screen[11]

1. In the last year, have your ever drunk or used drugs more than you meant to?
2. Have you ever felt you wanted or needed to cut down on your drinking or drug use in the last year?

In primary care patients, at least one affirmative answer to these two questions is nearly 80% sensitive and specific for substance abuse.

Reprinted with permission from Sunrise Press

     b)   The TICS tool has been used in primary care to identify substance abuse in general although it is not specific to opioid use it may be helpful in identifying patients at risk. (see Table 3)

6.   Specific tools to evaluate risk of prescription drug misuse include PDUQ (Prescription Drug Use Questionnaire), ORT (Opioid Risk Tool), SOAPP (Screener and Opioid Assessment for Patient with Pain, and SIASP (Screening Instrument for Substance Abuse Potential).[8,11,13]

     a)   The ORT is useful because it is brief, easy to use, self-administered tool, which has been shown to accurately measure patients risk for displaying aberrant drug related behaviors. Specifically this tool was designed for the initial visit for pain treatment before opioids are prescribed. For the palliative care practitioner, it may offer valuable history of substance abuse and risk factors that can predispose a patient to substance abuse.[11,13] This validated tool identifies the risk level for the patient and can guide appropriate monitoring for the patient who receives opioid therapy. (see Table 4)

7.   The SOAPP, PDUQ, and SIASP instruments screen for misuse/abuse in chronic pain patients who may already be taking opioids.

D.   State prescription monitoring programs may offer additional information regarding a patient's prescription history. Many states have prescription databases, which health practitioners, law enforcement authorities, and regulatory agencies can access to determine prescribing and dispensing patterns. Because these are state based programs, there are many variations of the information contained at these sites and some states limit access to these sites to only specific clinicians. These programs may help identify a patient who has more than one provider writing prescriptions, or using many pharmacies to obtain their medications and further assist with risk stratification.[11,13]

33

Table 4: Opioid Risk Tool[11]

Item	Mark each box that applies	Item score if female	Item score if male
Family history of substance abuse	[ ]		
Alcohol	[ ]	1	3
Illegal drugs	[ ]	2	3
Prescription drugs	[ ]	4	4
Personal history of substance abuse	[ ]	3	3
Illegal drugs	[ ]	4	4
Prescription drugs	[ ]	5	5
Age (mark box if 16-45)	[ ]	1	1
History of preadolescent sexual abuse	[ ]	3	0
Psychologic disease	[ ]		
Attention deficit disorder, obsessive-compulsive disorder, bipolar disorder, schizophrenia	[ ]	2	2
Depression	[ ]	1	1
Total		____	____
Total score risk category Low risk—0–3 Moderate risk—4-7 High risk—8 or higher			

Reprinted with permission from Sunrise Press

V. CARE FOR THE PATIENT

A. "Cure sometimes, treat often, comfort always" (Hippocrates)…clinicians need to collect assessment data and determine the patient's risk profile. The following classifications will assist in the design of the individualized monitoring plan for your patient

1. Low

- No history of substance abuse
- No prescription abuse/misuse
- Minimum or no significant risk factors

2. Medium

- History of substance abuse/misuse
- No prescription abuse
- Significant risk factors

3. High

- Active substance abuse
- Prescription opioid abuse
- Significant risk factors

33

4. After determining your patient risk, it is important to evaluate if the use of opioid medications is appropriate considering the following questions

- Is there a clear medical condition producing the symptom?

- Does the patient have a condition that contributes to the pain?

- Is there a physiological reason for the patient complaint of pain?

- Is the patient's self report consistent with symptoms?
    - Have you thoroughly investigated the risk and previous substance abuse history?
    - Has there been a trial of nonpharmacological interventions?
    - What medications have been previously used to alleviate or manage pain including dosage, frequency, and duration of trail?
    - Has there been a trial of non-opioid medications that was unsuccessful?
    - Does the severity of the pain warrant the use of opioids?
    - Is the patient opioid naive?
    - Is the patient requesting one specific type or brand of medication, stating that all others will fail?

B. Need for Team Approach

1. The use of a multidisciplinary approach is necessary to deal with the complex issues these patients experience. For effectiveness, it is suggested that the team include palliative care physicians, APRNs, registered nurses, social workers, psychologist or psychiatrist and, if possible, a mental health provider with expertise in the area of addiction medicine.[3,11]

2. It is important to utilize experts outside of palliative care team to assist with treatment of substance abuse and facilitate management of psychological conditions that may escalate medication misuse.[2,14]

3. The support of a mental health provider/addiction specialist can also support the staff in dealing with their own feelings and perceptions in dealing with this population.

4. Other helpful resources to provide comprehensive care include psychiatry and/or counseling

5. Concomittent treatment inlcudes participation in a 12-step, smoking cessation, and detoxification programs and support groups.[2,11]

6. If the patient is in a substance disorder program, collaboration with program staff assures consistency across settings.

33

C. Communication Skills

Therapeutic communication is essential to develop a relationship with the patient and establish trust.[15] Conveying the dual goals of treating a serious or life-threatening illness and its associated symptom, while addressing the substance abuse and or addiction is essential. Questions regarding substance use must be nonjudgmental. Aberrant behaviors must be addressed compassionately but with firm limitations. Trust is an important part of the clinician/patient relationship and is positively related to patient compliance with treatment recommendations, medication regimes, and improved patient outcomes. This trusting relationship between patient and clinician can in itself have healing effects.[16]

D. Customized Care Plan

An individualized plan of care that considers the patient's previous history and current needs will set realistic goals for therapy.[2] Careful management of pain and other symptoms can actually help reduce aberrant drug use behaviors. Limit setting, intensive social, and emotional support may help the patient minimize relapse. If the patient is utilizing medications to treat other conditions such as anxiety or depression, collaboration with mental health/psychiatry to optimize use of antidepressants and nonbenzodiazepine anxiolytics may stabilize the use of pain medications.[11] All of these factors again emphasize the need for a team approach.

E. Pharmacological and Pain Management Principles

Prudent prescribing for this population warrants awareness of the concepts of tolerance and physical dependence. Patients who have history of substance abuse may require higher drug doses to achieve the desired therapeutic effect. Consider the possibility of pseudoaddiction when increasing doses to achieve symptom management goals while concurrently evaluating for aberrant behaviors, and functional ability as appropriate to disease status.

The principles of pain management, as described in Chapter 6, *Pain*, still apply to the substance abuse patient but with the added considerations to avoid further harm. The patient with serious or life-threatening disease and comorbid abuse, misuse/addiction can be successfully treated with careful documentation, team work, and planning.[3]

F. Reassessment and Monitoring

Ongoing monitoring is essential in treating the patient who is an active substance abuser or one at risk for substance abuse.

1. Patients receiving opioid medications require regular visits to monitor pain, functional status, mood, medication usage, and well being.[17] Frequency of the visits is determined by the level of assessed risk and the patient's adherence to the clinical plan.

2. The ongoing monitoring can be guided by assessing the effectiveness of the interventions using the 4 A's (analgesia, activity, adverse events, aberrant behavior).[8,11] Asking questions related to the 4 A's guides the clinician in evaluating symptom management and the need for dose adjustments. S. Passik suggests the following considerations.[13]

    a) Analgesia

        i.   What was your average pain level during the past week?

        ii. What was your worst pain level during the past week?

        iii. What percentage of your pain has been relieved?

        iv. Does your current level of pain control make a real difference in your life? (This question should be specific for your patient and assess if they can function within their prescribed role within the family, work, etc.).

33

b) Activity

In addition to pain relief, functional improvement can be another measurement of successful interventions. The difference, between proper use of the medications and misuse, may be identified by change in patient functional status taking into account disease status. Corroboration with family is helpful.

c) Adverse effects

Side effects influence a patient's willingness to utilize and continue with therapeutic regimen. Severe constipation, nausea, or other side effects may detract from the benefits of the current therapy.

d) Aberrant behavior

i. Use of the medication other than as directed, requests for early refills, use of other substances or nonprescribed medications, reports of missing pills and failure to show up for scheduled appointments may all be indicators of aberrant behaviors.

ii. These incidents should be documented and the discrepancies confronted in a nonjudgmental manner. Review of these behaviors can offer opportunities for additional discussion regarding patients' rights and responsibilities in proper use of medications.

iii. Evidence of aberrant behaviors direct the level of monitoring required to manage increased risk.[2]

3. Although these parameters are helpful, they cannot replace the expert clinical judgment and assessment on the benefit versus burden of any symptom management therapy.

G. Pain Management Agreements—Considerations for Use

1. Pain management agreements clearly state goals, expectations, and limitations of the pain treatment plan in an effort to avoid misuse of prescription drugs.

2. Although pain management specialists strongly promote the use of pain agreements, palliative care providers may express reservations about use of these tools in the medically ill populations. Frequent concerns about agreement use are—if the clinician does not trust the patient, will the patient trust the clinician?[16] Will requiring use of these agreements for all patients using opioids further stigmatize opioids and contribute to under treatment of pain with the population who may already be resistant to taking medications for fear of addiction?

3. The challenge is protecting both the prescribing provider and the patient. The goal of relieving physical and emotional symptoms must not blind one to the problems and suffering that exists with substance abuse and diversion. Selective use of these agreements may provide safe management of symptoms with at risk individuals.

4. The content of the pain agreement must be written in a language that is easily understood, at an appropriate reading level and be educational in nature. The tone of the agreement must not be punitive or threatening. See Appendix 33-A for an example.

33

5. The following are suggested elements for inclusion in the agreement

    a) Designated single prescriber/practice to write prescriptions for opioids and/or other controlled substances.

    b) Use of a single designated pharmacy for all prescriptions.

    c) Timely communication between patient and prescriber for any changes in medication doses or medication changes.

    d) Random monitoring of medication, which may include pill counts.

    e) Random urine and blood toxicology screening.

    f) Expectation that prescription medications will only be used by the patient, used as prescribed, and be kept safe and secure to prevent loss and theft.

    g) Use of illegal substances may compromise patient's ability to obtain further opioids.

    h) Clear consequences stated for aberrant behavior, lost prescriptions, and requests for early refill or the like.[8,11]

6. Consider individual and unique practice issues, as well as the organization, when designing the agreement. Seeking legal counsel to review content and wording of the document.

7. Do not use the agreement as punishment, but as ongoing dialogue as to mutual plan for pain management including evidence based pain principles and appropriate medical interventions.

H. Drug Use Monitoring

1. Patients may underreport or conceal use of illicit drugs or nonprescribed medications. Drug testing can verify use of prescribed medications, while also detecting the presence of non prescribed medications or illicit drugs.

2. Different monitoring methods provide drug use information but also have limiting factors that may interfere with practical applications in measuring patient compliance.

    a) Blood or serum samples can detect low levels of substances but only reveal current drug use, not representing long-term adherence. These tests are very effective in emergency medicine to assist appropriate interventions. However, they tend to be expensive and invasive rendering them impractical in the pain management setting.[18]

    b) Oral fluid testing provides ease of obtaining samples but has a short detection window of only 4 hours. This method is gaining popularity because the sampling procedure is easily monitored.[18]

    c) Hair analysis offers the advantage of detecting substances for up to 6 months but is considered inefficient and prone to false-negative results.

    d) Urine drug testing (UDT) provides the most practical testing and is a better method for detection of opioids than blood plasma.[19] In contrast to forensic results, this test is designed to detect positive presence of prescribed substances. It is important to note that while this test detects the presence of a medication, it does not provide quantitative information that verifies the amount of drug in the patient's system.[11]

33

i. The two most common types of UDT are immunoassay and gas chromatography-mass spectrometry (GC-MS).

    (a) The immunoassay uses antibodies to detect the presence of specific drugs or metabolites of the drugs and is considered to be an initial, but not confirmatory, method of screening. Because this type of screening can produce false positive results, it is considered to be presumptive until confirmed by other methods.

    (b) The screening method GC-MS is considered the standard for confirmatory testing but is time consuming, costly, and requires a high level of expertise to perform. It can still fail to identify presence of some substances.[17]

ii. UDTs were originally designed for forensic use, not for verification of therapeutic medication regimes.

    (a) An initial screening usually includes testing for the "Federal Five," which includes amphetamines, cocaine, opiates, marijuana, and phencyclidine.

    (b) To screen for barbiturates, benzodiazepines, fentanyl, or oxycodone one may need to specifically request screening for these medications. It is interesting to note that specific substances are difficult to detect, especially the synthetic opioids.

    (c) Other medications may contain metabolites that register as false positives for opioids.[20]

    (d) To ensure that the prescribed medications are being covered by your screening test, include a list of the medications prescribed with the dosage and the time the patient reported taking the medications and send this along with the specimen.[11]

iii. Careful technique must be instituted in collecting and processing of urine. Note the color, temperature, and appearance of the specimen. Be aware that patients avoiding detection of drug use may adulterate, substitute, tamper, or dilute the specimen. If adulteration of the sample is suspected, repeat sampling is recommended in a controlled environment.

iv. When tests are positive, the APRN can confirm the results with the head of the lab. The laboratory can answer questions related to unexpected results and offer additional information and guidance. A repeat test may be performed.

    (a) False positive readings are common and clinical decisions should not be based only on preliminary findings. Urine test results are often misinterpreted. Expert advice and confirmatory testing are recommended. Confirmatory tests repeat screening and/or requesting testing for specific substances can offer additional information.

    (b) Be aware that other medications including over the counter products and foods (e.g., morphine may be detected in urine within 6-12 hours of ingesting bakery products containing poppy seeds)[21] can affect urine test results, further complicating

33

interpretation of the results. Note that the cut off scores established for industry and government needs are not necessary for clinical purposes. Use of forensic rather than therapeutic cut off scores, may result in a false negative.[11]

(c) When using urine testing to monitor drug usage, work closely with the laboratory and request assistance in interrupting results. Do not rely only on urine screenings alone in making clinical decisions to direct your prescriptive practice for symptom management.[11]

(d) Test results should be shared with the patient. Consider the patient's explanation of an abnormal UDT when determining your plan of action.[10] Open communication about purpose and use of these tests can help direct a comprehensive treatment plan. It is suggested to prepare an action plan in advance, based screening results and other information related to the patient's medication use.[20]

VI. ETHICAL PRINCIPLES OF PAIN MANAGEMENT AND THE SUBSTANCE MISUSE/ABUSE PATIENT

Persons with substance abuse history are less likely to receive effective pain management due to concerns about clinical and legal pressures related to substance misuse.[17] The following ethical principles support universal access to pain treatment.

1. Autonomy—self determination within treatment options. Patients treated with opioids are informed of low risk abuse but this risk is increased in the presence of family history of abuse or previous personal history of abuse.

2. Nonmalficence—do no harm. Determine the risk of addiction to avoid harming the patient with use of these substances. Monitor patient use and response. Prescribe limited quantities to patients with substance abuse issues.

3. Beneficence—a deliberate action performed for a patient's welfare. Opioid prescriptions are used with intent to reduce pain and suffering.

4. Justice—the treatments for pain are offered in an equitable fashion for intended patient benefit. The clinician performs a detailed examination of the indication for opioids in the substance abuse patient, while considering the role of non-opioids, interventional pain procedures and complementary therapies.[22]

VII. LEGAL AND REGULATORY CONSIDERATIONS

A. Use of controlled substance is regulated by federal and state laws. In the event of a difference between the state and federal law, the more stringent law is upheld. Each prescribing practitioner must act responsibly when prescribing controlled substances and prevent misuse. Knowledge of the federal laws and regulations as those in the state in which one practices should guide prescribing practice.

B. The Controlled Substances Act[23] is used by the federal government to discourage and enforce rules to prevent drug abuse. The Act does not set medical standards. A patient who is under treatment for addiction can receive opioids for analgesia. However, unless one holds a specific license for treating opioid addiction, one

33

cannot provide controlled substances to treat patients for addiction. It is important to write the prescription specifically for pain and document the indication for use of the medication in the prescription "for pain."[11]

C. Drug Enforcement Administration (DEA) Opioid Regulations

1. A small percentage of prescribing practitioners come under scrutiny of the DEA for their opioid prescribing practices.

2. Actions imposed against prescribers are usually related to those who knew or should have known their patients were diverting or abusing drugs. The DEA recognizes that under treatment of pain is a serious problem and that effective pain management is necessary. However they will seek out discrepancies and aberrant behavior by prescribers and pharmacists.

3. Documentation of patient care, including prescribing controlled substances, must reflect that

   a) Medication is given for a specific condition

   b) Closely monitoring of the patient

   c) Medications are not dispensed to those who are reselling the drugs

   d) Detailed and frequent oversight to prevent diversion or misuse in the known addicted patient.[11]

D. Risk Evaluation and Mitigation Strategies (REMS)[24]

1. Risk evaluation and mitigation strategies (REMS) are designed to minimize risks associated with use of medications, while optimizing benefit. These regulations are designed not only for safe use of the medication but also in consideration of public health risks associated with the medication.

2. There are REMS for many medications. Sustained release/long acting opioids, and immediate release transmucosal fentanyl products have approved REMS. (See Chapter 34, *Medications Commonly Used in Palliative Care*)

3. Goals of REMS includes access of the medications to a population who will derive benefit from the medication, while deterring misuse that will minimize overdose, morbidity, and mortality.

4. REMS may include

   a) Clinician training prior to prescribing medications including guidelines that the clinician must follow when prescribing a particular medication (i.e., newer long acting or higher dose opioids cannot be used for opioid naïve patients). Although these may seem cumbersome to the prescriber, their purpose is to minimize risk and promote safe and appropriate use of medications.[25]

   b) Patient education materials

   c) Pharmacy participation

E. Future Initiatives

Medications that focus on analgesia without promoting craving, absence of euphoria, and prevention of withdrawal symptoms would be ideal. New drug formulations are being designed to decrease the pleasure effect in medications.

33

thereby deterring the development of addiction. "Tamper proof" opioid formulations are being developed to help prevent the use of the medication by a route other than prescribed. Some manufactures have experimented with combining opioid agonists and antagonists but additional research is needed before these formulations are widely available.[11] Keeping abreast of new formulations released for use by the Food and Drug Administration (FDA) and note special considerations needed with these new products, such as REMS is imperative.

VIII. CONCLUSION

Comprehensive practical care is required for the patient who needs symptom management for serious or life-threatening diseases in the face of a known history of substance abuse. Concurrent treatment of the addictive disorder and comorbid mental health disorders may improve patient outcomes, while decreasing suffering. The most effective way to provide comprehensive care to this population is a team approach. This aides the clinician in caring for the patient, and offers a multidimensional approach to care including collaboration with experts in the field of substance abuse and community agency support. This same approach may benefit patients assessed to be at risk of substance misuse/abuse.

Careful assessment, utilization of risk management strategies (use of pain agreements or random urine testing) tailored to patient's needs, clinician's level of concern, close monitoring of drug use, and awareness of possible aberrant drug related behaviors can promote quality care of the individual who is also dealing with a serious or life-threatening disease. Each case requires individualized attention to care for the patients with substance misuse/abuse to promote safe and effective approaches to reduce pain and suffering for the patients, families and society as a whole.

33

Appendix A: **Example of Agreement for Long-term Opioid Use**

The purpose of this agreement is to protect your access to controlled substances and to protect our ability to prescribe for you. The long-term use of such substances as opioids (narcotic analgesics), benzodiazepine tranquilizers, and barbiturate sedatives is controversial because of uncertainty regarding the extent to which they provide long-term benefit. In people with a prior addiction, there is also the risk of the development of an addictive disorder or a recurrence of drug abuse. The extent of that risk is uncertain.

Because these drugs have potential for abuse or diversion, strick accountability is necessary when use is prolonged. For this reason, the following policies are agreed to by you (the patient) as a condition of the willingness of the provider whose signature appears below to consider the initial and/or continued prescription of controlled substances to treat your chronic pain.

1. Unless specific authorization is obtained for an exception, all controlled substances must come ONLY from the physicians or advanced practice registered nurse (APRN) at _____. You will not attempt to get pain medication from any other healthcare provider without telling him or her that you are taking pain medication prescribed by this clinic. You understand that failing to provide that information to a prescriber is against the law. If your primary care physician is willing to prescribe your medications, this clinic will have to approve the arrangements to ensure that there is no duplication. You will discontinue all previously used pain medications unless you are told to continue them. All controlled substances must be obtained at the same pharmacy, if possible. If the need to change pharmacies arises, our office must be informed. The pharmacy that you have selected is:

_____

Phone: _____

2. You are expected to inform our office of any new medications or medical conditions and of any adverse effects you experience from any of the medications that you take.

3. To maintain accountability, the prescribing physician has permission to discuss all diagnostic and treatment details with dispensing pharmacists or other professionals who provide your healthcare information. You agree to waive any applicable privilege or right of privacy or confidentiality with respect to the prescribing of your pain medication, and you authorize the clinic and your pharmacy to cooperate fully with any city, state, or federal law enforcement agency in the investigation of any possible misuse, sale, or other diversion of your pain medication. You authorize the clinic to provide a copy of this agreement to your pharmacy.

4. You may not share, sell, or otherwise permit others to have access to these medications.

5. Do not stop taking these drugs abruptly, because abstinence syndrome will likely develop.

6. Unannounced urine or serum toxicology screenings may be requested, and your cooperation is required. The presence of an unauthorized substance may prompt an adjustment in your treatment and monitoring.

7. Prescriptions and bottles of these medications may be sought by individuals with chemical dependency and should be closley safeguarded. It is expected that you will take the highest possible degree of care with your medications and prescriptions. They should not be left where others might see or otherwise have access to them.

8. Original containers of medications may be required for you to bring to office visits.

9. Because these drugs may be hazardous or lethal to people (especially children) who are not tolerant of their effects, you must keep the drugs away from those people.

10. Medications may not be replaced if they are lost, get wet, are destroyed, are left on an airplane, etc. Such events may cause your treatment to be reassessed, and an alternative therapy may be prescribed.

11. Refills will be given only at the discretion of the provider. The preparation of all refills requires advance notice of three (3) business days. Early refills will not be given unless the provider feels that there is justficiation to do so.

12. Prescription renewals are contingent upon your keeping scheduled appointments. All prescriptions will be given on weekdays, Monday through Friday, from 9:00 AM to 4:00 PM. Prescriptions will NOT be given at any other time unless extreme extraordinary circumstances apply.

13. If the responsibile legal authorities have questions concerning your treatment (eg, whether you were obtaining medications at several pharmacies) all confidentiality is waived, and those authorities may be given full access to our records of controlled-substance administration (as stated in item #3).

14. It is understood that failure to adhere to these policies may result in the cessation of therapy with controlled-substance prescribing by this physician or referral for further specialty assessment.

15. It should be understood that any medical treatment is initially a trial and that continued prescribing is contingent upon evidence of benefit.

16. The risks and potential benefits of these therapies are explained elsewhere. You must acknowledge that you have received that explanation.

17. You affirm that you have full right and power to sign and be bound by this agreement and that you have read, understood, and accepted its terms.

18. You are advised not to drive while you are being treated with any medication we prescribe without having had an appropriate driver's test that indicates that it is safe for you to drive.

If any of the above conditions is violated, the provider may choose to wean you off opioid medication, and your painful condition will be managed without the use of opioids. Further opioids may not be prescribed for any chronic painful condition that may develop. Violations of the above-stated terms might also result in your being discharged from the clinic with appropriate written notice and warning and without receiving weaning medications or treatment from _____

_____
Physician/APRN signature

_____
Patient signature

_____
Date

_____
Patient name (printed)

33

CITED REFERENCES

1. Miaskowski C. The use of risk-management approaches to protect patients with cancer-related pain and their healthcare providers. *Oncol Nurs Forum.* 2008;35(Suppl):20-24.
2. Kirsch KL, Passik SD. Palliative care of the terminally ill drug addict. *Cancer Invest.* 2006;24(4):425-431.
3. Kirsch KL, Compton P, Passik SD. Caring for the drug-addicted patient at the end of life. In: Ferrell BR, Coyle N, ed. *Oxford Textbook of Palliative Nursing.* 3rd ed. New York, NY: Oxford University Press Inc; 2010:817-828.
4. Substance Abuse and Mental Health Services Administration. *Results from the 2009 National Survey on Drug Use and Health: Volume I. Summary of National Findings.* (Office of Applied Studies, NSDUH Series H-38, HHS Publication No. SMA 10-4586Findings). Rockville, MD; U.S. Department of Health and Human Services, 2010. Available at: oas.samhsa.gov/NSDUH/2k9NSDUH/2k9ResultsP.pdf. Accessed September 19, 2012.
5. Centers for Disease Control and Prevention. *Tobacco Use: Targeting the Nation's Leading Killer at a Glance 2011.* Available at: www.cdc.gov/chronicdisease/resources/publications/AAG/osh.htm. Accessed September 18, 2012.
6. Harwood HJ, The Lewin Group for the National Institute on Alcohol Abuse and Alcoholism. *Updating the Economic Costs of Alcohol Abuse in the United States: Estimates, Update Methods, and Data.* 2000. Available at: pubs.niaaa.nih.gov/publications/economic-2000/alcoholcost.PDF. Accessed September 18, 2012.
7. Center for Behavioral Health Statistics and Quality, Substance Abuse and Mental Health Services Administration. *The DAWN Report: Highlights of 2009 Drug Abuse Warning Network (DAWN) Findings on Drug-Related Emergency Department Visits.* 2010. Available at: www.samhsa.gov/data/2k10/dawnsr034edhighlights/edhighlights.htm. Accessed September 19, 2012.
8. Smith HS, Fine P, Passik SD. *Opioid Risk Management Tools and Tips.* New York, NY: Oxford University Press Inc; 2009.
9. American Academy of Pain Medicine, American Pain Society, and the Academy of Addiction Medicine. *Definitions Related to the Use of Opioids for the Treatment of Pain.* 2009. Available at: www.geriatricpain.org/Content/Resources/CPGuidelines/Documents/AAPM_Definitions_%20Opioid%20Treatment.doc. Accessed September 19, 2012.
10. Webster LR, Fine PG. Approaches to improve pain relief while minimizing opioid abuse liability. *J Pain.* 2010;11(7):602-611.
11. Webster LR, Dove B. *Avoiding Opioid Abuse While Managing Pain.* 1st ed. North Branch, MN: Sunrise River Press; 2007.
12. Starr TD, Rogak LJ, Passik SD. Substance abuse in cancer pain. *Curr Pain Headache Rep.* 2010;14(4):268-275.
13. Passik SD. Issues in long-term opioid therapy: unmet needs, risks, and solutions. *Mayo Clin Proc.* 2009;84(7):593-601.
14. Penson RT, Nunn C, Younger J, et al. Trust violated: analgesics for addicts. *Oncologist.* 2003;8(2):199-209.
15. Burton-Macleod S, Fainsinger RL. Cancer pain control in the setting of substance abuse: establishing the goals of care. *J Palliat Care.* 2008;24(2):122-125.
16. Collen M. Opioid Contracts and random drug testing for people with chronic pain - think twice. *J Law Med Ethics.* 2009;37(4):841-845.
17. Savage SR, Kirsh KL, Passik SD. Challenges in using opioids to treat pain in persons with substance abuse disorders. *Addict Sci Clin Pract.* 2008;4(2):4-25.
18. Pesce A, West C. Drug-of-abuse testing and therapeutic drug monitoring. *MLO Med Lab Obs.* 2011;43(3):42,44,46.
19. Vadivelu N, Chen IL, Kodmundi V, Ortigosa E, Gudin MT. The implications of urine drug testing in pain management. *Curr Drug Saf.* 2010;5(3):267-270.
20. Moeller KE, Lee KC, Kissack JC. Urine drug Screening: practical guide for clinicians. *Mayo Clin Proc.* 2008;83(1):66-76.
21. Mayo Clinic Medical Laboratories. *Opiates.* 2012. Available at: www.mayomedicallaboratories.com/articles/drug-book/opiates.html. Accessed September 19, 2012.
22. Cohen JM, Jasser S, Herron PD, Margolis CG. Ethical perspectives: opioid treatment of chronic pain in the context of addiction. *Clin J Pain.* 2002;18 (4 Suppl):S99-S107.
23. U.S. Food and Drug Administration. *Controlled Substances Act.* 2009. Available at: www.fda.gov/regulatoryinformation/legislation/ucm148726.htm. Accessed September 19, 2012.
24. U.S. Food and Drug Administration. *Risk Evaluation and Mitigation Strategy (REMS) for Extended Release and Long-Acting Opioids.* 2012. Available at: www.fda.gov/Drugs/DrugSafety/InformationbyDrugClass/ucm163647.htm. Accessed September 19, 2012.

33

25.   Wright C, Schnoll S, Berstein D. Risk evaluation and mitigation strategies for drugs with abuse liability:
      public interest, special interest, conflicts of interest, and the industry perspective. *Ann NY Acad Sci.*
      2008;1141:284-303.

ADDITIONAL RESOURCES

Breitbart W, Passik SD, Casper DJ. Psychological and psychiatric interventions in pain control. In: Hanks G,
      Cherny NI, Christakis NA, Fallon M, Portenoy RK, eds. *Oxford Textbook of Palliative Medicine.* 4th ed.
      New York, NY: Oxford University Press; 2005:784-800.
Brennan MJ, Stanos S. Strategies to optimize pain management with opioids while minimizing risk of abuse.
      PM R. 2010;2(6):544-557.
Center to Advance Palliative Care (www.capc.org)
Rohsenow DJ, Colby SM, Martin RA, Monti PM. Nicotine and other substance interaction expectancies
      questionnaire: relationship of expectancies to substance use. *Addict Behav.* 2005;30(4):629-641.
Rosenblum A, Marsch LA, Joseph H, Portenoy RK. Opioids and the treatment of chronic pain: controversies,
      current status, and future directions. *Exp Clin Psychopharmacol.* 2008;16(5):405-416.
Zacharoff KL, Menefee Pujol LA, Corsini E. *The PAINEDUorg. Manual: A Pocket Guide to Pain Management.*
      Available at: www.painedu.com/manual.asp. 2010.

PART V

RESOURCES

CHAPTER 34

MEDICATIONS COMMONLY USED IN PALLIATIVE CARE

Victor Phantumvanit, PharmD, BCPS, BCOP

This chapter reviews the various classes of medications most commonly used in palliative care. The indications, dosages, side effects, and important notes regarding each specific medication have been provided. The medication cost is an estimate from the average whole sale price, and might vary by venue and location. Cost information should be assumed to be for the generic form (if available) unless otherwise stated. The availability of each medication may be affected by FDA Risk Evaluation and Mitigation Strategies (REMS) programs and medication shortage. Please contact your local pharmacy for more information.

List of table

Table 1—Lists the medications commonny used in palliative caret by class in the sequence below. See the key at the end of Table 1 for explanations of abbreviations found in the table

• Opioids • Nonsteroidal antiinflammatory drugs (NSAIDs) • Non-acetylated salicylates • Other analgesics	• Anticonvulsants • Tricyclic antidepressants • Benzodiazepines • Antidepressants • Antipsychotics • Psychostimulants	• Anticoagulant • Sedatives • Anticholinergic • Antidiarrheal • Laxatives

Table 2—Initial dosing recommendations for Actiq®.

Table 3—The Transmucosal Immediate Release Fentanyl (TIRF) Risk Evaluation and Mitigation Strategy (REMS) Program

Table 4—Listing of additional tables and appendices providing information on pharmacological therapies in other chapters.

34

Table 1: Medications Commonly Used in Palliative Care

Medication Generic (brand)/ Palliative Care Indications	Usual Doses	How Supplied	Major Side Effects	Comments	Cost $-$$$[1,2] Dose (quantity)
Opioids					
• For all opioids—consider opioid-naïve vs. opioid-tolerance • Doses should be titrated to desired effect and symptom control					
Morphine (MS Contin®, Oramorph SR®, Roxanol®, Avinza®, Kadian®) • Pain • Dyspnea	**Oral:** immediate release 10-30 mg every 4 hr **Parenteral:** 2.5-15 mg IV/SC every 2-6 hr **Rectal:** 10-20 mg every 4 hr	Oral tablet: 15 mg, 30 mg Oral tablet, extended release: 15 mg, 30 mg, 60 mg, 100 mg, 200 mg Avinza® (ER capsule): 30 mg, 45 mg, 60 mg, 75 mg, 90 mg, 120 mg Kadian (ER capsule): 10 mg, 30 mg, 50 mg, 60 mg, 80 mg, 100 mg, 200 mg Injection solution: 0.5 mg/mL, 1 mg/mL, 2 mg/mL, 4 mg/mL, 5 mg/mL, 8 mg/mL, 10 mg/mL, 15 mg/mL, 25 mg/mL, 50 mg/mL Rectal suppository: 5 mg, 10 mg, 20 mg, 30 mg	Constipation, pruritus, N/V, respiratory depression	Avinza® and Kadian® are 24 hours capsules that can be opened and sprinkled (not crushed) on food or via g-tube without losing SR profile, dose reduction in renal impairment	$-$$ Solution: 20 mg/5 mL (500 mL) = $65.03 12 hr tablets: 15 mg (30) = $28.05 30 mg (30) = $48.99 60 mg (30) = $89.99 100 mg (30) = $129.99 Tablets: 15 mg (20) = $12.99 30 mg (20) = $12.99 24 hr capsules: Avinza® 30 mg (20) = $97.99 60 mg (20) = $170.00 90 mg (20) = $268.00 120 mg (20) = $276.00 Kadian® 20 mg (20) = $95.17 50 mg (20) = $162.75 60 mg (20) = $191.08 100 mg (20) = $338.58
Hydromorphone (Dilaudid®, Exalgo®) • Pain • Dyspnea	**Oral tablet:** immediate release 2-4 mg every 4-6 hr; Extended release 8-64 mg every 24 hrs **Oral solution:** 2.5-10 mg every 3-6 hr **Parenteral:** 1-2 mg SC/IV every 4-6 hr **Rectal:** 3 mg every 6-8 hr Oral tablet: 2mg, 4 mg, 8 mg	Oral tablet: 2 mg, 4 mg, 8 mg Oral tablet, extended release: 8 mg, 12 mg, 16 mg Injection solution: 1 mg/mL, 2 mg/mL, 4 mg/mL, 10 mg/mL Rectal suppository: 3 mg	Constipation, N/V, somnolence	Dose reductions with renal impairment: Injection - ↓ initial dose by ¼ to ½ Oral - ↓ initial dose for moderate impairment (CrCl 40-60mL/min); use alternative analgesic in severe impairment (CrCl < 30 mL/min) Note: ER form should only be used in opioid tolerant patients; Exalgo® requires REMS training for prescribers	$ Tablets: 2 mg (20) = $1,5.33 4 mg (20) = $1,6.01 8 mg (20) = $2,9.51 Solution: 4 mg/mL (20 mL) = $42.99

34

Medication Generic (brand)/ Palliative Care Indications	Usual Doses	How Supplied	Major Side Effects	Comments	Cost $-$$$[1,2] Dose (quantity)
Oxycodone (OxyContin®, Oxy IR®, Roxicodone®) • Pain • Dyspnea	**Oral:** immediate release 5-20 mg every 4-6 hr PRN	Oral solution: 5 mg/5 mL, 20 mg/mL Oral tablet: 5 mg, 10 mg, 15 mg, 20 mg, 30 mg Oral tablet, extended release: 10 mg, 20 mg, 40 mg, 80 mg	Pruritus, constipation, N/V, dizziness, somnolence	Long acting OxyContin® is brand name only, therefore, insurances may not cover until cheaper long-acting opioid has failed (i.e., morphine)	$$-$$$ <u>12 hr tablets:</u> OxyContin® 10 mg (20) = $50.61 20 mg (20) = $85.34 40 mg (20) = $153.50 60 mg (20) = $211.44 80 mg (20) = $287.10 <u>Tablets:</u> Oxycodone 5 mg (20) = $22.76 10 mg (20) = $15.99 15 mg (20) = $20.78 30 mg (20) = $27.71
Oxymorphone (Opana®, Opana ER®) • Pain • Dyspnea	**Oral:** immediate release 5-20 mg every 4-6 hr PRN; extended release 5 mg every 12 hr	Oral Tablet: 5 mg, 10 mg Oral Tablet, extended release: 7.5 mg, 15 mg	Pruritus, constipation, N/V, dizziness, somnolence	Take on empty stomach	$$$ <u>Tablets:</u> 5 mg (20) = $71.99 <u>12 hr tablets:</u> 5 mg (20) = $47.99 7.5 mg (20) = $65.99 10 mg (20) = $84.99 15 mg (20) = $114.99 20 mg (20) = $145.99 40 mg (20) = $250.00
Fentanyl (Duragesic®, Sublimaze®, Fentora®, Actiq®, Lazanda®, Abstral®, Onsolis®, SUBSYS®) • Non-IV administration: chronic, moderate to severe pain Continued on next page	**Do not use non-IV in opioid-naïve patients.** Please note: only the most commonly used agents & doses have been listed **Transdermal:** dose based on patient's current 24-hr oral morphine equivalent. Replaced every 72 hrs **Fentora® buccal tablet:** initially 100 mcg (titrate by 100 mcg). Dissolve tablet in buccal cavity. No more than 2 doses per pain episode with at least 4 hrs between treating pain episodes	Injection solution: 0.05 mg/mL Intravenous solution: 0.05 mg/mL, 50 mcg/mL Transdermal patch, extended release: 12 mcg/hr, 25 mcg/hr, 50 mcg/hr, 75 mcg/hr, 100 mcg/hr Buccal tablet: 100 mcg, 200 mcg, 300 mcg, 400 mcg, 600 mcg, 800 mcg	Pruritus, sweating, N/V, asthenia, confusion, somnolence, urinary retention	A 25 mcg/hr transdermal patch is equianalgesic to ~50 mg of oral morphine/day **Black Box warning:** Non-IV fentanyl containing products are for pain management in patients who are opioid tolerant to at least the equivalent of a 25 mcg patch. Use for acute or post-op pain is contraindicated. **Black box warning:** do not convert on a mcg to mcg basis from any other fentanyl products to FENTORA®[3]	$$$ <u>Tablets:</u> Fentora® 200 mcg (28) = $791.02 Fentanyl citrate 400 mcg (30) = $599.93 1,200 mcg (30) = $799.93 <u>72 hr patches:</u> Fentanyl 100 mcg/hr (5) = $215.99 75 mcg/hr (5) = $201.97 50 mcg/hr (5) = $129.99 12 (12.5) mcg/hr (5) = $95.27

34

Medication Generic (brand)/ Palliative Care Indications	Usual Doses	How Supplied	Major Side Effects	Comments	Cost $-$$$[1,2] Dose (quantity)
Fentanyl —continued	**Actiq® lozenge:** initially 200 mcg for breakthrough pain episode; may repeat once per episode. Must wait at least 4 hrs before treating another pain episode. Dose may be titrated			Initial Fentora® dose is always 100 mcg except if a patient has already been using Actiq® (see table 2)[3] Fentora® may cause mouth sores in patients with dry mouth *Access of the following formulations is restricted according to REMS program[2]: – Abstral® (fentanyl SL tablet) – Actiq® (fentanyl lozenge) – Fentora® (fentanyl buccal tablet) – Lazanda® (fentanyl nasal spray) – SUBSYS® (fentanyl sublingual spray) *Access to the following is restricted to enrollment in the FOCUS™ program: - Onsolis™ (fentanyl buccal film)	Lozenge: Actiq® 200 mcg (20) = $927.31 400 mcg (20) = $1,194.94 600 mcg (20) = $1,436.93 800 mcg (20) = $1,671.84 1,600 mcg (20) = $2,627.02
Methadone (Dolophine®, Methadose®) • Pain	**Oral:** initial dose 2.5-10 mg every 8-12 hr (based on patient 24-hr oral morphine equivalents)	Oral Solution: 5 mg/5 mL, 10 mg/5 mL, 10 mg/mL Oral Tablet: 5 mg, 10 mg Oral Tablet for Suspension: 40 mg used only in methadone maintenance programs Injection Solution: 10 mg/mL	Cardiac dysrhythmia, hypotension, diaphoresis, constipation, N/V, asthenia, dizziness, respiratory depression	Long half life, accumulates with repeated doses; needed dose adjustment should be made every 3-5 days. Multiple drug interactions.	$ Tablets: 5 mg (20) = $11.99 10 mg (20) = $11.99 Dispersible tablets: 40 mg (20) = $16.99

34

Medication Generic (brand)/ Palliative Care Indications	Usual Doses	How Supplied	Major Side Effects	Comments	Cost $-$$$[1,2] Dose (quantity)
Tramadol (Ultram®)[4] • Pain	**Oral:** immediate release 50-100 mg every 4-6 hr (max 400 mg/day; 300 mg/day for elderly)	Oral Tablet: 50 mg Oral Tablet, extended release: 100 mg, 200 mg	Pruritus, constipation, N/V, dizziness, headache, somnolence	50 mg tramadol is equianalgesic to ~60 mg of oral codeine Risk of seizures has been reported in patients using tramadol at recommended and high doses, but risk is greater during concurrent antidepressant use[4]	$-$$$ Tablets: 50 mg (30) = $16.99 24 hr tablets: 100 mg (30) = $109.99 200 mg (30) = $145.99
Tapentadol (Nucynta®) • Pain	**Oral:** immediate release, Day 1: 50-100 mg every 4-6 hr (max 700 mg/day), Day 2 (Max 600 mg/day)	Oral Tablet: 50 mg, 75 mg, 100 mg Oral Tablet, extended release: 50 mg, 100 mg, 150 mg, 200 mg, 250 mg	Constipation, N/V, dizziness, somnolence	Currently no generic available	$$ Tablets: 50 mg (20) = $65.99
NSAIDS					
Aspirin • Pain	**Oral:** 325-650 mg every 4-6 hr (max 4 g/day)	Oral tablet: 81 mg, 325 mg Oral tablet, chewable: 81 mg Oral tablet, enteric coated: 81 mg, 325 mg, 500 mg, 650 mg Rectal suppository: 120 mg, 300 mg, 600 mg	GI ulcer, bleeding, tinnitus, bronchospasm, angioedema, Reye's syndrome	High risk of bleeding, particularly GI. Use with caution in preexisting liver disease and avoid in severe liver disease. Least potent inhibitor of renal prostaglandins	$ Tablets: 325 mg (100) = $11.99 Chewable: 81 mg (36) = $11.99
Diclofenac (Voltaren®, Voltaren XR®) • Pain • Inflammation	**Oral:** immediate release 50 mg TID (max 150 mg/day)	Oral tablet, enteric coated: 25 mg, 50 mg, 75 mg Oral tablet, extended release: 75 mg, 100 mg	Blood coagulation disorder. Burning sensation in the eye, lacrimation, keratitis. CHF, hypertension, GI bleed	Arthrotec: combination product containing either 50 or 75 mg of enteric coated diclofenac and 200 mcg of misoprostol Flector[5]: 1.3% patch (180 mg) applied to most painful site BID (VERY minimal systemic absorption)	$$-$$$ Tablets: 50 mg (60) = $39.99 24 hr tablets: 100 mg (60) = $153.98 EC tablets: 25 mg (60) = $75.99 75 mg (60) = $47.99

34

Medication Generic (brand)/ Palliative Care Indications	Usual Doses	How Supplied	Major Side Effects	Comments	Cost $-$$$[1,2] Dose (quantity)
Ibuprofen (Motrin®, Advil®) • Pain • Inflammation	**Oral:** 200-400 mg every 4-6 hr (max 1.2 g/day)	Oral capsule, liquid-filled: 200 mg Oral suspension: 100 mg/5 mL, 50 mg/1.25 mL Oral tablet: 200 mg, 400 mg, 600 mg, 800 mg Oral tablet, chewable: 100 mg	Hypotension, Rash, Hypernatremia, Flatulence, N/V, Thrombocytosis, GI bleed	Low risk of inducing hepatotoxicity but should be avoided in severe hepatic impairment Possible increase in nephrotoxicity Use caution with concomitant use in patients on low-dose aspirin for cardioprotection	$ <u>Tablets:</u> 400 mg (30) = $11.99 600 mg (30) = $13.99 800 mg (30) = $12.99
Indomethacin (Indocin®) • Pain • Inflammation	**Oral:** 25-50 mg BID to TID (max 200 mg/day)	Oral capsule: 25 mg, 50 mg Oral capsule, extended release: 75 mg	Headache, tinnitus, dizziness, GI side effects, nephrotoxicity	Higher risk of nephrotoxicity vs. other NSAIDS. May aggravate depression or other psychological disturbances secondary to CNS penetration	$-$$ <u>Capsules:</u> 25 mg (30) = $15.99 50 mg (30) = $15.99 <u>CR capsules:</u> 75 mg (30) = $82.15
Ketorolac (Toradol®) • Pain • Inflammation	**IM:** 60 mg single dose or 30 mg every 6 hr (max 120 mg/day) **IV:** 30 mg single dose or 30 mg every 6 hr (max 120 mg/day) **Oral:** 20 mg, followed by 10 mg every 4-6 hr (max 40 mg/day)	Intramuscular solution: 30 mg/mL Injection: 15 mg/mL, 30 mg/mL Oral tablet: 10 mg	High incidence of headache, increased nephrotoxicity, GI complications	Use no longer than 5 days Use 15 mg in patients older than 65 years of age, less than 50 kg, or with renal impairment	$$ <u>Tablets:</u> 10 mg (30) = $24.99
Nabumetone (Relafen®) • Pain • Inflammation	**Oral:** 1,000 mg/day (max 2,000 mg/day)	Oral tablet: 500 mg, 750 mg	Edema, pruritus, abdominal pain, constipation, indigestion, N/V, occult blood in stools, increased LFTs, dizziness headache, tinnitus	Less GI bleeding and side effects (vs. COX 2 inhibitors) Reduce dose in hepatic dysfunction to daily or BID dosing	$$ <u>Tablets:</u> 500 mg (60) = $40.99 750 mg (60) = $68.99
Naproxen (Aleve®, Naprosyn®) • Pain • Inflammation	**Oral:** initial 500 mg, then 250 mg every 6-8 hr (max 1,250 mg/day)	Oral suspension: 25 mg/mL Oral tablet: 250 mg, 375 mg, 500 mg Oral tablet, enteric coated: 375 mg, 500 mg	Edema, pruritus, rash, constipation, ototoxicity, tinnitus, dyspnea	Increased hepatotoxicity (decrease dose 50% in hepatic disease) and possible nephrotoxicity, high tissue penetration, potent inhibitor of leukocyte function	$-$$$ <u>Suspension:</u> 25 mg/mL (500 mL) = $51.49 <u>Tablets:</u> 250 mg (90) = $15.99 375 mg (90) = $18.99 500 mg (60) = $19.99 <u>EC tablets:</u> 375 mg (60) = $39.99 500 mg (60) = $64.99

34

Medication Generic (brand)/ Palliative Care Indications	Usual Doses	How Supplied	Major Side Effects	Comments	Cost $-$$$$[1,2] Dose (quantity)
Mefenamic acid (Ponstel®) • Pain • Inflammation	**Oral:** initial 500 mg, then 250 mg every 4 hr (max therapy duration 1 week)	Oral capsule: 250 mg	Increased GI side effects		$$$$ Capsules: 250 mg (30) = $429.99
Meloxicam (Mobic®) • Pain • Inflammation	**Oral:** initial 7.5 mg once daily (max 15 mg/day)	Oral suspension: 7.5 mg/5 mL Oral tablet: 7.5 mg, 15 mg	Edema, abdominal pain, constipation, diarrhea, indigestion, N/V, headache, upper respiratory infection, fever	Decreased GI bleeding and side effects (vs. COX 2 inhibitors)	$-$$ Suspension: 7.5 mg/5 mL (100 mL) = $86.99 Tablets: 7.5 mg (30) = $15.99 15 mg (30) = $12.99
Piroxicam (Feldene®) • Pain • Inflammation	**Oral:** 10-20 mg once daily (max dose 20 mg/day)	Oral capsule: 10 mg, 20 mg	Doses > 20 mg associated with increased GI side effects. Hepatotoxicity	High risk of serious GI adverse effects vs. other NSAIDS. Daily to BID dosing	$$-$$$ Capsules: 10 mg (30) = $77.68 20 mg (30) = $134.28
Sulindac (Clinoril®) • Pain • Inflammation	**Oral:** 150-200 mg BID (max 400 mg/day)	Oral tablet: 150 mg, 200 mg	GI side effects: abdominal cramps, abdominal pain, constipation, diarrhea, flatulence, indigestion, loss of appetite, N/V	High risk of hepatotoxicity vs. other NSAIDS, use caution and low doses in cirrhosis, marketed as "renally sparing" but reports of renal failure exist, caution in renal insufficiency	$ Tablets: 150 mg (60) = $18.99 200 mg (60) = $27.98
Celecoxib (Celebrex®) • Pain	**Oral:** initial 400 mg, additional 200 mg can be given on day 1 if needed, maintenance dose 200 mg twice daily	Oral capsule: 50 mg, 100 mg, 200 mg, 400 mg	Hypertension, diarrhea, headache, myocardial infarction	Decreased incidence of GI ulcerations, minimal to no inhibition of platelet function, cross allergy with sulfonamides, similar renal effects to traditional NSAIDS, use 100 mg daily dose if possible because of adverse CV effects with long term use No generic available	$$$ Capsules: 100 mg (30) = $90.99 200 mg (30) = $140.99 400 mg (30) = $208.98

34

Medication Generic (brand)/ Palliative Care Indications	Usual Doses	How Supplied	Major Side Effects	Comments	Cost $-$$$[1,2] Dose (quantity)
Non-Acetylated Salicylates					
Salsalate (Disalcid®) • Pain • Inflammation	**Oral:** 3,000 mg/day in 2-3 divided doses	Oral tablet: 500 mg, 750 mg	Rash, nausea, tinnitus, hypertension, renal impairment, hepatic impairment, GI bleed		$ Tablets[5]: 500 mg (100) = $39.99 750 mg (100) = $76.65
Other Analgesics					
Acetaminophen (Tylenol®, APAP®, Paracetamol®) • Pain • Antipyretic	**Oral:** 650 to 1,000 mg every 4-6 hr as needed (max 3,000-4,000 mg/day 3000 mg/day in elderly) **Rectal:** 650 mg every 4-6 hr as needed (max 6 suppositories/day) **IV:** (≥ 50 kg) 1,000 mg every 6 hr or 650 mg every 4 hr, (< 50 kg) 15 mg/kg every 6 hr or 12.5 mg/kg every 4 hr; minimum dosing interval 4 hrs, max single dose 15 mg/kg or 750 mg; max daily dose 75 mg/kg/day or 3750 mg/day	Oral capsule: 500 mg Oral elixir/liquid/syrup: 160 mg/5 mL Oral solution: 160 mg/5 mL, 80 mg/0.8 mL, 500 mg/5 mL Oral suspension: 160 mg/5 mL, 80 mg/0.8 mL Oral tablet: 325 mg, 500 mg Oral tablet, chewable: 80 mg, 160 mg Oral tablet, extended release: 650 mg Rectal suppository: 120 mg, 325 mg, 650 mg Intravenous solution: 10 mg/ml	Pruritus, constipation, N/V, headache, insomnia, agitation, atelectasis, liver failure	Doses of more than 4 grams/day can lead to liver failure Found in many over the counter preparation	$(oral form)-$$ (IV form) Tablets: 500 mg (100) = $16.99 Injection: 1,000 mg (1) = $10.27

34

Medication Generic (brand)/ Palliative Care Indications	Usual Doses	How Supplied	Major Side Effects	Comments	Cost $-$$$[1,2] Dose (quantity)
Anticonvulsants					
Gabapentin (Neurontin®) • Neuropathic pain	**Oral:** initial: 100 mg TID, increase by 100 mg TID every 3 days, common dosage range 300-3,600 mg/day in 3 divided doses	Oral capsule: 100 mg, 300 mg, 400 mg Oral solution: 250 mg/5 mL Oral tablet: 100 mg, 300 mg, 400 mg, 600 mg, 800 mg	Peripheral edema, N/V, viral disease, ataxia, dizziness, nystagmus, somnolence, hostile behavior, fatigue	Adjust dose for renal dysfunction (CrCl < 60 mL/min) No significant documented drug-drug interactions Do not stop abruptly	$-$$$ Capsules: 100 mg (90) = $43.99 300 mg (90) = $18.99 400 mg (90) = $74.99 Solution: 250 mg/5 mL (470 mL) = $139.99 Tablets: 600 mg (90) = $97.99 800 mg (90) = $99.99
Pregabalin (Lyrica®) • Neuropathic pain • Fibromyalgia	**Oral:** initial 150 mg/day in divided BID or TID (max 300 mg/day in 2-3 divided doses)	Oral capsule 25 mg, 50 mg, 75 mg, 100 mg, 150 mg, 200 mg, 225 mg, 300 mg	Angioedema Peripheral edema Increased appetite and, weight gain. Constipation, xerostomia, ataxia, dizziness, headache, Incoordination, blurred vision, disturbance in thinking, euphoria	Adjust dose for renal dysfunction (CrCl < 60 mL/min) No significant documented drug-drug interactions Do not stop abruptly Doses up to 600 mg have been studied with no significant additional benefit and an increase in adverse effects Currently no generic available	$$$ Capsules: Any strength (30) = $91.99
Oxcarbazepine (Trileptal®) • Neuropathic pain	**Oral:** 300 mg BID, increase by 300 mg/day every 3 days, common dosage range 600-2,400 mg/day	Oral suspension: 300 mg/5 mL Oral tablet: 150 mg, 300 mg, 600 mg	Hyponatremia, abdominal pain, N/V, abnormal gait, dizziness, headache, nystagmus, fatigue	Anecdotal data: less adverse effects than carbamazepine Renal dose: start at 150 mg BID and titrate slowly	$$-$$$ Suspension: 300 mg/5 mL (250 mL) = $147.99 Tablets: 150 mg (60) = $79.99 300 mg (60) = $131.00 600 mg (60) = $259.98
Lamotrigine (Lamictal®) • Neuropathic pain	**Oral:** 25 mg QOD x 2 weeks, increase to 25 mg daily x 2 weeks, increase by 25-50 mg/day every 1-2 weeks, common dosage range 50-400 mg/day	Oral tablet: 25 mg, 100 mg, 150 mg, 200 mg Oral tablet, chewable: 5 mg, 25 mg	Rash, abdominal pain, diarrhea, N/V, ataxia, dizziness, headache, somnolence, diplopia	Do not stop abruptly	$-$$ Tablets: 25 mg (60) = $17.99 100 mg (60) = $17.99 150 mg (60) = $31.99 200 mg (60) = $31.99 Chewable: 25 mg (60) = $179.99

34

Medication Generic (brand)/ Palliative Care Indications	Usual Doses	How Supplied	Major Side Effects	Comments	Cost $-$$$[1,2] Dose (quantity)
Topiramate (Topamax®) • Migraine • Neuropathic pain	**Oral:** 25-50 mg daily, increase by 25-50 mg every week (max 1,600 mg/day)	Oral capsule: 15 mg, 25 mg Oral tablet: 25 mg, 50 mg, 100 mg, 200 mg	Flushing, diarrhea, loss of appetite, altered sense of taste, weight loss, confusion, dizziness, paraesthesia, somnolence, upper respiratory infection, fatigue	Limited data for use in neuropathic pain	$-$$ Capsules: 15 mg (60) = $70.99 25 mg (60)= $85.99 Tablets: 25 mg (60) = $29.99 50 mg (60) = $39.99 100 mg (60) = $49.99 200 mg (60) = $49.99
Zonisamide (Zonegran®) • Neuropathic pain	**Oral:** 100 mg at bedtime, increase every 2 weeks, common dosage range 200-400 mg at bedtime	Oral capsule: 25 mg, 50 mg, 100 mg	Loss of appetite, ataxia, confusion, dizziness, somnolence, agitation	Cross sensitivity with sulfa allergy. Limited data regarding weight loss	$$ Capsules: 25 mg (100) = $49.99 50 mg (100) = $91.99 100 mg (100) = $188.86
Levetiracetam (Keppra®) • Partial seizures • Neuropathic pain	**Oral:** 500 mg BID-TID, increase every 2 weeks, usual dosage range 1-3 g/day	Intravenous: 100 mg/mL Oral solution: 100 mg/mL Oral tablet: 250 mg, 500 mg, 750 mg, 1,000 mg Oral tablet, extended release: 500 mg, 750 mg	Loss of appetite, infections, asthenia, headache, somnolence, nasopharyngitis, fatigue	Used for neuropathic pain and migraines Dose reduce in renal insufficiency (CrCl < 80 mL/min)	$$-$$ Oral solution: 100 mg/mL (473mL) = $259.99 24 hr tablets: 500 mg (30) = $32.99 Tablets: 500 mg (30) = $29.99 1,000 mg (30) = $122.00
Carbamazepine (Tigerton®, Tegretol®) • Trigeminal & glosso-pharyngeal neuralgia	**Oral:** 100 mg BID, usual dosage range 200 mg BID-QID	Oral tablet: 200 mg Oral tablet, chewable: 100 mg Oral tablet, extended release: 200 mg, 400 mg Oral capsule, extended release: 100 mg, 200 mg, 300 mg Oral suspension: 100 mg/5 mL	Hypertension, hypotension, N/V, dizziness, nystagmus, somnolence, blurred vision, atrioventricular block, CHF, liver failure, renal failure, agranulocytosis	Monitor CBC, LFTs, serum therapeutic levels (4-12 mcg/mL) Multiple drug-drug interactions via enzyme induction levels increased by enzyme inhibitors, high plasma protein binding	$-$$ Tablets: 200 mg (90) = $14.99 Chewable: 100 mg (60) = $14.99 12 hr tablets: 200 mg (60) = $54.99 400 mg (60) = $106.65 12 hr capsules: 100 mg (60) = $105.98 300 mg (60) = $105.98 Suspension: 100 mg/5 mL (450 mL) = $67.95

34

Medication Generic (brand)/ Palliative Care Indications	Usual Doses	How Supplied	Major Side Effects	Comments	Cost $-$$$[1,2] Dose (quantity)
Valproic acid (Depakene®, Divalproex®, Depakote®) • Migraine • Neuropathic pain	**Oral:** 125 mg TID, usual dosage range 500-1,000 mg TID	Valproic acid: Oral capsule, liquid-filled: 250 mg Oral syrup: 250 mg/5 mL Divalproex®: Oral capsule, delayed release sprinkles: 125 mg Oral tablet, delayed release: 125 mg, 250 mg, 500 mg Oral tablet, extended release: 250 mg, 500 mg	Liver dysfunction, pancreatitis, low platelets, N/V	Monitor serum therapeutic levels (50-100 mcg/mL), CYP450 enzyme inhibitor	$-$$$ Capsules: Valproic acid 250 mg(60)=$39.98 Syrup: Valproate® sodium 250 mg/5 mL (150 mL) = $17.99 Capsule sprinkles: Divalproex® sprinkles 125 mg(60)=$51.98 24 hr tablets: Divalproex® sodium 250 mg(60)=$83.99 500 mg(60)=$35.99 EC tablets: Divalproex® sodium 125 mg(60) = $15.00 250 mg(60) = $18.00 500 mg(60) = $29.99
Phenytoin (Dilantin®) • Neuropathic pain	**Oral:** 300 mg daily or 100 mg TID, usual dosage range 300-400 mg/day	Oral suspension: 100 mg/4 mL, 125 mg/5 mL Oral tablet, chewable: 50 mg	Pruritus, constipation, gingival hyperplasia, N/V, osteomalacia, ataxia, confusion, nephrotoxicity, low platelets	Monitor serum levels: (10-20 mcg/mL therapeutic range) Decreased efficacy vs. other agents	$-$$ Suspension: 125 mg/5 mL (237 mL) = $28.98 Chewable: Dilantin® Infatabs 50 mg (90) = $63.99 Capsules: Dilantin® 30 mg (90) = $54.99 100 mg (90) = $58.99 ER Capsules: 100 mg (90)= $31.99
Tricyclic Antidepressants (TCAs)					
Amitriptyline (Elavil®) • Neuropathic pain	**Oral:** 25 mg at bedtime (10 mg if patient is frail or elderly); may increase at weekly intervals to a max dose of 150 to 200 mg/day	Oral tablet: 10 mg, 25 mg, 50 mg, 75 mg, 100 mg, 150 mg	Somnolence, weight gain, anticholinergic effects, arrhythmias, worsening depression	Monitor BP	$ Tablets: 10 mg (30) = $11.99 25 mg (30) = $12.99 50 mg (30) = $12.99

34

Medication Generic (brand)/ Palliative Care Indications	Usual Doses	How Supplied	Major Side Effects	Comments	Cost $-$$$[1,2] Dose (quantity)
Nortriptyline (Pamelor®) • Neuropathic pain	**Oral:** 25 mg at bedtime (10 mg if patient is frail or elderly); may increase at weekly intervals to a max dose of 150 mg/day	Oral capsule: 10 mg, 25 mg, 50 mg, 75 mg Oral solution: 10 mg/5 mL Oral tablet: 25 mg	Somnolence, weight gain, anticholinergic effects, arrhythmias, worsening depression	Monitor BP	$ Capsules: 10 mg (30) = $17.99 25 mg (30) = $12.99 50 mg (30) = $19.99 Solution: 10 mg/5 mL (473 mL) = $53.99
Desipramine (Norpramin®) • Neuropathic pain	**Oral:** 25 mg at bedtime (10 mg if patient is frail or elderly); may increase at weekly intervals to a max dose of 100 to 200 mg/day	Oral tablet: 10 mg, 25 mg, 50 mg, 75 mg, 100 mg, 150 mg	Somnolence, weight gain, anticholinergic effects, arrhythmias, worsening depression	Monitor BP	$$ Tablets: 10 mg (30) = $36.99 25 mg (30) = $38.99 50 mg (30) = $62.50
Benzodiazepines					
Lorazepam (Ativan®) • Anxiety • Insomnia	**Oral:** Anxiety: initially, 2 to 3 mg/day divided into 2 to 3 daily doses Maintenance: 2 to 6 mg/day divided into 2 to 3 doses. Insomnia: 2 to 4 mg at bedtime	Oral solution: 2 mg/mL Oral tablet: 0.5 mg, 1 mg, 2 mg Injection: 2 mg/mL, 4 mg/mL	Asthenia, dizziness, sedation, unsteadiness, transient amnesia	Elimination half-life: 12-14 hrs	$-$$ Solution: 2 mg/mL (30 mL) = $44.99 Tablets: 2 mg (30) = $21.99
Clonazepam (Klonopin®) • Anxiety • Insomnia	**Oral:** Anxiety: 0.25 mg BID; may increase to 1 mg/day after 3 days Insomnia: 0.25-0.5 mg at bedtime	Oral tablet: 0.5 mg, 1 mg, 2 mg Oral tablet, disintegrating 0.125 mg, 0.25 mg, 0.5 mg, 1 mg, 2 mg	Somnolence, abnormal coordination, ataxia, depression, dizziness, memory impairment, seizures, increased salivation	Elimination half-life: 30-40 hrs	$-$$$ ODT: 0.25 mg (30) = $38.49 0.5 mg (30) = $37.50 1 mg (30) = $46.99 2 mg (30) = $55.99 Tablets: 0.5 mg (30) = $13.99 1 mg (30) = $11.99
Diazepam (Valium®) • Anxiety • Insomnia • Skeletal muscle spasm	**Oral:** Anxiety: 2-10 mg BID/QID Muscle spasm: 2-10 mg BID-QID **IV/IM:** Anxiety: 2-10 mg every 3-4 hr (max 30 mg/8 hours) Muscle spasm: 5-10 mg every 3-4 hr PRN	Oral solution: 5 mg/5 mL Oral tablet: 2 mg, 5 mg, 10 mg Injection: 5 mg/mL	Ataxia, euphoria, incoordination, somnolence, diarrhea, hypotension, rash, muscle weakness, respiratory depression	Elimination half-life: 20-50 hrs, prolonged in elderly	$-$$$ Solution: 1 mg/mL (60 mL) = $16.47 Tablets: 2 mg (30) = $13.99 5 mg (30) = $11.99 10 mg (30) = $12.99

34

Medication Generic (brand)/ Palliative Care Indications	Usual Doses	How Supplied	Major Side Effects	Comments	Cost $-$$$[1,2] Dose (quantity)
Oxazepam (Serax®) • Anxiety • Insomnia	**Oral:** Mild/moderate: 10-15mg TID-QID PRN Severe, agitation or associated with depression: 15-30 mg TID-QID PRN	Oral capsule: 10 mg, 15 mg, 30 mg	Dizziness, headache, sedation, somnolence, drug dependence, withdrawal sign or symptom		$$ Capsules: 10 mg (30) = $17.99 15 mg (30) = $45.99 30 mg (30) = $43.72
Temazepam (Restoril®) • Anxiety • Insomnia	**Oral:** 7.5 to 30 mg at bedtime	Oral tablet: 7.5 mg, 15 mg, 22.5 mg, 30 mg	Hypotension, somnolence, blurred vision		$ Capsules: 15 mg (30) = $12.99 30 mg (30) = $14.99
Alprazolam (Xanax®) • Anxiety • Insomnia	**Oral:** 0.25 to 0.5 mg TID, may increase every 3 to 4 days if necessary (max 4 mg in divided doses)	Oral tablet: 0.25 mg, 0.5 mg, 1 mg, 2 mg Oral tablet, disintegrating: 0.25 mg, 0.5 mg, 1 mg, 2 mg Oral tablet, extended release: 0.5 mg, 1 mg, 2 mg, 3 mg Oral solution: 1 mg/mL	Drowsiness, depression, headache, constipation, diarrhea, dry mouth	Elimination half-life: 11 hrs	$-$$ 24 hr tablets: 1 mg (30) =$69.99 2 mg (30) = $75.99 3 mg (30) = $109.98 ODT: 0.25 mg (30) = $11.99 0.5 mg (30) = $12.99 1 mg (30) = $12.99 2 mg (30) = $15.99 Tablets: 0.25 mg (30) = $11.99 0.5 mg (30) = $12.99 1 mg (30) = $12.99 2 mg (30) = $15.99
Midazolam (Versed®) • Sedation	**Oral:** 10 to 20 mg at bedtime (doses may vary depending on individual patient needs)	Oral solution: 2 mg/mL Oral syrup: 2 mg/mL Injection solution: 1 mg/mL, 5 mg/mL	Excessive somnolence, headache, hiccups		$ Inj. Solution (1 mg/mL): Package of 25 x 2 mL = $12.95

34

Medication Generic (brand)/ Palliative Care Indications	Usual Doses	How Supplied	Major Side Effects	Comments	Cost $-$$$[1,2] Dose (quantity)
Antidepressants					
Fluoxetine (Prozac®) • Depression	**Oral:** initially 20 mg daily in the morning. May increase after several weeks if inadequate response (max dose 80 mg daily) OR 90 mg once a week (weekly capsule), starting 7 days after the last daily dose of 20 mg	Oral capsule: 10 mg, 20 mg, 40 mg Oral capsule, delayed release: 90 mg Oral solution/syrup: 20 mg/5 mL Oral tablet: 10 mg, 20 mg	Headache, nausea, vomiting, insomnia, anorexia, anxiety, asthenia, diarrhea, nervousness, somnolence, dizziness, dry mouth, dyspepsia, sweating, tremor, decrease libido		$-$$$ Capsule (delayed release): 90 mg (4) = $123.99 Capsules: 10 mg (30) = $14.99 20 mg (30) = $24.99 40 mg (30) = $40.99 Solution: 20 mg/5 mL (120 mL) = $19.99 Tablets: 10 mg (30) = $13.99 20 mg (30) = $27.99
Sertraline (Zoloft®) • Depression	**Oral:** 50 mg daily; may be increased at intervals of at least 1 week to a (max dose of 200 mg/day)	Oral solution: 20 mg/mL Oral tablet: 25 mg, 50 mg, 100 mg	Diarrhea, nausea, headache, insomnia, ejaculation disorder, dizziness, dry mouth, fatigue, somnolence, agitation, anorexia, constipation, dyspepsia, decrease libido		$-$$ Solution: 20 mg/mL (60) = $59.99 Tablets: 50 mg (30) = $12.99 100 mg (30) = $15.99
Citalopram (Celexa®) • Depression	**Oral:** 20 mg daily; dose increases should usually occur in increments of 20 mg at intervals of no less than one week (max dose 40 mg/day)	Oral solution: 10 mg/5 mL Oral tablet: 10 mg, 20 mg, 40 mg	Diaphoresis, constipation, diarrhea, nausea, vomiting, xerostomia, dizziness, headache, insomnia, sedation, tremor, agitation, disorder of ejaculation, fatigue		$$$ Solution: 10 mg/5 mL (240 mL) = $99.99 Tablets: 10 mg (30) = $16.99 20 mg (30) = $39.99 40 mg (30) = $26.99
Mirtazapine (Remeron®) • Depression • Insomnia	**Oral:** 15 mg daily; may increase in dose every 1-2 weeks (max dose of 45 mg/day)	Oral tablet: 7.5 mg, 15 mg, 30 mg, 45 mg Oral disintegrating tablet: 15 mg, 30 mg, 45 mg	Somnolence, weight gain, xerostomia, increased appetite, constipation, asthenia, weight gain, dizziness, increased serum triglycerides, dream disorder, ALT increased		$$ Tablets: 7.5 mg (30) = $49.99 15 mg (30) = $ 55.99 30 mg (30) = $49.99 45 mg (30) = $45.99 ODT: 15 mg (30) = $70.99 30 mg (30) = $79.99 45 mg (30) = $71.49

34

Medication Generic (brand)/ Palliative Care Indications	Usual Doses	How Supplied	Major Side Effects	Comments	Cost $-$$$[1,2] Dose (quantity)
Duloxetine (Cymbalta®) • Diabetic peripheral neuropathy • Fibromyalgia • Depression	**Oral:** 20-60 mg /day (daily-BID)	Oral capsule, Delayed Release: 20 mg, 30 mg, 60 mg	Nausea, headache, xerostomia, somnolence, insomnia	Avoid abrupt discontinuation of therapy; taper the dose to avoid withdrawal; if intolerable symptoms, resume the previous dose followed by smaller decreases	<u>Capsule (delayed Release):</u> 30 mg (30) = 181.98 60 mg (30) = 181.98 (20 mg capsule's price is not available via drugstore.com)
Antipsychotics					
Haloperidol (Haldol®) • Delirium • Nausea & vomiting	**IM, IV, Oral:** <u>Nausea:</u> 0.5-2 mg (no PO) every 4-8 hr PRN[6] <u>Delirium:</u> Mild: 0.25-0.5 mg every 4-8 hr PRN Moderate: 1-2 mg every 4-8 hr PRN Severe: 2-5 mg every 4-8 hr PRN	Oral solution: 2 mg/mL Oral tablet: 0.5 mg, 1 mg, 2 mg, 5 mg, 10 mg, 20 mg	Hypotension, constipation, xerostomia, akathisia, dystonia, extrapyramidal symptoms, somnolence, blurred vision, prolonged QT interval		$-$$ <u>Tablets:</u> 0.5 mg (60) = $14.99 1 mg (60) = $13.33 2 mg (60) = $19.99 5 mg (60) = $17.99 10 mg (60) = $72.99 20 mg (60) = $124.99
Olanzapine (Zyprexa®) • Delirium • Nausea & vomiting	**Oral:** <u>Delirium:</u> 5 mg daily for up to 5 days <u>Chemotherapy-associated delayed N/V</u> (unlabeled use; in combination with a corticosteroid and serotonin [5HRT$_3$] antagonist): 10 mg daily for 3-5 days	Oral disintegrating tablet: 5 mg, 10 mg, 15 mg, 20 mg Oral tablet: 2.5 mg, 5 mg, 7.5 mg, 10 mg, 15 mg, 20 mg	Orthostatic hypotension, peripheral edema, hypercholester-olemia, hyperglycemia, increased appetite, increased prolactin level, serum triglycerides raised, weight gain, constipation, xerostomia, dizziness, somnolence tremor	ODT is currently not available as generic	$$$ <u>ODT:</u> Zyprexa® Zydis®: 5 mg (30) = $470.01 10 mg (30) = $659.97 <u>Tablets:</u> 10 mg (30) = $379.98 15 mg (30) = $490.03
Quetiapine (Seroquel®) • Delirium • Insomnia	**Oral:** <u>Delirium:</u> 50 mg BID; may increase as necessary on a daily basis in increments of 50 mg BID (max dose 400 mg/day) <u>Insomnia:</u> 25 mg at bedtime	Oral tablet: 25 mg, 50 mg, 100 mg, 200 mg, 300 mg, 400 mg Oral tablet, extended release: 50 mg, 150 mg, 200 mg, 300 mg, 400 mg	Hypertension, orthostatic hypotension, tachycardia, serum cholesterol & triglyceride increase, weight gain, abdominal pain, constipation, increased appetite, indigestion, increased liver enzymes, dizziness, tremor, lethargy, agitation, fatigue		$$$ <u>Tablets:</u> 25 mg (60)= $212.09 50 mg (60) = $375.00 100 mg (60) = $364.98 200 mg (60) = $683.97 <u>24 hr tablet:</u> 50 mg (60) = $337.99 150 mg (60)= $597.99 200 mg (60) = $673.99

34

Medication Generic (brand)/ Palliative Care Indications	Usual Doses	How Supplied	Major Side Effects	Comments	Cost $-$$$[1,2] Dose (quantity)
Psychostimulants					
Methylphenidate (Ritalin®, Methylin®) • Counter opioid related sedation • Counter cancer related fatigue • Depression[6]	**Oral:** 7.5 mg BID, may start from 2.5-5 mg and titrate up (max 60 mg/day)	Oral solution: 5 mg/5 mL, 10 mg/5 mL Oral tablet: 5 mg, 10 mg, 20 mg Oral tablet, extended release: 10 mg, 18 mg, 20 mg, 27 mg, 36 mg, 54 mg	Headache, tics, decreased appetite, insomnia, nausea, vomiting, abdominal pain, anorexia, dizziness, insomnia, vomiting, anorexia		$-$$ Tablets: 5 mg (20) = $29.99 10 mg (20) = $15.99 20 mg (20) = $20.99 CR tablets: 20 mg (20) = $35.99
Dextroamphetamine (Dexedrine®) • Counter opioid related sedation • Counter cancer related fatigue	**Oral:** immediate-release 5 to 60 mg in 2 to 3 divided daily; sustained-release 5 to 60 mg daily	Oral tablet: 5 mg, 10 mg Oral capsule, extended release: 5 mg, 10 mg, 15 mg	Loss of appetite, xerostomia, insomnia, feeling nervous, irritability, restlessness		$-$$ Tablets: 5 mg (20) = $12.99 10 mg (20) = $18.46 24 hr capsule: 5 mg (20) = $41.29 10 mg (20) = $59.20 15 mg (20) = $69.49
Modafinil (Provigil®) • Counter opioid related sedation • Counter disease related fatigue	**Oral:** 200 mg daily in the morning; doses up to 400 mg have been used	Oral tablet: 100 mg, 200 mg	Rash, nausea, dizziness, headache, insomnia, anxiety, feeling nervous		$$$ Tablets: 100 mg (30) = $528.98 200 mg (30) = $723.02
Steroids					
Dexamethasone (Decadron®)[6] • Acute spinal cord compression • Increased intracranial pressure • Pain related to nerve compression, visceral distension, bone metastases • Nausea • Anorexia	**Oral:** Nerve compression, visceral distention: 4-8 mg every 8-12 hr Nausea/bone pain: 4-12 mg daily **IV:** Spinal cord compression: 40-100 mg or equivalent as loading doses or every 6 hours x 1st 24-72 hours Nausea/bone pain: 4-12 mg daily	Oral elixir: 0.5 mg/5 mL Oral solution: 0.5 mg/5 mL, 1 mg/mL Oral tablet: 0.5 mg, 0.75 mg, 1 mg, 1.5 mg, 2 mg, 4 mg, 6 mg	Adrenal suppression, psychosis insomnia, vertigo, acne, osteoporosis, myopathy, delayed wound healing	Increased risk of infection due to immune suppression	$ Elixir: 0.5 mg/mL (120 mL) = $49.99 Solution: 4 mg/mL (25 mL) = $37.99 Tablets: 0.5 mg (30) = $12.99 0.75 mg (30) = $13.99 1 mg (30) = $19.99 1.5 mg (30) = $12.99 2 mg (30)= $21.99 4 mg (30) = $19.99 6 mg (30) = $22.99

34

Medication Generic (brand)/ Palliative Care Indications	Usual Doses	How Supplied	Major Side Effects	Comments	Cost $-$$$[1,2] Dose (quantity)
Prednisone (Deltasone®, Predicort®, Sterapred®) • Asthma • Disorders of respiratory, nervous, & immune systems	**Oral:** 5-60 mg daily; varies based on patient response	Oral tablet: 1 mg, 2.5 mg, 5 mg, 10 mg, 20 mg, 50 mg Oral solution: 5 mg/5 mL	Adrenal suppression, psychosis, agitation insomnia, vertigo, acne, osteoporosis myopathy, delayed wound healing, cushingoid appearance	Increased risk of infection due to immune suppression	$ Tablets: 1 mg (30) = $14.99 2.5 mg (30) = $12.99 5 mg (30) = $12.99 10 mg (30) = $11.99 20 mg (30) = $11.99 50 mg (30) = $17.99 Solution: 5 mg/5 mL (30 mL) = $14.99
Anticoagulants					
Warfarin (Coumadin®) • Venous thromboembolic event (VTE)	**Oral:** 2 to 5 mg PO/IV daily; adjust dose based on the results of INR; usual maintenance, 2 to 10 mg PO/IV once a day	Oral tablet: 1 mg, 2 mg, 2.5 mg, 3 mg, 4 mg, 5 mg, 6 mg, 7.5 mg, 10 mg	Intraocular hemorrhage, cholesterol embolus syndrome, tissue necrosis, blood dyscrasias, fever, "purple toe" syndrome	Requires monitoring of INR	$ Tablets: 1 mg (30) = $13.99 2 mg (30) = $14.99 2.5 mg (30) = $14.99 3 mg (30) = $15.99 4 mg (30) = $14.99 5 mg (30) = $13.99 7.5 mg (30) = $23.99 10 mg (30) = $24.99
Enoxaparin (Lovenox®) • PE • DVT treatment & prophylaxis	**Injection:** DVT treatment: 1 mg/kg SC every 12 hr OR 1.5 mg/kg SC every 24 hr DVT prophylaxis: 40 mg SC every 24 hr	Subcutaneous solution: 30 mg/0.3 mL, 40 mg/0.4 mL, 60 mg/0.6 mL, 100 mg/mL, 80 mg/ 0.8 mL, 150 mg/mL, 120 mg/ 0.8 mL	Diarrhea, nausea, anemia, bleeding, major thrombocytopenia, increased liver function test, fever		$$$$ Injection: 30 mg/0.3 mL (3) = $65.97 40 mg/0.4 mL (3) = $80.97 60 mg/0.6 mL (3) = $127.97 80 mg/0.8 mL (3) = $174.96 100 mg/mL (3) = $208.97 150 mg/mL (3) = $337.99
Dalteparin (Fragmin®) • VTE in patient with cancer • DVT prophylaxis	**Injection:** VTE: 200 IU/kg (max 18,000 IU) SC every 24 hr for 30 days; then 150 IU/kg SC every 24 hr for 2-6 months; dosing not established after 6 months. DVT prophylaxis: 5,000 IU SC every 24 hr	Subcutaneous solution: 10,000 IU/mL, 2,500 IU/0.2 mL, 15,000 IU/0.6 mL, 5,000 IU/0.2 mL, 7,500 IU/0.3 mL, 18,000 IU/0.72 mL, 12,500 IU/0.5 mL, 25,000 IU/mL	Hematoma, injection site pain, irritation		$$$$ Injection: 2,500 IU/0.2 mL (0.2) = $29.77 5,000 IU/0.2 mL (0.2) = $39.99 10,000 IU/mL (1) = $77.16

34

Medication Generic (brand)/ Palliative Care Indications	Usual Doses	How Supplied	Major Side Effects	Comments	Cost $-$$$[1,2] Dose (quantity)
Fondaparinux (Arixtra®) • DVT treatment	**Injection:** 5 mg (< 50 kg), 7.5 mg (50 to 100 kg), or 10 mg (>100 kg) SC daily	Subcutaneous solution: 2.5 mg/0.5 mL, 5 mg/0.4 mL, 7.5 mg/0.6 mL, 10 mg/0.8 mL	Injection site reaction, rash, fever	Currently no generic available	$$$-$$$$ Injection: 2.5 mg/0.5 mL (10) = $593.04 7.5 mg/0.6 mL (1) = $1,354.14

Sedatives

Medication Generic (brand)/ Palliative Care Indications	Usual Doses	How Supplied	Major Side Effects	Comments	Cost $-$$$[1,2] Dose (quantity)
Zolpidem (Ambien®) • Insomnia	**Oral:** immediate release 10 mg once immediately before bedtime (max 10 mg/day); extended release 12.5 mg immediately before bedtime; oral spray 10 mg (2 sprays directly into mouth over the tongue) immediately before bedtime (max 10 mg/day); sublingual 10 mg immediately before bedtime	Oral tablet: 5 mg, 10 mg Oral tablet, extended release: 6.25 mg, 12.5 mg Sublingual tablet: 5 mg, 10 mg Mucous membrane spray: 5 mg/0.1 mL	Diarrhea, nausea, allergy, dizziness, drugged state, headache, somnolence, visual disturbance		$-$$ Tablets: 5 mg (30) = $17.99 10 mg (30) = $17.99 CR tablets: 6.25 mg (30) = $155.99 12.5 mg (30) = $155.99
Trazodone (Desyrel®) • Antipepressant • Insomnia	**Oral:** immediate release 150 mg/day in divided doses; may increase dosage by 50 mg/day every 3 to 4 days (max 400 mg/day for outpatients and 600 mg/day for inpatients); extended release 150 mg once daily in the evening, preferably at bedtime; may increase by 75 mg/day every 3 days (max 375 mg/day)	Oral tablet: 50 mg, 100 mg, 150 mg, 300 mg Oral tablet, extended release: 150 mg, 300 mg	Blurred vision, dizziness, drowsiness, dry mouth, fatigue, headache, nausea/vomiting constipation, confusion, edema, weight change, tremor	When used for insomnia, dose at bedtime only	$ Tablets: 50 mg (30) = $11.99 100 mg (30) = $13.99 150 mg (30) = $20.87 300 mg (100) = $402.20
Pentobarbital (Nembutal®) • Sedation	**IM:** 150 to 200 mg **IV:** 100 mg IV initially; after 1 min, may give additional small doses at 1 min. intervals, if necessary, up to total of 500 mg	Injection solution: 50 mg/mL	Confusion, dizziness, somnolence, agitation		$$$ Injection: 50 mg/mL (20 mL) = $594.64

34

Propofol (Diprivan®) • Sedation	**IV:** 1 mg/kg followed by 0.5 mg/kg every 3 to 5 min as needed for sedation	Intravenous emulsion: 10 mg/mL	Injection site pain, nausea, vomiting, involuntary movement, bradyarrhythmia, heart failure, hypertension		$ Emulsion: Package of 25x20 mL = $180.00 ($7.20/vial)
Phenobarbital (Luminal®) • Sedation	**Oral:** Daytime sedation: 30-120 mg divided into 2 or 3 doses (max 400 mg/day) Hypnotic: 100-320 mg as a single dose (solution) or 100-200 mg/day (max 400 mg/day)	Oral elixir: 20 mg/5 mL Oral solution: 20 mg/5 mL Oral tablet: 15 mg, 16.2 mg, 30 mg, 32.4 mg, 60 mg, 64.8 mg, 97.2 mg, 100 mg	Respiratory depression, somnolence	Available in suppository form via compounding pharmacy	$ Elixir: 20 mg/5 mL (473 mL) = $26.96 Tablets: 16.2 mg (30) = $14.99 32.4 mg (30) = $15.99 64.8 mg (30) = $17.99
Anticholinergic					
Hyoscyamine (Levsin®)[7] • Excessive respiratory secretions	**Sublingual:** 0.125 mg TID to QID	Oral tablet: 0.125 mg, 0.15 mg Oral tablet, disintegrating: 0.125 mg Oral capsule, extended release: 0.375 mg Sublingual tablet: 0.125 mg Oral elixir: 0.125 mg/5 mL Oral liquid: 0.125 mg/mL	Diminished sweating, xerostomia, dizziness, somnolence, blurred vision, mydriasis, delay when starting to pass urine		$$ Tablet: 0.125 mg (30) = $31.99 ODT: 0.125 mg (30) = $26.99 12 hr tablet: 0.375 mg (30) = $37.99 SL tablet: 0.125 mg (30) = $26.99 Liquid: Levsin® 0.125 mg/mL (15 mL) = $45.99
Scopolamine patch[6] (Transderm-Scop®) • Nausea & vomiting • Excessive respiratory secretions	**Transdermal:** 1 patch behind ear every 3 days (steady state in 24 hours)	Transdermal patch, extended release: 0.33 mg/24 hr	Xerostomia, somnolence, blurred vision	Currently not available as generic	$$$ 72 hr patch: 1.5 mg (4) = $69.00
Glycopyrrolate (Robinul®)[7] • Excessive respiratory secretions	**IV:** 0.1-0.2 mg TID PRN	Injection solution: 0.2 mg/mL Oral Tablet: 1 mg, 2 mg	Flushing, constipation, vomiting, xerostomia, nasal congestion		$$ Tablets: 1 mg (30) = $31.50 2 mg (30) = $45.33

34

Medication Generic (brand)/ Palliative Care Indications	Usual Doses	How Supplied	Major Side Effects	Comments	Cost $-$$$[1,2] Dose (quantity)
Atropine eye drops[8] • Excessive respiratory secretions	**Oral:** 1-2 drops every 4-6 hr PRN	Ophthalmic solution: 1 %	Tachycardia, constipation, xerostomia, blurred vision, photophobia		$$ Solution: 1% (5 mL) = $23.99
Antidiarrheals					
Diphenoxylate + Atropine (Lomotil®) • Diarrhea	**Oral:** 2 tablets or 10 mL QID (20 mg/day of diphenoxylate) until control achieved, then reduce dosage to amount necessary to maintain bowel control (max dose 20 mg/day of diphenoxylate)	Oral solution: 0.025-2.5 mg/5 mL Oral tablet: 0.025-2.5 mg	Abdominal discomfort, nausea, vomiting, dizziness, sedation, somnolence, euphoria, malaise		$ Liquid: 0.025-2.5 mg/5 mL (60 mL) = $20.60 Tablets: 0.025-2.5 mg (30) = $14.99
Loperamide (Imodium®) • Diarrhea	**Oral:** 4 mg followed by 2 mg after each loose stool (max 16 mg/day)	Oral capsule/tablet: 2 mg Oral liquid/solution: 1 mg/5 mL	Dizziness, fatigue, abdominal pain, constipation, nausea, dry mouth		$ Capsules: 2 mg (30) = $12.99
Tincture of opium, deodorized (DTO®) • Diarrhea	**Oral:** 0.6 mL QID (max 6 mL daily)	Tincture: 10 mg/mL	Nausea, vomiting, lightheadedness, dizziness, drowsiness, constipation	Contains alcohol	$$$ Tincture: 10 mg/mL (118 mL) = $542.00
Laxatives					
Methylnaltrexone (Relistor®) • Opioid-induced constipation	**Subcutaneous:** (< 38 kg or > 114 kg) 0.15 mg/kg (round dose up to nearest 0.1 mL of volume) (38 to < 62 kg) 8 mg (62-114 kg) 12 mg; administer 1 dose every other day as needed (max 1 dose/24 hours)	Injection solution: 12 mg/0.6 mL	Diaphoresis, abdominal pain, flatulence, nausea, dizziness	Dosed according to body weight (kg)	$$ Injection: 1 vial = $55.20
Sennosides (Senokot®) • Constipation	**Oral:** 1-2 tablets (8.6-17.2 mg) BID (max 4 tablets BID)	Oral tablet: 8.6 mg, 17 mg, 25 mg Solution/syrup: 176 mg/5 mL 8.8 mg/5 mL	Abdominal pain, diarrhea, excessive bowel activity, melanosis coli, nausea, hypokalemia, yellow-brown urine discoloration, nephritis		$ Tablets: 8.6 mg (100) = $11.99

34

Medication Generic (brand)/ Palliative Care Indications	Usual Doses	How Supplied	Major Side Effects	Comments	Cost $-$$$[1,2] Dose (quantity)
Polyethylene Glycol (Miralax®) • Constipation	**Oral:** 17 g (1 Tbsp) in 8 oz. water	Oral powder for solution: 17 g/dose	Abdominal distension and cramping, flatulence, excessive bowel activity, nausea		$$ Oral Powder: 17 g/dose (527 g) = $39.99
Bisacodyl (Dulcolax®) • Constipation	**Oral:** 5-15 mg daily (max 30 mg/day) **Rectal:** 10 mg suppository daily	Oral tablet, enteric coated: 5 mg Rectal suppository: 10 mg Rectal enema: 10 mg/1.25 oz	Abdominal cramping, excessive diarrhea, nausea, vomiting		$ Suppository: 10 mg (100) = $25.99 Tablets: 5 mg (100) = $9.99
Magnesium Citrate • Constipation	**Oral:** 150-300 mL once, may repeat as needed	Oral solution: 1.75 g/30 mL	Diarrhea, asthenia, dizziness		$ Oral solution: 1.75 g/30 mL (296 mL) = $1.92
Lactulose (Enulose®, Kristalose®) • Constipation • Encephalopathy	**Oral:** 15-30 mL daily; may increase to 60 mL (40 grams lactulose)/day, if needed	Oral solution/syrup: 10 g/15 mL Kristalose® (oral powder for suspension): 10 g/packet, 20 g/packet	Bloating, diarrhea, epigastric pain, flatulence, nausea, vomiting, muscle cramping		$$ Solution: 473 mL = $19.98 Oral Powder: Kristalose® pack 10 g (30) = $57.57 20 g (30) = $79.86

Key:

BID—2 times per day
CR—controlled release
CV—cardiovascular
DVT—deep vein thrombosis
EC—enteric coated
ER—extended release
GI—gastrointestinal
hr—hour(s)
IM—intramuscular
IR—immediate release
IV—intravenous

LFT—liver function test
N/V—nausea & vomiting
ODT—orally disintegrating tablet
oz—ounce
PRN—as needed
QID—4 times per day
SR—sustained release
TID—3 times per day
Tbsp—tablespoon
VTE—venous thromboembolism
XR—extended release

34

Table 2: Initial Fentora® Dosing Recommendations for Patients on Actiq®[1,2]

Current Actiq® Dose (mcg)	Initial Fentora® Dose*
200	100 mcg tablet
400	100 mcg tablet
600	200 mcg tablet
800	200 mcg tablet
1200	2 x 200 mcg tablets
1600	2 x 200 mcg tablets

* From this initial dose, titrate patient to effective dose.

Table 3: The Transmucosal Immediate Release Fentanyl (TIRF) Risk Evaluation and Mitigation Strategy (REMS) Program[8]

- An FDA-required program designed to ensure informed risk-benefit decisions before initiating treatment, & while patients are treated to ensure appropriate use of TIRF medicines
- The purpose of the TIRF REMS Access program is to mitigate the risk of misuse, abuse, addiction, overdose & serious complications due to medication errors with the use of TIRF medicines
- You must enroll in the TIRF REMS Access program to prescribe, dispense, or distribute TIRF medicines

- Included medications
  - Abstral® (fentanyl sublingual tablet)
  - Actiq® (fentanyl oral transmucosal lozenge)
  - Fentora® (fentanyl buccal tablet)
  - Lazanda® (fentanyl nasal spray)
  - Onsolis™ (fentanyl buccal soluble film)
  - Subsys® (fentanyl sublingual spray)
  - Approved generic equivalents of these products are also covered under this program

- TIRF medicines are indicated only for the management of breakthrough pain in adult cancer patients 18 years of age and older (16 years of age and older for Actiq® brand and generic equivalents) who are already receiving and who are tolerant to around-the-clock opioid therapy for their underlying persistent cancer pain.
  Patients considered opioid-tolerant are those who are taking:
  - At least 60 mg of oral morphine/daily
  - At least 25 mcg transdermal fentanyl/hour
  - At least 30 mg of oral oxycodone daily
  - At least 8 mg oral hydromorphone daily
  - At least 25 mg oral oxymorphone daily
  - Or an equianalgesic dose of another opioid daily for a week or longer

- TIRF medicines are contraindicated
  - In opioid non-tolerant patients
  - In the management of acute or postoperative pain, including headache/migraine and dental pain
  - For use in the emergency room

- For further information call 1-866-822-1483 or visit online at www.TIRFREMSaccess.com

34

Table 4: List of Additional Medication Tables by Chapter

Chapter	Table/Appendix Number—Title
6: Pain	4—Considerations in the Use of NSAIDs and Acetaminophen 6—Selective Co-Analgesics for Pain Appendix 6-B—Opioid Titration Guidelines Appendix 6-C—Opioid Equianalgesics Appendix 6-D—Guidelines for Opioid Rotation Appendix 6-E—Guide for the Use of Methadone
9: Insomnia	3—Pharmacological Management of Insomnia
10: Constipation	2—Pharmacological Management of Constipation
11: Nausea and Vomiting	3—Antiemetic Drugs In Palliative Care
12: Delirium	3—Suggested Dosing Of Common Antipsychotics
15: Psychosocial Aspects	3—Anxiety-Inducing Medications 4—Pharmacological Management of Anxiety 5—Commonly Prescribed Benzodiazepines: A Comparison Chart 8—Pharmacological Management of Depression 9—Selected Herbal Preparation and Dietary Supplements for Depression 10—Atypical Anti-Psychotic Medications Used for the Treatment of Schizophrenia and Bipolar Disorder 11—Mood-Stabilizing Medications
17: HIV/AIDS	Appendix 17-A—FDA Approved Antiretroviral Medications
19: Heart Failure	5—Common Pharmacological Management for Heart Failure 6—Common Pharmacological Management of Heart Failure Symptoms In Pediatric Palliative Care
20: Pulmonary	3—COPD Treatment Management 4—Pharmacological Management of COPD 5—Pulmonary Medication Delivery Systems 8—Pharmacological Management of Pulmonary Hypertension
21: Renal	3—Clinical Algorithm and Preferred Medications To Treat Pain in Dialysis Patients
23: Neurological Conditions	1—Summary of Dementia Medications 2—Summary of Antiparkinson Medications 3—Common Side Effects of Levodopa
24: Diabetes	3—Types of Insulin
25: Hypercalcemia	3—Treatment Measures to Reverse Hypercalcemia
26: SIADH	4—Pharmacological Management of SIADH
28: Pediatrics	7—Analgesic Doses for Children 6 Months To 50 kg Appendix 28-A—Pediatric Symptom Management
29: The Older Adult Population	4—Principles of Pain Management in the Older Adult 6—Common Pharmacological Changes with Aging Influencing Pain Management 9—Drugs Commonly Causing Delirium In The Older Adult With Cancer
32: Care of the Actively Dying Patient	4—Medications Commonly Used for Palliative Sedation

34

CITED REFERENCES

1. Drugstore.com. 2012. Available at: www.drugstore.com/. Accessed April 16, 2012.
2. Micromedex® 2.0. *Truven Health Analytics.* 2012. Available at: www.micromedex.com. Accessed January 26, 2012.
3. Cephalon, Inc. *Fentora—Prescribing Information.* 2011. Available at: www.fentora.com/pdfs/pdf100_prescribing_info.pdf. Accessed January 26, 2012.
4. Sansone RA, Sansone LA. Tramadol: seizures, serotonin syndrome, and coadministered antidepressants. *Psychiatry.* 2009;6(4):17-21.
5. King Pharmaceuticals, Inc. *Flector—Prescribing Information.* 2011. Available at: nccs-dailymed.nlm.nih.gov/dailymed/drugInfo.cfm?id=60126#section-14.3. Accessed January 26, 2012.
6. Abrahm JA. *Physician's Guide to Pain and Symptom Management in Cancer Patients.* 2nd ed. Baltimore, MD: Johns Hopkins University Press; 2005: 200-204,338,368,410.
7. Back IN, Jenkins K, Blower A, Beckhelling J. A study comparing hyoscine hydrobromide and glycopyrrolate in the treatment of death rattle. *Palliat Med.* 2001;15(4):329-636.
8. De Simone GG, Eisenchlas JHR, Junin M, Pereyra F, Brizuela R. Atropine drops for drooling: a randomized controlled trial. *Palliat Med.* 2006;20:665-671.
9. Federal Food and Drug Administration. *The Transmucosal Immediate Release Fentanyl (TIRF) Risk Evaluation and Mitigation Strategy (REMS) Program.* Available at: www.TIRFREMSaccess.com. Accessed October 23, 2012.

34

CHAPTER 35

OXYGEN: FROM SUPPLEMENTAL THERAPY TO MECHANICAL VENTILATION

Sterling R Bouxman, RRT, RN, ACNP BC, MSN

I. **INTRODUCTION**

The use of oxygen and mechanical ventilation is often necessary in the setting of compromised cardiopulmonary function and oxygenation. Conditions include neurological, musculoskeletal, rheumatologic, oncological, cardiac, pulmonary, as well as trauma. The benefits and burdens of oxygen therapy should always be weighed with an inclination toward providing therapy than withholding it. Patients, their respective families, or caregivers are often unaware of the specifics of care, lifestyle restrictions, and quality-of-life issues imposed by oxygen therapies.

Oxygen may be delivered by several methods. The goal is to utilize the lowest oxygen concentration possible to achieve oxygenation. Delivery systems vary from very low supplemental oxygen to the provision of 100% oxygen, meeting all of the patient's ventilatory requirements. Systems include low flow, high flow, heated humidified therapy, noninvasive positive pressure ventilation, and invasive ventilation. This chapter will discuss various types and forms of supplemental oxygen, providing a basic introduction to the terms and the processes of oxygen therapy and both noninvasive and invasive ventilation. Additionally, the implications and requirements imposed by ventilatory support, including equipment and lifestyle limitations, particularly for end-of-life care are presented. The palliative APRN assists in decision-making and patient and family support. Collaboration with respiratory therapists, pulmonologists, and other members of the interdisciplinary team optimizes the use of these technologies.

II. **SUPPLEMENTAL OXYGEN**

  A. Goal of oxygen therapy is to achieve a resting oxygen saturation (Spo_2) of > 90% (although a goal of > 88% may be used in patients with severe disease), or partial pressure of oxygen in the blood (Pao_2) of $\geq$ 60 mm Hg.[1]

  B. Benefits

  1. Supplemental oxygen may decrease hypoxic vasoconstriction, thereby reducing pulmonary artery pressure and development of cor pulmonale.

  2. Oxygen reduces respiratory and heart rate, thereby conserving the body's energy stores, diminishing cardiac demands.

  3. In states of hypoxia, oxygen improves cognition, perfusion of oxygen to organs and tissues, sleep quality, and exercise tolerance.

  4. Currently, oxygen is the only treatment shown to provide a survival benefit in chronic obstructive pulmonary disease (COPD).[2-4]

35

C. The a need for supplemental oxygen is determined by clinical signs and symptoms such as dyspnea, heart rate, blood pressure, respiratory rate, use of accessory muscles of breathing, changes in respiratory pattern, restlessness, pallor, headache, diaphoresis, cyanosis, and changes in cognition. Pulse oximetry, arterial blood gas analysis, pulmonary function testing, and a 6-minute walk test establish baseline oxygen and carbon dioxide levels and baseline functional capacity.[1]

D. Complications

1. Physiologically, even the use of low oxygen concentrations, while generally safe, may result in absorption atelectasis and, although rare, hypercapnia resulting in respiratory acidosis.[5]

2. High concentration oxygen $\geq$ 50% is associated with oxygen. Oxygen toxicity is generally associated with concentrations greater than or equal to 50%.[5] Oxygen damage caused by free radical formation may decrease lung compliance, damage to the small airways, and a reduced diffusion capacity across the alveolar membrane.[5] Therefore, whenever possible, reduction of Fio_2 (fraction of inspired oxygen) is advised.[5]

E. Long-term oxygen therapy is always indicated in individuals with a Pao_2 of $\leq$ 55 mm Hg and oxygen saturation of $\leq$ 88% and in individuals with a Pao_2 of 55-59 in the presence of pulmonary hypertension, sequelae of right heart failure, cor pulmonale, and erythrocytosis.[1]

F. Oxygenation Monitoring

In order to promote optimal care, an understanding of oxygen monitoring is essential.

1. Pulse oximetry is an inexpensive, quick assessment of oxygenation status. Of note, pulse oximetry does not directly measure oxygen saturation (Spo_2). The probe placed on the finger measures two wavelengths of infrared light and applies the absorbed light reaching the probe sensor to an algorithm in the unit. Low blood flow as with reduced cardiac output; elevated serum levels of methemoglobin, carboxyhemoglobin, and bilirubin; some fingernail polishes; and strong ambient sunlight may adversely affect the accuracy of the oximeter.

2. Arterial blood gas (ABG) more accurately measures direct oxygen saturation.

3. The use of transcutaneous carbon dioxide ($Ptcco_2$) is increasing. This method uses a transcutaneous sensor, which measures carbon dioxide in the blood. Prior to its use, an ABG should be drawn to correlate the results with that of the $Ptcco_2$ to ensure accuracy.

III. OXYGEN DELIVERY SYSTEMS

35

A. Supplemental oxygen is available in multiple forms and delivery devices. The delivery system is determined by the patient's oxygen requirement based on tidal volume, respiratory rate, oxygen saturation, clinical status, and setting of care. Currently, the maximum amount of oxygen available in the home for long-term use is 10 liters per minute (L/min) via oxygen concentrator. Transient higher flow rates are attainable via compressed gas systems but are not suitable for long-term use at higher flow rates.

B. There are 2 classifications of oxygen delivery systems—low flow and high flow. Table 1 delineates commonly used low flow and high flow devices

    1. High flow systems meet all of the patient's respiratory requirements. These systems deliver precise concentrations of oxygen to the patient and are generally available in the acute care and LTAC (long-term acute care) setting.

    2. Low flow systems deliver a set liter flow and the oxygen concentration delivered depends on the patient's inspiratory rate, tidal volume, and mask fit.

        a) Mostly used for mild to moderate hypoxemia.

        b) Low flow is appropriate in the skilled and home setting as well as inpatient settings.

Table 1: Low Flow and High Flow Oxygen Delivery Systems[1,6]

Low Flow	High Flow
• Nasal cannula (1-6 L/min, Fio_2 24-40%) • Non-rebreather (10+ L/min, Fio_2 60-100%) • Simple face mask (5-10 L/min, Fio_2 35-50%) • Nasal cannula with reservoir • Oxymizer® (0.5-12 L/min, Fio_2 varies with liter flow) • Large volume nebulizer (28-98%); used in inpatient settings	• High flow nasal cannula (up to 100%) • Venturi mask (range from 24-50%) • Dual large volume nebulizers (varies)

C. Low Flow Oxygen Devices

    1. The nasal cannula is designed for a liter flow of 1-6 L/min. One liter per minute will provide approximately 24% oxygen, and each additional liter per minute will provide an additional 4% oxygen concentration, giving a range of 25-40%.[7]

        a) Nasal cannulas that have small reservoirs built into the system (e.g., Oxymizer® mustache and pendant) and provide higher concentrations of oxygen and utilize a higher flow rate than a standard nasal cannula.

        b) Pulse-dose nasal administration via nasal cannula is an oxygen conservation device that delivers oxygen only upon inspiration. It is available in the outpatient setting using a portable oxygen concentrator with pulse-dose capabilities.[8]

    2. A non-rebreather mask achieves high oxygen concentrations in an emergency transport setting, emergency department, and medical or intensive care units. It provides from 60-90% oxygen and should be used with a liter flow of ≥ than 10 L/min. Proper mask fit, respiratory rate, tidal volume, and liter flow affect the actual concentration delivered.[9]

        a) Transtracheal oxygen is a relatively uncommon, low flow oxygen delivery system. Oxygen is delivered by a catheter that is surgically placed into the trachea between the second and third tracheal rings. It can be used in tandem with other oxygen delivery systems. Only clinicians with specialized training should manipulate the catheter unless there is a life-threatening emergency.

D. High Flow Devices

    1. These devices use wall mounted oxygen delivery from a centrally located liquid oxygen source. The most commonly used high flow systems are the heated high flow system, and the air entrainment mask

35

a) Heated high flow device—similar in appearance to a nasal cannula, but accommodates a higher gas flow rate. The oxygen,delivered via wall source, passes through humidification and mixing system is a precise oxygen concentration. This enables delivery of high concentrations of oxygen (up to 100%) and allows the patient to eat and speak unencumbered while wearing this device.

b) The air entrainment—used exclusively for inpatient or emergent settings. The mask fits over the mouth and nose, with a sized or adjustable port that draws room air into a specific mixing ratio to deliver a precise preset concentration of oxygen. The faster the oxygen flow, the more ambient air drawn into the system. The mask has a range of oxygen concentration of 24-50% depending upon the size of the entrainment port. Obstructed entrainment ports or tubing (e.g., water, kinked tubing) decrease the flow rate, but increase oxygen concentration.

IV. SOURCES OF OXYGEN

1. Oxygen sources and their associated benefits and detriments are listed in Table 2. Of note, all oxygen, regardless of delivery system used, supports combustion, but will not explode.

2. In the home setting, there are 3 basic sources of supplemental oxygen— compressed gas, liquid reservoirs, and oxygen concentrators. Determination of system utilization is based on multiple factors including cost, portability, availability, weight, home electrical source, patient's ambulatory status, patient/families' ability to refill tanks, and oxygen requirements of the patient.

3. Oxygen delivery in the inpatient setting is generally from central liquid systems. When the oxygen system is used, the gas passes through a flowmeter, which regulates the pressure and delivers a set liter flow into the tubing, which connects to the delivery device.

Table 2: Benefits and Negative Aspects for Home Oxygen Delivery Systems[1,8,10]

Oxygen Source	Benefits	Negative Aspects	Liter Flow
Oxygen concentrator	• Steady supply • No refilling required • Limited liter flow • Low cost • Available in larger home units & smaller lighter-weight portable units • Available in pulse-dose mode or continuous & pulse-dose mode	• Requires electricity in either wall source or battery— backup oxygen system is needed in case of power outages • Less accurate at higher flow rates • High noise levels	Up to 10 L/min— home units only
Compressed gas	• Can be used at higher liter flows • Not dependent upon electricity • Low cost	• Damage to tank may cause tank to be a projectile • Requires frequent refilling • Portable tanks are larger & heavier than liquid systems and have less capacity	Up to 15+ L/min
Liquid reservoir	• Easy of portability for ambulatory use • Reduced tank weight • Requires less frequent filling than compressed gas	• Potential of thermal burns during refilling portable tanks as oxygen is at −222.65 °C • Higher costs	Up to 6 L/min

35

4. Compressed gas is used for transporting patient within the hospital or outside the hospital. All oxygen tanks are green in color. Green oxygen tanks with colored bands representing different oxygen-gas mixture. Yellow tanks contain compressed air only.

5. Air compressors are available for home use. They do not provide supplemental oxygen but utilize room air to power a medication nebulizer. There are portable compressors that run on battery, as well as the more familiar electric air compressor models.

V. INTRODUCTION TO MECHANICAL VENTILATION

A. When palliative care consultations are requested, mechanical ventilation may already be in place or it may be the focus of an advance care planning discussion. Its use in hospice settings may be limited by expense and its life prolonging intent. Mechanical ventilation (MV) is a common artificial method of providing gas exchange in a patient with respiratory failure, with the inability to adequately oxygenate, eliminate carbon dioxide, or to preserve and/or protect the airway. Unlike a natural breath that occurs because of the negative pressure within the lungs produced by the action of respiratory musculature, MV forces air into the lungs with positive pressure. There are non-invasive and invasive or conventional forms of MV.[11]

B. Non-invasive positive pressure ventilation (NIPPV) is a form of MV that uses only a face mask interface. It is frequently used for respiratory failure during an exacerbation of COPD or heart failure, in patients who have expressed wishes to forgo intubation, or as temporary measure for patients and families considering long-term mechanical ventilation. NIPPV is commonly used for obstructive and central sleep apnea in the home setting. A disadvantage of NIPPV is that it may not meet the patient's ventilatory requirements and offers no airway protection. NIPPV may assist the patients' respiratory requirements in 2 modes—continuous positive airway pressure (CPAP) or bilevel positive airway pressure (BiPAP).

1. CPAP is not appropriate for some patients. It provides the same level of preset pressure to the patient during the inspiratory and expiratory phase of respiration, and is most frequently used in sleep apnea.

2. BiPAP delivers 2 levels of preset pressure, a higher level for inspiration, and a lesser and a residual pressure during expiration. It creates a more natural feeling breath for the patient, and may be better tolerated.

C. Invasive mechanical ventilation involves delivery of positive pressure to force air into the lungs via an endotracheal or tracheostomy tube.[11]

1. Ventilators have evolved from the original negative pressure "body box" of the 1950's to the positive pressure mechanical ventilators used today. A rarely used negative pressure ventilator that seals the upper body at the waist and neck, known as a cuirass or "shell," is available.[12]

2. Indications for invasive mechanical ventilation include hypoxemic or hypercarbic respiratory failure. Neuromuscular, neurological, and cardiac disease among others may be underlying etiologies for respiratory failure. Invasive mechanical ventilation improves oxygenation, decreases the work of breathing, or reverses respiratory acidosis.[12] It is used in settings or trauma to maintain a patent airway.

35

3. Invasive mechanical ventilation is used for surgical procedures and airway protection.

4. Patients with COPD or other pulmonary impairments may frequently retain serum CO_2. Over time, the kidneys may compensate through retention of bicarbonate, offsetting the elevated $Paco_2$ and normalizing the pH. This is considered chronic respiratory failure, or compensated respiratory acidosis. When there is an acute rise in the $Paco_2$ and acidosis in a patient that has chronic respiratory failure, it is known as acute on chronic respiratory failure.

5. Assessment—there are critical considerations to initiation of invasive MV. Will the MV be short-term or long-term? Can the underlying etiology or disease process be resolved? Is the use of MV for a progressive and irreversible condition such as neuromuscular diseases or pulmonary disease? Could the patient be "bridged," or the underlying medical issues ameliorated by a trial of non invasive positive pressure ventilation (NIPPV)? Does the patient want or can the patient tolerate NIPPV?

6. The decision to pursue invasive mechanical ventilation requires careful, thoughtful information and education of the patient and family regarding risks, benefits, and care requirements. It is far more difficult emotionally, and sometimes legally, to stop the process once it has been initiated. Therefore, it is incumbent upon the APRN to discuss its indications, reasonable expectations of its use, possible outcomes, and futile care. Education should include description of placement and maintenance of a tracheostomy, suctioning, as well as quality of life and physical limitations imposed by long-term invasive mechanical ventilation.

7. Utilizing the correct terminology in regard to MV allows for better education of patients and families. The term mechanical ventilator, or ventilator should be used, and not a "respirator." A respirator is a face mask type device that is used to block particulate matter from entering the upper airway, such as caring for patients with tuberculosis.

8. There are many methods of mechanical ventilation, and the patient's physical characteristics, underlying disease process, reasons for instituting the mechanical ventilation, and respiratory requirements, are taken into consideration prior to initiating a given mode of ventilation and setting the ventilator parameters.

D. Providing Invasive Mechanical Ventilation

1. To provide invasive mechanical ventilation, a patient must be intubated using an endotracheal tube (ETT) or tracheostomy tube. The ETT is initially used. Once the ETT is placed, mechanical breaths are delivered via a bag valve mask, often called an Ambu Bag®. The stomach and lungs should be auscultated to insure that there is proper ETT placement. A CO_2 detector is frequently used to assess proper placement. A chest radiograph is obtained to confirm ETT placement.

35

2. All of the parameters for each delivered breath by the ventilator are preset by the clinician, discussed below, as are alarms settings. A full set of backup parameters are also set based upon the goals and modes of ventilation.

3. The essential ventilator settings are the mode of ventilation (discussed below), tidal volume, respiratory rate, percentage of oxygen delivered with

each breath, trigger sensitivity, inspiratory flow rate, and positive end expiratory pressure.[11]

a) The fraction of inspired oxygen, referred as the Fio_2, is the percentage of oxygen delivered with each breath. It is expressed as a decimal with 1.0 representing 100% oxygen, and as examples, an Fio_2 of 30% and 50% are expressed as 0.3 and 0.5 respectively.

b) Trigger sensitivity is the level of effort required to trigger the ventilator to deliver a breath. It detects either the negative pressure generated by the patient's inspiratory effort, or a reduction in the flow of gas within the circuit when the patient attempts to take a breath. Too high or low a trigger setting may significantly increase the patient effort required to take a breath, or cycle the ventilator to provide breaths too rapidly.

c) Inspiratory flow rate (IFR) is the speed at which the breath is delivered, expressed in liters per minute. If the IFR is set too low for a given patient, the time the breath takes to be delivered is extended, causing patient discomfort. It also affects airway pressures and possible air trapping within the lungs.

d) The respiratory rate is the number of breaths that will be delivered in one minute.

e) The positive end expiratory pressure is set, and is referred to as PEEP. This is the residual pressure remaining in the system following the delivery of the mechanical breath, and transmitted to the patient's airways and alveoli. PEEP is used to keep the airways and alveoli pneumatically splinted open, thereby providing for improved oxygenation and gas exchange. Optimal PEEP is the lowest PEEP required to provide the most efficacious oxygenation. Airway pressures should always be the lowest possible to meet the patient's oxygenation and ventilation requirements. Excessive airway pressures in mechanical ventilation may affect hemodynamic stability.

4. The most commonly used modes of providing mechanical ventilation are pressure controlled mechanical ventilation/pressure assist control (P/CMV-PAC) and volume controlled mechanical ventilation/volume assist control (V/CMV-VAC).

a) Volume CMV is volume controlled ventilation. The patient is unable to breathe on their own and the breathing is done by the ventilator.

b) Volume assist control (AC) allows the patient to breath spontaneously between preset parameters. VAC delivers a preset tidal volume such that the patient initiated breath may be assisted or unassisted by the ventilator.

c) Pressure controlled ventilation delivers a pressure preset by the clinician. The volume delivered with each breath is variable, and may vary from breath to breath. Pressure controlled ventilation is used commonly when volume controlled ventilation does not meet the parameters required to meet oxygenation or ventilation goals.

d) Pressure assist control (PAC) also has preset parameters, and the patient may breath spontaneously between mechanically delivered breaths assisted or unassisted by the ventilator.

35

5. When a patient is started on invasive mechanical ventilation, the endotracheal tube is connected to a large bore flexible tubing that, in turn, is connected to the ventilator. The tubing has both an inspiratory and expiratory limb, which join at a "Y" shaped tubing near the endotracheal tube. When the patient attempts to take a breath, there is a slight decrease in either flow or pressure within the ventilator circuit that is sensed by the ventilator, which then almost instantaneously delivers the breath within the parameters preset by the clinician. Exhalation is a passive process allowing for release of gas through an exhalation valve. The patient however, may breathe spontaneously, and depending upon the parameters selected, the spontaneous breaths may be either assisted or unassisted by the ventilator.

E. Monitoring—to ensure that the patient is being appropriately oxygenated and ventilated post initial monitoring includes blood pressure, heart rate, respiratory rate, oxygen saturation (Spo_2), and arterial blood gases.

1. PEEP may be increased to improve oxygenation providing for increased alveolar recruitment, and Fio_2 may be titrated upward (or downward) until oxygenation targets are reached. The goals of oxygenation are to meet the oxygenation criteria determined by the clinician, and are dependent upon the disease process.

2. It is always desirable to use the lowest Fio_2 possible to reach oxygenation goals. High concentrations of oxygen should be avoided when possible as concentrations greater than Fio_2 of 0.50 for extended periods is associated with lung injury due to oxygen toxicity via free radical damage.[13]

3. Parameters for pressures and gas exchange targets vary widely depending on underlying condition and degree of respiratory compromise. Traumatic brain injury, chest trauma, acute respiratory distress syndrome (ARDS), and COPD as examples, have widely differing parameters.

4. If the patient is not being appropriately ventilated as evidenced by an increase in the carbon dioxide ($Paco_2$) level, the respiratory rate, and/or tidal volumes may be adjusted depending upon the disease process and mode of ventilation. Goals are generally to keep the pH in range of 7.35-7.45, and the $Paco_2$ in the 35-45 mm Hg range.

5. There are many disease processes in which normal parameters cannot be met without causing lung injury from the invasive mechanical ventilation, thus there are acceptable limits outside of normal ranges that are appropriate for individual disease processes.

6. If the patient has been paralyzed (either by trauma or deliberately with a paralytic agent), the patient will appear quiet and resting comfortably, with the work of breathing fully assumed by the invasive mechanical ventilation. If not paralyzed or appropriately sedated, the respiratory pattern of the patient and ventilator may be mismatched, causing discomfort, restlessness, and agitation, This is known as asynchrony, dyssynchrony, or "fighting the ventilator."[14] This may occur with disconnections, insufficient tidal volumes, respiratory patterns, too low or too high of an inspiratory flow rate, oxygenation status, and incompatibility with the mode of ventilation, ventilator interface, or a variety of other factors.

35

F. Complications—invasive mechanical ventilation forces gas into the lungs, as opposed to natural breaths, which are created by negative pressure in the lungs in relation to ambient atmospheric pressure.

1. Excessive pressures required in invasive mechanical ventilation are sometimes too great and cause distention within the lungs, resulting in lung injury called barotraumas (rupture of alveoli caused by increased pressure in the lung).[15] Airway pressures are measured on a breath by breath basis and monitored continuously. Of note, airway and ventilatory pressures are measured in centimeters of water pressure, not millimeters of mercury.

2. Excessive intrapulmonary pressures may also cause hemodynamic instability and decrease venous return. Settings are titrated to keep airway pressures to the lowest possible while meeting the patient's ventilatory requirements.

3. Invasive mechanical ventilation is an abnormal process and may be quite uncomfortable for the patient. Anxiolytics, paralytics, sedatives, and pain medications may be administered and titrated for patient comfort. These agents are generally titrated downward prior to and during the normal weaning and extubation process.

4. In severe ARDS, the lung compliance (volume of gas delivered per unit of pressure increase) may be so restricted, (frequently called "stiff" lungs") that volume controlled ventilation will likely cause lung injury if the tidal volume required to normalize blood gas derangements are delivered. In this case, pressure controlled ventilation is utilized along with lower tidal volumes.

5. A condition known as "permissive hypercapnia" is employed in conditions such as ARDS, whereby the ventilator parameters cannot be met without causing injury, and the $Paco_2$ is allowed to be more elevated than would normally be acceptable to reduce the possibility of barotrauma.

G. If long-term invasive mechanical ventilation is likely, the endotracheal tube is generally replaced with a tracheostomy to reduce risk of laryngeal injury and improve patient comfort.[16]

1. Family members can be taught to suction, manage the tracheostomy appliance, and basics of managing a ventilator at home.

2. Patients may be mobile at home while on a ventilator via appropriate equipment, such as wheelchair designed to accommodate a ventilator, but it is a very limiting and cumbersome (despite the small size of the home mechanical ventilators), and requires a large degree of adjunct equipment and support. Back up plans for power failures need to be in place before the patient goes home.

VI. WEANING FROM INVASIVE MECHANICAL VENTILATION

There are several generally accepted parameters that need to be met prior to discontinuing ventilation and extubation. The actual decision-making process is based upon many factors and clinical judgment, with a global view of the patient's condition and overall clinical status.

A. A primary issue in determining readiness to wean is reversal or resolution of the condition that necessitated MV. Traditional criteria to determine weaning ability include, but are not limited to: adequate oxygenation with the lowest Fio_2, minute ventilation, lung compliance, hemodynamic stability, and electrolyte correction.[12,17]

35

B. Additional factors that may interfere with the weaning process or the ability to wean from MV include fever affecting ventilatory status by its metabolic sequelae and increased oxygen requirements; nutritional status, patient's ability to protect their airway from secretions; or the inability to clear excess secretions. Weaning to the point of patient exhaustion should be avoided.

C. In addition to the aforementioned parameters, a rapid shallow breathing index (RSBI) may be performed during spontaneous breathing trials. The respiratory rate is divided by the tidal volume (expressed in liters) and a score of less than 105 is desirable. This is only a tool and should be used in combination with clinical judgment and the patient's clinical status.

D. Another tool used for weaning is the measurement of the patient's ability to generate appropriate inspiratory pressure. This is measured by occlusion of the tracheal tube with a pressure manometer and assessment of the respiratory muscle capacity to generate appropriate inspiratory force.

E. Methods of Weaning Process

When weaning is initiated, there are 3 methods—pressure support with PEEP, invasive mechanical ventilation, and T-piece ventilation. Sedation must be assessed and minimized, and all paralytics discontinued.

1. Pressure support—this mode provides 2 levels of pressure during inhalation. When the patient initiates a breath, the ventilator is triggered to provide a preset level of inspiratory pressure to insure an adequate tidal volume to provide sufficient ventilation. A preset level of PEEP may be used to keep the alveoli pneumatically splinted open and provide sufficient oxygenation. Fio_2 is gradually adjusted downward to meet the Pao_2 and ventilation goals, as is the level of pressure support. Pressure support with PEEP is basically NIPPV via an endotracheal tube.

2. Invasive mechanical ventilation—synchronized intermittent mechanical ventilation(SIMV). This mode provides a low preset respiratory rate, and in between the mechanically delivered breaths, the patient may breathe spontaneously. The mechanically delivered breaths are synchronized with the patient's inspiratory efforts, delivering partial support. The level of ventilatory support with this method can be adjusted from 0-100%, and are titrated downward as the patients pulmonary status improves. Use of SIMV is a common practice and is thought to rest the musculature. However, there is little evidence to support its use[18]

3. T-piece—a "T" shape piece of ventilatory circuit tubing is inserted into the ventilator circuit allowing the patient to breathe spontaneously. Ventilatory parameters are monitored to determine ability to wean. T-piece weaning is also referred to as a spontaneous breathing trial.[18] The spontaneous breathing trial may include minimal assistance by the ventilator in the form of CPAP or pressure support.

F. Weaning may be a rapid process or a prolonged process requiring days to weeks, or longer. If the condition that necessitated ventilator support has been resolved, the patient may be extubated without significant weaning trials. This is commonly done when the mechanical ventilator is used for a surgical procedure.

G. Failure to wean is defined as the need for re-intubation within 24 hours of discontinuance of mechanical ventilation, although this time frame may vary.

Initially after extubation, the patient may require, or benefit from a period of supportive ventilation in the form of NIPPV, which may minimize the need for re-intubation.

H. Patients with chronic pulmonary disease or other pathological processes may have significant difficulty weaning and require an extended period of ventilatory support. If after a period of 10-14 days, ventilatory support is still required, then a decision to place a tracheostomy must be considered. However, in palliative situations, this time may be lengthened with respect to benefits and burdens of doing so. Mechanical ventilation may be continued for months to years via tracheostomy tube, even in the home setting.

I. Extubation

1. Extubation is the process whereby the endotracheal tube is removed. It differs from weaning in that weaning refers to the slow withdrawal of mechanical ventilatory support.

2. For extubation to be successful

a) The patient should be conscious, neurologically intact, have a patent airway with minimal secretions, and be able to protect the airway.

b) Resolution of the factors that precipitated the need for mechanical ventilation, attainment of oxygenation goals with $Fio_2 < 0.4$ to 0.5, evidence of adequate respiratory muscle strength, and PEEP in the 5-8 cm H_2O range or less are also required.[18]

c) A cuff leak should be present. Presence of a cuff leak (air escaping between the tracheal wall and ETT when the ETT cuff is deflated) indicates normal airflow around the ETT. The absence of a cuff leak may indicate laryngeal edema.

3. Prior to extubation, the head of bed is elevated to 90 degrees, and the airway is suctioned. The patient is then instructed to take a deep inhalation while the tracheal cuff is deflated and the tube removed as the patient exhales. Suctioning and hemodynamic monitoring should be continuous after extubation. NIPPV may be helpful or required.[19]

4. Extubation in a patient that has a tracheostomy tube is called decannulation.

VII. WITHDRAWAL OF MECHANICAL VENTILATION AND OXYGEN THERAPY

A. The purpose of MV and oxygen therapy is to support respiratory functioning; however there complications and burdens associated with them. When the burdens exceed the benefits with a negative impact on quality of life for patients and families, healthcare providers may consider discontinuation.[20]

B. The procedures for withdrawal are often delineated by individual healthcare organizations and may vary from the hospital setting or the home setting under hospice. General guidelines include

1. Clinical staff should have a meeting to review what the policies and procedures are, and to make sure everyone is in agreement with the process.

a) Any clinician may excuse him/herself from participation.

b) Medications (opioids and benzodiazepines) and the process of withdrawal should be reviewed.

35

    c) Some staff may need support in the process of stopping these therapies terminal extubation. (See Chapter 4, *Ethical Considerations*)

    d) The designated of a healthcare provider to a specific task should be completed.

2. Assure patient and families that dyspnea will be minimized and that vigilant monitoring and staff presence will be provided.

3. A terminal wean or terminal extubation may occur whereby the patient is not expected to survive. The patient is extubated, or ventilatory support is titrated downward to a point that it will no longer sustain life.

    a) The decision to withdraw ventilatory support, when survival is not expected, is very difficult. Consideration is given to the wishes of the patient and family, potential irreversibility of the disease process requiring mechanical ventilation, clinical status, and overall prognosis for potential recovery. Many organizations have policies for ventilation withdrawal and should be referenced.

    b) The endotracheal tube may or may no remain in place during a terminal wean. Oral secretions should be suctioned to minimize breath sounds distressing to the patient, family, or caregivers.

    c) Appropriate opioids and anxiolytics for dyspnea and respiratory distress should be administered prior to extubation/weaning. Dosing and type of medications used will vary depending upon the setting, patient's opioid naïvety, level of discomfort, tolerance to specific medications, etc. In an acute or rehabilitation setting, opioids are usually administered intravenously. In the home settings, opioids may be administered intravenously, subcutaneously, via a nasogastric or gastronomy tube, and/or rectally. Paralytics are discontinued to monitor for respiratory distress, which is then managed appropriately.

4. During the process, social services and spiritual support should be present to support both the family and the caregivers. Bereavement counseling should be available.

VIII. ROLE OF THE PALLIATIVE CARE NURSE PRACTITIONER

A study by Cox, et al[21] observed that there were differing expectations of outcomes of care and perspectives among patients, families, home caregivers, and the respective clinicians in the intensive care unit. Regardless of the underlying disease process, expectations of favorable outcomes in survival, functional status, and quality of life were significantly higher for the family, patient, and home caregivers than for their clinicians. The APRN provides patient and families with education, and supports their informed decision-making processes. This includes reasonable expectations and plans of care that are in accordance with the patient's wishes.

The use of supplemental oxygen and mechanical ventilation in the management of serious or progressive life-threatening illness may be required. While oxygen may improve patient survival, function, and quality of life, it will not reverse the disease process for which is was prescribed. Mechanical ventilation may be a temporary or long-term intervention. As a long-term therapy, issues of expectations and after hospital care will arise. Disposition is an essential domain for the APRN to explore. If the patient initiates mechanical ventilation, and is then found to be unable to wean, where will this ventilator dependent patient receive long-term care? Is a permanent long-term care facility with a severely restricted lifestyle acceptable to the patient? If the patient wants the ventilator to be discontinued in the future, would the facility allow it? Do the patient's and family's financial resources allow for 24/7 care? Is the home environment, financial, and social supports adequate for home care? Have caregiving issues and requirements been discussed with the potential caregivers and are there appropriate backup plans in place?

End-of-life conversations regarding determination of wishes for resuscitation, mechanical ventilation, and advance directives are essential. The discussion of end of life care should include the benefits, expectations, and quality of life for a patient that requires mechanical ventilation. (See Chapter 5, *Communication*)

CITED REFERENCES

1. American Thoracic Society. *Home Oxygen Therapy.* Available at: www.thoracic.org/clinical/COPD-guidelines/for-health-professi...ment-of-stable-copd/long-term-oxygen-therapy/home-oxygen-therapy.php. Accessed May 24, 2012.
2. Arim Q, Wilt TJ, Weinberger SE, et al. Diagnosis and management of stable chronic obstructive pulmonary disease: a clinical practice guideline update from the American College of Chest, American College of Chest Physicians, American Thoracic Society, and European Respiratory Society. *Ann Intern Med.* 2011;155:179-191.
3. Katsenos S, Constantopoulas SH. Long term oxygen therapy in COPD; factors affecting and ways of improving patient compliance. *Online Pulmonary Medicine.* 2011 article ID 325362. Available at: www.hindawi.com/journals/pm/2011/325362/. Accessed March 19, 2012.
4. Global Initiative for Chronic Lung Disease. *Global Strategy for the Diagnosis, Management, and Prevention of Chronic Obstructive Pulmonary Disease.* 2011. Available at: www.goldcopd.org/uploads/users/files/GOLD_Report_2011_Feb21.pdf. Accessed October 4, 2011.
5. American Thoracic Society. *Hazards of Oxygen.* Available at: www.thoracic.org/clinical/copd-guidelines/for-health-professio...gement-of-stable-copd/long-term-oxygen-therapy/hazards-of-oxygen.php. Accessed May 22, 2012.
6. Kacmarek RM. Delivery systems for long-term oxygen therapy. *Respir Care.* 2000:45(1):84-92.
7. Bailey P. Oxygen delivery for infants, children, and adults. *UpToDate.* 2012. Available at: www.uptodate.com/contents/oxygen-delivery-systems-for-infants-children-and-adults?source=search_result&search=oxygen+therapy&selectedTitle=4%7E150#H2427423. Accessed August 27, 2012.
8. Dunne PJ. The clinical impact of new long-term oxygen therapy technology. *Respir Care.* 2009;54(8):1100-1111.
9. American Thoracic Society. *COPD Guidelines: Oxygen Delivery Methods.* 2012. Available at: www.thoracic.org/clinical/copd-guidelines/for-health-professionals/exacerbation/inpatient-oxygen-therapy/oxygen-delivery-methods.php#2. Accessed August 17, 2012.
10. Vines DL. Navigating the respiratory pyramid of care. Presentation at: Massachusetts Society for Respiratory Care 33rd Annual Conference; September 22-23, 2010; Sturbridge, MA.
11. Courey AJ, Hyzy RC. Overview of mechanical ventilation. *UpToDate.* 2012. Available at: www.uptodate.com/contents/overview-of-mechanical-ventilation?source=search_result&search=mechanical+ventilation&selectedTitle=1%7E150. Accessed August 27, 2012.
12. Celli BR. Mechanical ventilatory support. In: Longo DL, Fauci AS, Kasper DL, Hauser SL, Jameson JL, Loscalzo J, eds. *Harrison's Principles of Internal Medicine (online).* 18th ed. Columbus, OH: McGraw-Hill Companies, Inc. 2012. Available at: www.accessmedicine.com/content.aspx?aid=9105809. Accessed May 3, 2012.
13. Malhorta A, Schwartz DR, Schwartzstein RM. Oxygen toxicity. *UpToDate.* 2012. Available at: www.uptodate.com/contents/oxygen-toxicity?source=related_link. Accessed August 27, 2012.
14. Kaufman DA, Fuchs B, Lipschik G. Assessment of respiratory distress in mechanically ventilated patients. *UpToDate.* 2010. Available at: www.uptodate.com/contents/assessment-of-respiratory-distress-in-the-mechanically-ventilated-patient?source=see_link. Accessed August 27, 2012.
15. Hyzy RC. Pulmonary barotraumas in mechanical ventilation. *UpToDate.* 2011. Available at: www.uptodate.com/contents/pulmonary-barotrauma-during-mechanical-ventilation?source=see_link. Accessed August 27, 2012.

35

16.   Hyzy RC. Overview of tracheostomy. *UpToDate.* 2011. Available at:
       www.uptodate.com/contents/overview-of-tracheostomy?source=see_link&anchor=H14#H2. Accessed
       August 27, 2012.

17.   Hess D, Kacmarek R. Modes of mechanical ventilation. In: Hess D, Kacmarek R. *Essentials of
       Mechanical Ventilation.* New York, NY: McGraw-Hill; 1996:17-19.

18.   MacIntyre NR, Branson RD. Discontinuing mechanical ventilation. In: MacIntyre NR, Branson RD.
       Mechanical Ventilation. 2nd ed. St. Louis, MO: Saunders; 2009:317-320.

19.   Bauman KA, Hyzy RC. Extubation management. *UpToDate.* 2012. Available at:
       www.uptodate.com/contents/extubation-management?source=see_link#H7. Accessed August 27, 2012.

20.   Campbell ML. Mechanical ventilation. In: Nelson P, ed. *Withdrawal of Life-Sustaining Therapies.*
       Pittsburgh, PA: Hospice and Palliative Nurses Association; 2010:35-43.

21.   Cox CE, Martinu T, Sathy SJ, et al. Expectations and outcomes of prolonged mechanical ventilation. *Crit
       Care Med.* 2009;37(11):2888-2894.

CHAPTER 36

NATIONAL GUIDELINES AND APRN PRACTICE

Constance M. Dahlin, APRN-BC, ACHPN®, FPCN, FAAN
Judy Lentz, RN, MSN, NHA

Preface—There are two national documents that delineate expectations, guidelines, and preferred practices for palliative care. These are The National Consensus Project for Quality Palliative Care, *Clinical Practice Guidelines for Quality Palliative Care,*[1] and the National Quality Forum, *A National Framework and Preferred Practices for Palliative and Hospice Care Quality: A Consensus Statement.*[2] Both provide a comprehensive framework to evaluate quality palliative care. They serve as the basis for the performance measures used in Palliative Care Certification by The Joint Commission. This resource offers the APRN specific line by line recommendations on applying the *Clinical Practice Guidelines* and the 38 Preferred Practices (PP) to promote the highest provision of quality advanced practice palliative nursing.

DOMAIN 1: STRUCTURE AND PROCESSES OF CARE

Guideline 1.1—A comprehensive and timely interdisciplinary assessment of the patient and family forms the basis of the plan of care.

Criteria

1. Assessment reflects advanced assessment by APRN consistent with master's education in a specific population focus, scope of practice, and within the limits of licensure. Assessment is reviewed on a regular basis and systematically documented reflecting coordinated interdisciplinary perspectives.

2. The APRN, within state statutes of scope of practice, completes an initial comprehensive assessment and subsequent reevaluation through patient and family interviews, review of medical and other available records, discussion with other providers, physical examination and assessment, and relevant laboratory and/or diagnostic tests or procedures. The APRN may perform a consultative evaluation that includes the patient's current medical status; adequacy of diagnosis and treatment consistent with review of past history, diagnosis and treatment; and responses to past treatments.

3. The APRN assessment process includes documentation of disease status, including diagnoses and prognosis; comorbid medical and psychiatric disorders; physical and psychological symptoms; functional status; social, cultural, and spiritual strengths, values, practices, concerns, and goals; advance care planning concerns, preferences, and documents; and appropriateness of hospice referral including Physical Aspects of Care, Domain 3: Psychological and Psychiatric Aspects of Care, Domain 4: Social Aspects of Care, Domain 5: Spiritual, Religious, and Existential Aspects of Care, and Domain 8: Ethical and Legal Aspects of Care.

36

4. The APRN performs appropriate assessment of children with consideration of age and stage of neurocognitive development and within scope of practice.

5. The APRN documents assessment of the patient and family perception and understanding of the serious or life-threatening illness including patient and family expectations of treatment, goals for care, quality of life, as well as preferences for the type and site of care.

6. The APRN performs a comprehensive assessment of the elements of quality of life defined by the 4 domains of physical, psychological, social, and spiritual aspects of care. Interventions are focused to alleviate distress in any of these domains.

7. This APRN performs comprehensive assessment on a regular basis and in subsequent intervals or in response to significant changes in the patient's or family's status or goals.

> ** Preferred Practice Example for APRN under DOMAIN/GUIDELINE 1.1**

PP1—The APRN provides palliative and hospice care as part of the interdisciplinary team who collaborates with primary healthcare professional(s).

PP2—The palliative APRN seeks certification as an Advanced Certified Hospice and Palliative Nurse (ACHPN®), commits to continuing education, and assures provision of care by an interdisciplinary team 24/7.

Guideline 1.2—The care plan is based on the identified and expressed preferences, values, goals, and needs of the patient and family and is developed with professional guidance and support for patient-family decision-making. *Family* is defined by the patient.

Criteria

1. The APRN formulates a care plan based upon an ongoing assessment and reflects goals set by the patient and family or surrogate in collaboration with the interdisciplinary team (IDT). Such goals reflect the changing potential benefits and burdens of various care options at critical decision points during the course of illness.

2. In collaboration with the patient, family, and other involved healthcare providers, the APRN develops the care plan with the additional input, when indicated, of other providers in the community, such as school professionals, community service providers, and spiritual leaders.

3. The ARPN changes the care plan based on the evolving needs and preferences of the patient and family and recognizes the complex, competing, and shifting priorities in goals of care. The evolving care plan is documented over time.

4. The APRN provides support for patient-family decision-making and develops, implements, and coordinates the care plan in collaboration with the patient and family. The APRN promotes patient and family education of the care plan and assures communication of the care plan to all involved health professionals. Particular attention is necessary when a patient transfers to a different care setting to communicate with the receiving provider. The APRN is an important collaborator in this.

5. The ARPN documents treatment and care setting alternatives and communicates with the patient and family in a manner that promotes informed decision-making.

6. The APRN assures that treatment decisions are based on goals of care established by the patient, family, and IDT; assessment of risk and benefit; and best evidence. Reevaluation of treatment efficacy, patient-family goals, and choices is documented.

** Preferred Practice Example for APRN under DOMAIN/GUIDELINE 1.2**

PP3— The APRN regularly reviews a timely care plan based on values, preferences, goals and needs of patient/family and communicates with the entire interdisciplinary team.

PP4—The APRN promotes a seamless patient transfer through various care settings with communication of patient values, preferences, and beliefs and refers to hospice when appropriate. The APRN educates patient, family and co-team members as needed to make informed decisions

Guideline 1.3—An interdisciplinary team (IDT) provides services to the patient and family consistent with the care plan. In addition to chaplains, nurses, physicians, and social workers, other therapeutic disciplines who provide palliative care services to patients and families may include child-life specialists, nursing assistants, nutritionists, occupational therapists, pharmacists, physical therapists, psychologists, and speech and language pathologists. Complementary and alternative therapies may be included.

Criteria

1. An APRN provides specialist-level palliative care delivered as a member of an IDT.

2. The APRN is part of a team that includes palliative care professionals with the appropriate patient-population-specific education, credentialing, and experience, and the skills to meet the physical, psychological, social, and spiritual needs of both patient and family. The APRN has graduate nursing training and is certified by NBCHPN® in advanced hospice and palliative nursing. APRNs should be expected to have current certification as an ACHPN® or seek certification within 1 year of employment.

3. The interdisciplinary palliative care team involved in the care of children, whether the child is a patient or a family member of either an adult or pediatric patient, has expertise in the delivery of services for such children. The APRN has the appropriate education to match the population he or she is serving.

4. The APRN is part of the team that provides palliative care expertise and staff 24 hours a day, 7 days a week. The APRN is knowledgeable about access to respite services available for the families and caregivers of children or adults with serious or life-threatening illnesses.

5. The patient and family have access to palliative care expertise and staff 24 hours a day, 7 days a week. Respite services are available for the families caring for either children or adults with serious or life-threatening illnesses

6. The APRN participates in regular IDT communication (at least weekly or more often as required by the clinical situation) to plan, review, evaluate, and update the care plan, with input from both the patient and family. The APRN is an essential part of quality care, policy development, and creation of clinical practices.

** Preferred Practice Example for APRN under DOMAIN/GUIDELINE 1.3**

36

PP5—The APRN is educated as appropriate for advanced practice, licensed accordingly, and experienced in hospice and palliative care. Certified as ACHPN®, the APRN demonstrates leadership according to standards of professional performance, assures availability of qualified nursing professionals 24/7 to meet the needs of the patient/family.

Guideline 1.4—The palliative care program is encouraged to use appropriately trained and supervised volunteers to the extent feasible.

Criteria

1. For programs utilizing volunteers, the APRN participates in the development of policies and procedures to ensure safe and quality volunteer programs, such as recruitment, screening (including background checks), training, job descriptions, role clarification, work practices, support, supervision, and performance evaluation, in addition to clarity of the responsibilities of the program to its volunteers.

2. A program that uses volunteers has policies and procedures outlining the program's responsibilities to its volunteers. The APRN assures appropriate use of volunteers.

3. The APRN may participate in screening, educating, coordinating, and collaborating with volunteers.

> ** Preferred Practice Example for APRN under DOMAIN/GUIDELINE 1.4**

PP6—The APRN may create such policies and procedures, develop volunteer programs, supervise appropriately screened volunteers, and provide education for volunteers.

Guideline 1.5 Support for education, training, and professional development is available to the interdisciplinary team.

Criteria

1. Orientation for the APRN includes the attitudes, knowledge, and skills in the domains of palliative care (i.e., pain and symptom assessment and management; communication skills; medical ethics; grief and bereavement; family and community resources; and hospice care including philosophy, eligibility, and core features of the Medicare Hospice Benefit).

2. APRN education and training occurs in various venues such as baccalaureate and graduate programs, preceptorships, practicums, or palliative APRN fellowships in compliance with federal and state licensure and credentialing regulations.

3. The palliative care program supports the ARPN's professional development through mentoring, preceptorship, and supervision.

4. APRNs participate in essential continuing palliative care education, and their participation is documented accordingly. Educational resources, focused on the domains listed in this document, are available and provided to APRNs or sought out in a number of venues.

5. Palliative care programs ensure appropriate education for APRNs, specifically graduate degrees in clinical nursing, and appropriate professional experience.

6. Palliative care programs encourage APRN discipline-specific certification, or other recognition of competence, as part of the educational support for the interdisciplinary team. Educational resources, education, and support are provided specifically to enhance IDT communication and collaboration.

7. Education regarding effective team management, human resource management, budgets, and strategic planning is available to support APRN leadership.

** Preferred Practice Example for APRN under DOMAIN/GUIDELINE 1.5**

PP7—The APRN is expected to participate in educational programming based on their level of care responsibilities and with the financial support by the organization of these efforts.

Guideline 1.6—In its commitment to quality assessment and performance improvement, the palliative care program develops, implements, and maintains an ongoing data driven process that reflects the complexity of the organization and focuses on palliative care outcomes.

Criteria

1. The palliative care program commits to the pursuit of excellence and the highest quality of care and support for all patients and their families. The program determines quality by providing regular and systematic measurement, analysis, review, evaluation, goal setting, and revision of the processes and outcomes of care. The APRN participates in the quality process.

2. Quality care follows the national quality strategy set out by the U.S. Department of Health and Human Services in carrying out the provisions of the Affordable Care Act. The strategy states

   - "Making care safer by reducing harm caused in the delivery of care.

   - Ensuring that each person and family is engaged as partners in their care.

   - Promoting effective communication and coordination of care.

   - Promoting the most effective prevention and treatment practices for the leading causes of mortality, starting with cardiovascular disease.

   - Working with communities to promote wide use of best practices to enable healthy living.

   - Making quality care more affordable for individuals, families, employers, and governments by developing and spreading new healthcare delivery models."[3]

3. The APRN coordinates care continually focused on the illness trajectory, which offers the right care at the right time in the course of an individual's disease or condition.

4. The APRN participates in the quality assessment and performance improvement (QAPI) review done across all the domains including organizational structure, education, team utilization, assessment and effectiveness of physical, psychological, psychiatric, social, spiritual, cultural, and ethical assessment and interventions.

5. The ARPN participates in QAPI process in which the palliative care program establishes quality improvement policies and procedures.

36

6. A process for quality improvement is documented and leads to change in clinical practice. The APRN participates in or develops quality improvement projects that might include the development and testing of screening, history, and assessment tools, and appropriate protocols for diagnoses, interventions, and outcomes. Some examples may include

    •   Structure and Processes—development of outcomes for program development, education and training, development of quality measures, cost analysis

    •   Physical Aspects of Care—education and training, development and testing of evidence based therapies

    •   Psychological and Psychiatric Aspects of Care—education and training, development and testing of bereavement and grief screening, assessment tools of types of grief, and development and testing of evidence based therapies

    •   Social Aspects of Care—education and training, development and testing of social screening, assessment, and intervention tools; identification and enhancement of the evidence base within the social domain

    •   Spiritual, Religious, and Existential Aspects of Care—education and training, development and testing of spiritual screening, history and assessment tools; and appropriate protocols for spiritual diagnoses, interventions and outcomes.

    •   Cultural Aspects of Care—education and training, development and testing of cultural assessment tools and culturally appropriate interventions; evaluation of outcomes within and across cultural and linguistic communities

    •   Care of the Imminently Dying Patient—education and training, appropriate protocols for the imminently dying patient

    •   Ethical and Legal Aspects of Care—education and training, appropriate protocols for ethical and legal occurrences, best practices for advance care planning

7. Quality improvement activities are routine, regular, reported, and are shown to influence clinical practice. Designated staff, with experience in QAPI planning including an APRN, operates the QAPI process in collaboration with leaders of the palliative care program.

8. The clinical practices of the APRN reflect the integration and dissemination of research and evidence of quality process.

9. Quality improvement activities for clinical services are collaborative, interdisciplinary, and focused on meeting the identified needs and goals of patients and their families.

10. Patients, families, health professionals, and the community participate in evaluation of the palliative care program.

> ** Preferred Practice Example for APRN under DOMAIN/GUIDELINE 1.6**

PP8—The APRN participates in quality improvement policies and procedures for the palliative care program and evaluates the outcomes. The APRN ensures all nursing staff members comply routinely as per policies.

Guideline 1.7—The palliative care program recognizes the emotional impact on the palliative care team providing care to patients with serious or life-threatening illnesses and their families.

Criteria

1. The program provides emotional support to APRNs to facilitate coping with the stress of caring for individuals and families affected by serious or life-threatening illness.

2. Support structure of APRNs includes regular meetings where review, impact, and processes of the provision of palliative care are discussed.

3. The program and IDT implements interventions to promote resiliency and sustainability of APRN Team members.

> ** Preferred Practice Example for APRN under DOMAIN/GUIDELINE 1.4**

PP9—The APRN serves as an emotional support to staff and volunteers. In addition, the APRN identifies and accesses further resources for emotional support per organizational policies.

Guideline 1.8—Community resources ensure continuity of the highest quality palliative care across the care continuum.

Criteria

1. Palliative care programs support and promote continuity of care throughout the trajectory of illness across all settings. The APRN plays a role in continuity and consistency across settings.

2. Non-hospice palliative care programs have a relationship with one or more hospices and other community resources to ensure continuity of the highest-quality palliative care across the care continuum.

3. Non-hospice palliative care programs and APRNs routinely inform patients and families about hospice and other community based healthcare resources when such resources are consistent with the patient's and family's values, beliefs, preferences, and goals of care. APRNs make referrals only with patient and family consent.

4. Referring clinicians, as described by Centers for Medicare and Medicaid Services (CMS), including other APRNs, are routinely informed about the availability and benefits of hospice, as well as other appropriate community resources for their patients and families. The APRN understands these services and offers early discussion of these services and early referral to such services as hospices and community resources.

5. The APRN participates and facilitates the work of hospice programs, non-hospice palliative care programs, and other major community service providers involved in the patient's care to establish policies for formal written and verbal communication about all domains in the plan of care.

6. The APRN is aware of policies to enable timely and effective sharing of information among teams while safeguarding privacy.

7. When possible, hospice and palliative care program staff, including APRNs, participate in each other's team meetings to promote regular professional communication, collaboration, and an integrated plan of care on behalf of patients and families.

36

8. Hospice and palliative programs, as well as other major community providers, routinely seek opportunities to collaborate and work in partnership to promote increased access to quality palliative care across the continuum.

> ** Preferred Practice Example for APRN under DOMAIN/GUIDELINE 1.8**

PP10—The APRN effectively collaborates with community resources to assure provision of quality palliative care.

Guideline 1.9—The physical environment in which care is provided meets the preferences, needs, and circumstances of the patient and family to the extent possible.

Criteria

1. When feasible, care occurs in the setting preferred by the patient and his/her family and this preference is elicited by the APRN.

2. When care is provided outside the patient's or family's home, the APRN negotiates and collaborates with residential service providers to maximize the patient's safety. Flexible visiting hours, as appropriate, promote social interaction for the patient. A space is arranged for families to visit, rest, and prepare or eat meals, as well as to meet with palliative care providers and other professionals, along with other needs identified by the family.

3. Providers in all settings address the unique care needs of children as patients, family members, or visitors.

> ** Preferred Practice Example for APRN under DOMAIN/GUIDELINE 1.9**

PP11—When feasible and safe, the APRN provides care as per the patient's preferences meeting the needs of safety, visitation, family, comfort, privacy, and other needs as identified by the patient and/or family. The APRN elicits and advocates for preferences for care, participates in planning to honor these preferences and provides care in accordance with the plan.

DOMAIN 2: PHYSICAL ASPECTS OF CARE

Guideline 2.1—The interdisciplinary team expertly assesses and manages pain and/or other physical symptoms and subsequent effects based upon the best available evidence.

Criteria

1. The goal of pain and symptom management is the safe and timely reduction of a physical symptom to an acceptable level to the patient, or surrogate if the patient is unable to report distress.

2. The APRN provides symptom assessment and treatment as part of the IDT.

3. APRNs demonstrate specialist-level skill in symptom control for all types of serious or life-threatening illnesses. Symptoms include, but are not limited to pain, shortness of breath, nausea, fatigue, anorexia, insomnia, and constipation.

4. It is essential that healthcare organizations develop and utilize symptom assessment, treatment policies, standards, and guidelines appropriate to the care of patients with serious or life-threatening illnesses that conform to best palliative care practices.

5. The APRN facilitates and promotes the use of such assessments, policies, standards, and guidelines.

6. The APRN documents regular, ongoing assessment of pain, other physical symptoms, and functional capacity. Validated symptom assessment instruments are utilized when available. Symptom assessment of adults with cognitive impairment and of children, is performed by appropriately trained professionals using validated instruments when available.

7. The APRN treats distressing symptoms and side effects, which includes the entire spectrum of effective pharmacological, interventional, behavioral, and complementary and interventions therapies that are supported as supported by research, and refers to appropriate specialists.

8. Symptom assessment, treatment, and treatment outcome information including side effects is recorded in the medical record by the APRN and transmitted across healthcare settings during transitions.

9. The APRN identifies barriers related to the use of opioid analgesics and addresses misconceptions of the risks of side effects, addiction, respiratory depression, and hastening death.

10. As opioid prescribers, APRNs develop and adopt opioid analgesic risk assessment and management plans consistent with state/federal regulations for use with patients requiring long term opioid therapy. The APRN instructs patients, families, and/or other involved health providers about safe usage of opioids including operation of machinery, driving, storage, inventory, and appropriate opioid disposal.

Guideline 2.2—The assessment and management of symptoms and side effects are contextualized to the disease status.

Criteria

1. The APRN develops treatment plans for physical symptoms in the context of the disease, prognosis, and patient functional limitations. The APRN assesses the patient, family or surrogate's understanding of the illness in relation to patient-centered goals of care.

2. The APRN assesses the patient or surrogate understanding of disease and its consequences, symptoms, side effects of treatments, functional impairment, and potentially beneficial treatments with consideration of culture, cognitive function, and developmental stage.

3. The APRN educates family and other healthcare providers to support safe and appropriate care of the patient. The APRN provides family with resources for response to urgent needs.

| ** Preferred Practice Example for APRN under DOMAIN/GUIDELINE 2.1** |

36

PP12—The APRN measures and documents all symptoms using available standardized scales.

PP13—The APRN assesses and manages symptoms and treatment side effects in a timely, safe, and effective manner with a goal of providing relief that is acceptable to the patient and family.

Guideline 3.1—The interdisciplinary team expertly assesses and addresses psychological and psychiatric aspects of care based upon the best available evidence to maximize patient and family coping.

Criteria

1. The APRN has training and skills to identify the potential psychological and psychiatric impact of serious or life-threatening illness, on both the patient and family including depression, anxiety, delirium, and cognitive impairment.

2. Based on patient and family goals of care, the APRN develops interventions that address psychological needs and psychiatric diagnoses, promote adjustment to the physical condition, and support opportunities for emotional growth, psychological healing, completion of unfinished business, and effective grieving.

3. The APRN performs and documents regular, ongoing assessment of psychological reactions related to the illness (including but not limited to stress, anticipatory grieving, and coping strategies) and psychiatric conditions. Whenever possible and appropriate, a validated and context-specific assessment tool are used.

4. The APRN psychological assessment that includes patient and family understanding of the disease or condition, symptoms, side effects, and their treatments, as well as assessment of caregiving needs, decision-making capacity, and coping strategies.

5. The APRN effectively treats and manages psychiatric diagnoses, with appropriate psychiatric collaboration, diagnoses such as severe depression, suicidal ideation, anxiety, delirium, or patients with comorbid psychiatric illness accompanying their serious or life-threatening illness.

6. The APRN provides family education that includes the provision of safe and appropriate psychological support measures to the patient.

7. The APRN skillfully communicates treatment alternatives, promoting informed decision-making by the patient and family and documents these discussions.

8. The APRN bases treatment decisions on assessment of risk and benefit, evidence informed practice, and patient/family preferences.

9. The APRN utilizes pharmacological, nonpharmacological, and complementary and interventional therapies for the treatment of psychological distress or psychiatric syndromes, as appropriate.

10. The APRN responds to psychological distress promptly, and effectively reflecting patient/family choice. The APRN documents regular reassessment of treatment efficacy, response to treatment, and patient-family preferences.

11. The APRN refers to appropriate healthcare professionals with specialized skills in age-appropriate psychological and psychiatric treatment (e.g., psychiatrists, psychologists, social workers). The APRN identifies psychiatric comorbidities present in family to ensure appropriate referral for treatment.

12. The APRN provides developmentally appropriate assessment and support to pediatric patients and children who are family members of pediatric or adult patients.

36

13. The APRN communicates with individuals using verbal, nonverbal, and/or symbolic means appropriate to the patient, with particular attention to patients with cognitive impairment and the developmental stage and cognitive capacity of children.

14. The APRN provides staff education regarding the recognition and treatment of anticipatory grief and common psychological and psychiatric syndromes (e.g. anxiety, depression, delirium, hopelessness, suicidal ideation, substance withdrawal symptoms), and professional coping strategies in managing difficult symptoms.

> ** Preferred Practice Example for APRN under DOMAIN/GUIDELINE 3.1**

PP14—The APRN measures and documents the presence of anxiety, depression, delirium, behavioral disturbances, and other psychological symptoms using available standardized scales.

PP15—The APRN manages anxiety, depression, delirium, behavioral disturbances in a timely, safe, and effective manner to achieve outcomes acceptable to the patient and family, and assess responses accordingly.

Guideline 3.2—A grief and bereavement program is a core component of the palliative care program available to patients and families, based on assessment of need.

Criteria

1. The APRN demonstrates patient-population-appropriate education and skill in the care of patients, families, and staff experiencing loss, grief, and bereavement.

2. The APRN identifies and recognizes loss and grief in patients and families living with serious or life-threatening illness at diagnosis. The APRN performs ongoing assessment and reassessment throughout the illness trajectory.

3. Staff and volunteers, including those who provide bereavement services, receive ongoing education, supervision, and support in coping with their own grief, and responding effectively to patients' and families' grief.

4. At time of admission to hospice or a palliative care, the APRN completes an initial developmentally appropriate professional assessment to identify patients and families at risk for complicated grief, bereavement, and comorbid complications, particularly among older adults.

5. The APRN ensures that identified patients and families receive intensive support, and prompt referral to appropriate professionals as needed.

6. Bereavement services and follow-up are available to the family for a minimum of 12 months, after the death of the patient.

7. The APRN ensures that culturally and linguistically appropriate information on loss, grief, and the availability of bereavement support services is routinely communicated to the family before and after the death of the patient. This includes community services such as support groups, counselors, and collaborative partnerships with hospice.

8. The APRN provides support and grief interventions in accordance with developmental, cultural, and spiritual needs and the expectations and preferences of the family, with attention to children family members of any patient.

36

> ** Preferred Practice Example for APRN under DOMAIN/GUIDELINE 3.2**

PP16—The APRN may assist in the development of, as well as offer, a grief and bereavement care plan to patients and families prior to, and for at least 13 months after the death of the patient.

DOMAIN 4: SOCIAL ASPECTS OF CARE

Guideline 4.1—The interdisciplinary team expertly assesses and addresses the social aspects of care to meet patient-family needs, promote patient-family goals, and maximize patient-family strengths and well-being.

Criteria

1. The APRN facilitates and enhances patient-family understanding of, and coping with, illness and grief; supports patient-family decision-making; discusses the patient's and family's goals for care; provides emotional and social support; and enhances communication within the family and between patient-family and the IDT.

2. The APRN collaborates with the IDT social worker with patient-population-specific skills in the assessment of, and interventions to address, social needs during a life-threatening or serious illness.

3. Health professionals, including APRNs, skilled in assessment and intervention of the developmental needs and capacities of children, are available. This includes both pediatric patients and children who are family members of pediatric or adult patients.

> ** Preferred Practice Example for APRN under DOMAIN/GUIDELINE 4.1**

PP17—The APRN conducts regularly scheduled patient and family conferences with the interdisciplinary team to provide information, discuss goals of care, disease prognosis, and advance care planning and offer support.

Guideline 4.2 A comprehensive, person-centered interdisciplinary assessment identifies the social strengths, needs, and goals of each patient and family.

Criteria

1. The APRN assesses and documents a social assessment including the following elements

   - Family structure and function—roles, communication, and decision-making patterns

   - Strengths and vulnerabilities—resiliency; social and cultural support networks; effect of illness or injury on intimacy and sexual expression; prior experiences with illness, disability, and loss; risk of abuse, neglect, or exploitation

   - Changes in family members' schooling, vocational roles, recreational activities, and economic security

   - Geographic location, living arrangements, and perceived suitability of living environment

36

- Patient's and family's perceptions about caregiving need, availability, and capacity

- Needs for adaptive equipment, home modifications, and transportation

- Access to medications (prescription and over-the-counter) and nutritional products

- Need for and access to community resources, financial support, and respite

- Advance care planning and legal concerns (see Domain 8: Ethical and Legal Aspects of Care, Guideline 8.1)

2. The APRN's social care plan reflects the patient's and family's culture, values, strengths, goals, and preferences, which may change over time.

3. The APRN implements interventions to maximize the social well-being and coping skills of both the patient and family, including education and family meetings.

4. The APRN refers the patient and family to appropriate resources and services, that address the patient's and family's identified social needs and goals, and support patient-family strengths.

> ** Preferred Practice Example for APRN under DOMAIN/GUIDELINE 4.2**

PP18—The APRN develops and implements a comprehensive social care plan, which addresses the social, practical, and legal needs of the patient and caregivers, including but not limited to relationships, communication, existing social and cultural networks, decision-making, and work.

DOMAIN 5: SPIRITUAL, RELIGIOUS, AND EXISTENTIAL ASPECTS OF CARE

Guideline 5.1—The interdisciplinary team assesses and addresses spiritual, religious, and existential dimensions of care.

Criteria

1. Spirituality is recognized as a fundamental aspect of compassionate patient and family centered care, honoring the dignity of all persons.

2. Spirituality is defined as, "the aspect of humanity that refers to the way individuals seek and express meaning and purpose and the way they experience their connectedness to the moment, to self, to others, to nature, and/or to the significant or sacred."[1] The APRN is responsible for recognizing spiritual distress and for attending to the patient's and the family's spiritual needs, within their scope of practice.

3. The interdisciplinary palliative care teams, in all settings, includes spiritual care professionals; specifically a board certified professional chaplain, with skill and expertise in assessing and addressing spiritual and existential issues frequently confronted by pediatric and adult patients with serious or life-threatening illnesses and their families.

4. The APRN communication with the patient and family is respectful of their religious and spiritual beliefs rituals, and practices. The APRN does not impose his/her own spiritual, religious, or existential beliefs and practices on their patients, patients' families, and colleagues.

36

> ** Preferred Practice Example for APRN under DOMAIN/GUIDELINE 5.1**

PP19—The APRN develops and documents a plan based on assessment of religious, spiritual, and existential concerns using a structured instrument and integrates the information obtained from the assessment into the palliative care plan.

Guideline 5.2—A spiritual assessment process, including a spiritual screening, history questions, and a full spiritual assessment as indicated, is performed. This assessment identifies the religious or spiritual/existential background, preferences, and related beliefs, rituals, and practices of the patient and family; as well as spiritual symptoms, such as spiritual distress and/or pain, guilt, resentment, despair, and hopelessness.

Criteria

1. Regular, ongoing exploration of spiritual and existential concerns occurs; including but not limited to life review, assessment of hopes, values, and fears, meaning, purpose, beliefs about afterlife, spiritual or religious practices, cultural norms, beliefs that impact understanding of illness, coping, guilt, forgiveness, and life-completion tasks. These spiritual themes are documented and communicated to the team. Whenever possible, a standardized instrument is used.

2. The APRN documents periodic reevaluation, of the impact of spiritual/existential interventions and patient and family preferences.

3. As a member of the IDT, the APRN addresses spiritual/existential care needs, goals, and concerns identified by patients, family members according to established protocols and documented in the interdisciplinary care plan, during transitions of care, and/or in discharge plans. The APRN offers support for issues of life closure, as well as other spiritual issues, in a manner consistent with the patient's and the family's cultural, spiritual, and religious values.

4. The APRN refers to appropriate community-based professionals with specialized knowledge or skills in spiritual and existential issues when appropriate (e.g., to a pastoral counselor or spiritual director). Spiritual care professionals are recognized as specialists who provide spiritual counseling.

5. The APRN supports and indicates the patient's spiritual sources of strength.

> ** Preferred Practice Example for APRN under DOMAIN/GUIDELINE 5.2**

PP20—The APRN assesses religious, spiritual, and existential concerns using a structured instrument and integrates the information obtained from the assessment into the palliative care plan.

Guideline 5.3—The palliative care service facilitates religious, spiritual, cultural, rituals or practices as desired by patient and family, especially at the time of death.

Criteria

1. Professional and institutional use of religious/spiritual symbols and language are sensitive to cultural and religious diversity.

36

2. The APRN supports the patient and family in their desires to display and use their own religious/spiritual and/or cultural symbols.

3. Healthcare chaplaincy and APRNs facilitate contacts with spiritual/religious communities, groups or individuals, as desired by the patient and/or family. Palliative care programs create procedures to facilitate patients' access to clergy, religious, spiritual, and culturally-based leaders, and/or healers in their own religious, spiritual, or cultural traditions.

4. APRNs acknowledge their own spirituality as part of their professional role. The APRN participates in opportunities to engage staff in self-care and self-reflection on their beliefs and values as they work with seriously ill and dying patients. It is expected that APRNs respect of spirituality and beliefs of all colleagues and the creation of a healing environment in the workplace.

5. Non-chaplain palliative care providers obtain training in basic skills of spiritual screening and spiritual care.

6. The APRN ensures follow up after the patient's death (e.g., phone calls, attendance at wake or funeral, scheduled visit) to offer support and identify any additional needs that require community referral, and help the family during bereavement

---

** Preferred Practice Example for APRN under DOMAIN/GUIDELINE 5.3**

PP21—The APRN provides information about the availability of spiritual care services and makes spiritual care available either through organizational spiritual counseling or through the patient's own clergy relationship.

PP22—The APRN assures that specialized palliative and hospice care teams include spiritual care professionals, who are appropriately educated and certified in palliative care. The APRN builds relationships with community clergy, and provides education and counseling related to end-of-life care.

DOMAIN 6: CULTURAL ASPECTS OF CARE

Guideline 6.1—The palliative care program serves each patient, family, and community in a culturally and linguistically appropriate manner.

Criteria

1. Culture is multidimensional.

2. Culture is far reaching and may include, many aspects such as race, ethnicity, and national origin; migration background, degree of acculturation, and documentation status; socioeconomic class; gender, gender identity, and gender expression; sexual orientation; family status; spiritual, religious, and political belief or affiliation; physical, psychiatric, and cognitive ability; literacy, including health and financial literacy; and age.

3. During the assessment process, the APRN elicits and documents the cultural identifications, strengths, concerns, and needs of the patient and family, recognizing that cultural identity and expression vary within families and communities.

36

4. The APRN creates a plan of care that addresses the patient's and family's cultural concerns and needs and maximizes their cultural strengths. APRNs consistently convey respect for the patient's and family's cultural perceptions, preferences, and practices regarding illness, disability, treatment, help seeking, disclosure, decision-making, grief, death, dying, and family composition.

5. The APRN communicates in a language and manner that the patient and family understand.

    -   APRNs tailor their communication to the patient's and family's level of literacy, health literacy, financial literacy, and numeracy.

    -   For patients and families who do not speak or understand English, or who feel more comfortable communicating in a language other than English, the palliative care program makes all reasonable efforts to use professional interpreter services, accessed either in person and/or by phone. When professional interpreters services are unavailable, other healthcare providers, preferably those trained in palliative care, may interpret for patients and families. In general, family members are not placed in the role of interpreter. However, in the absence of all other alternatives, the ARPN may use family members to interpret in an emergency situation if the patient and family agree to this arrangement.

    -   In addition to interpreter services, the palliative care program endeavors to provide written materials in each patient's and family's preferred language. When translated written materials are not available, the program utilizes professional interpreter services as described above, to facilitate patient and family understanding of information provided by the program.

6. The APRN respects and accommodates dietary and ritual practices of patients and their families.

7. The APRN identifies community resources that serve various cultural groups and refer patients and families to such services, as appropriate.

> ** Preferred Practice Example for APRN under DOMAIN/GUIDELINE 6.1**

PP23—The APRN incorporates cultural assessment as a component of comprehensive palliative and hospice care assessment, including, but not limited to locus of decision-making, preferences regarding disclosure of information, truth telling and decision-making, dietary preferences, language, family communication, desire for support measures such as palliative therapies and complementary and interventional therapies, perspectives on death, suffering and grieving, and funeral/burial rites.

PP24—The APRN provides professional interpreter services and education materials that are culturally sensitive and in the patient and family's preferred language.

Guideline 6.2—The palliative care program continually strives to enhance its cultural and linguistic competence.

36

Criteria

1. *Cultural competence* refers to the process by which APRNs respond respectfully and effectively to people of all cultures and languages in a manner that recognizes, affirms, and values the worth of individuals, families, and communities.

2. The palliative care program values diversity as demonstrated by creating and sustaining a work environment that affirms multiculturalism. The recruitment, hiring, retention, and promotion practices of the palliative care program reflect the cultural and linguistic diversity of the community it serves.

3. The APRN cultivates cultural self-awareness and recognizes personal cultural values, beliefs, biases, and practices inform perceptions of patients, families, and colleagues. APRNs strive to prevent value conflicts from undermining their interactions with patients, families, and colleagues.

4. To reduce health disparities within and among the communities it serves, the palliative care program provides education to help APRNs increase their cross-cultural knowledge and skills.

5. The palliative care program regularly evaluates and, if needed, modifies its services, policies, and procedures to maximize its cultural and linguistic accessibility and responsiveness to a multicultural population. Input from patients, families, and community stakeholders is elicited and integrated into this process.

DOMAIN 7: CARE OF THE IMMINENTLY DYING PATIENT

Guideline 7.1—The interdisciplinary team identifies, communicates, addresses, and skillfully manages the signs and symptoms of impending death to meet the physical, psychosocial, spiritual, social, and cultural needs of patients and families.

Criteria

6. The APRN recognizes the need for higher intensity and acuity of care during the active dying phase.

7. Prior to and at onset of the dying process, the APRN routinely elicits and honestly addresses concerns, hopes, fears, and expectations about the dying process in a developmentally appropriate manner, with respect for the social and cultural context of the family.

8. In collaboration with the patient and family and the IDT, the APRN provides care with respect for patient and family values, preferences, beliefs, culture, and religion.

9. The ARPN acknowledges the patient's imminent death, and communicates signs and symptoms of approaching death to the patient and family, in culturally and developmentally appropriate language, with attention to population specific issues and age appropriateness.

Guideline 7.2—An assessment of actual or potential symptoms, preferences for site of care, attendance of family and/or community members, treatments and procedures is performed and documented by the interdisciplinary team.

Criteria

1. The APRN assesses the patient for symptoms and proactively considers other potential symptoms and concerns.

2. With the patient and family, the APRN develops a plan to meet the unique needs of the patient and family during the actively dying phase and the needs of family immediately following the patient's death. The APRN reassesses and revises the plan in a timely basis.

36

3. The APRN documents in the medical record and communicates in a timely manner any inability to meet the patient's and family's expressed wishes for care immediately leading up to and following the death.

4. The APRN introduces or reintroduces a hospice referral, if such an option is congruent with the patient's and family's goals and preferences for patients who have not accessed hospice services.

5. Before the patient's death, the APRN sensitively addresses, as appropriate, autopsy, organ and tissue donation, and anatomical gifts, with respect to institutional and regional policies.

Guideline 7.3—Respectful post-death care is delivered honoring the patient and family culture and religious practices.

Criteria

1. The APRN assesses and documents cultural and religious practices particular to the post-death period, and delivers care honoring those practices and in accordance with both institutional practice and local laws and regulations.

Guideline 7.4—An immediate bereavement plan is activated post-death.

Criteria

1. The APRN formulates and activates a post-death bereavement plan based on a social, cultural, and spiritual grief assessment.

2. The APRN assures that a healthcare team member is assigned to the family in the post-death period to support the family and assist with religious practices, funeral arrangements, and burial planning.

> ** Preferred Practice Example for APRN under DOMAIN/GUIDELINE 7.1**

PP25—The APRN recognizes and documents the transition to the active dying phase and communicates to the patient, family, and staff the expectation of imminent death.

PP26—The APRN educates the family on a timely basis regarding signs and symptoms of imminent death in a developmentally-, age- and culturally-appropriate manner.

PP27—As part of the ongoing care planning process, the APRN routinely ascertains and documents patient and family wishes about the site of death, and fulfills patient and family preferences when possible.

PP28—The APRN provides adequate dosage of analgesics and sedatives as appropriate to achieve patient comfort during the active dying phase and addresses concerns and fears about use of opioids and analgesics and hastening death.

PP29—The APRN promotes post-death treatment of the body that is respectful and in accordance with the cultural and religious practices of the family and local law.

PP30—The APRN facilitates effective grieving by implementing in a timely manner a bereavement care plan after the patient's death when the family remains the focus of care.

36

DOMAIN 8: ETHICAL AND LEGAL ASPECTS OF CARE

Guideline 8.1—The patient or surrogate's goals, preferences, and choices are respected within the limits of applicable state and federal law and within current accepted standards of medical care, and professional standards of practice. These goals, preferences, and choices form the basis for the plan of care.

Criteria

1. The APRN includes professionals with knowledge and skill in ethical, legal, and regulatory aspects of medical decision-making in care planning.

2. The APRN educates the patient and family about advance care planning documents; including but not limited to, designation of a surrogate healthcare decision-maker for (except for minors) out of hospital do not resuscitate orders, and advance directives.

3. The APRN sensitively elicits the patient or surrogate's expressed values, care preferences, religious beliefs, and cultural considerations, in collaboration with the family to assist in understanding patient and family decision-making. The APRN confirms and routinely reviews these values, preferences, and considerations, with particular attention to changes in healthcare status or transitions of care, and assures they are documented.

4. The ARPN routinely documents all expressed wishes, preferences, and values including the completion of clinician orders such as inpatient resuscitation status, out of hospital do not resuscitate orders, and healthcare surrogate declaration documents for adult patients. The APRN assists in completion of documents to promote communication and understanding of the patient's preferences for care across the healthcare continuum, and/or the preferences of the patient's designated surrogate.

5. The APRN documents and addresses the failure to honor the patient's or surrogate's preferences to assure it is accessible to other healthcare providers

6. To determine decision-making capacity, the ARPN assesses the ability of the patient and family to secure and accept needed care and to cope with the illness and its consequences. The adult patient with decisional capacity determines the level of involvement of the family in decision-making and communication about the care plan. Patients with disabilities are assumed to have capacity unless determined otherwise.

7. In situations with pediatric patients, the ARPN documents the child's views and preferences for medical care, including assent for treatment (when developmentally appropriate), and assures it is given appropriate weight in decision-making. When the child's wishes differ from those of the adult decision-maker, the APRN assures appropriate professional staff members are available to assist the family.

8. The APRN advocates for the observance of previously expressed wishes of the patient or surrogate in these situations. For patients unable to communicate and have not previously expressed their values, preferences, or beliefs, the APRN seeks to identify advance directives, evidence of previously expressed wishes, values and preferences, and the designated surrogate decision makers.

9. The APRN provides assistance and guidance to surrogate decision makers about the legal and ethical basis for surrogate decision-making, including honoring the patient's known preferences, substituted judgment, and best-interest criteria.

36

10. The APRN routinely encourages patients and families to seek professional advice on creating or updating legal and financial documents such as property wills, guardianship agreements, and custody documents.

** Preferred Practice Example for APRN under DOMAIN/GUIDELINE 8.1**

PP31—The APRN documents the designated surrogate/decision-maker in accordance with state law for every patient in primary, acute, and long-term care and in palliative and hospice care.

PP32—The APRN documents the patient/surrogate preferences for goals of care, treatment options, and setting of care at first assessment and at frequent intervals as conditions change.

PP33—The APRN converts the patient treatment goals into medical orders and ensures that the information is transferable and applicable across care settings, including long-term care, emergency medical services, and hospitals, such as the Physician/Provider Orders for Life-Sustaining Treatment (POLST) programs.

PP34—For minors with decision-making capacity, the APRN documents the child's views and preferences for medical care, including assent for treatment, and assures that these are given appropriate weight in decision-making. The APRN makes appropriate professional staff members available to both the child and the adult decision-maker for consultation and intervention when the child's wishes differ from those of the adult decision-maker.

PP35—The APRN promotes advance directives and surrogacy designation availability and access across care settings, while protecting patient privacy and adherence to Health Insurance Portability and Accountability Act (HIPAA) regulations (e.g., by Internet-based registries or electronic personal health records).

PP36—The APRN develops healthcare and community collaboration to promote advance care planning and completion of advance directives for all individuals (e.g., Respecting Choices, Community Conversations on Compassionate Care).

Guideline 8.2—The palliative care program acknowledges and addresses the complex ethical issues arising in the care of people with serious or life-threatening illness.

Criteria

1. The APRN, as part of the palliative care team, aims to prevent, identify, and resolve ethical dilemmas common to the provision of palliative care such as withholding or withdrawing treatments, instituting do not resuscitate (DNR) orders, and the use of sedation in palliative care.

2. The APRN has education in ethical principles guiding the provision of palliative care.

3. Ethical concerns commonly encountered in palliative care are identified, recognized, and addressed to prevent or resolve these concerns, using the ethical principles of beneficence, respect for individuals and self-determination, justice and nonmaleficence with attention to avoidance of conflicts of interest.

4. The APRN documents ethical clinical issues and appropriately refers to ethics consultants or a committee for case consultation and assistance in conflict resolution.

36

5. Ethics committees are consulted in the appropriate manner to guide policy development, assist in clinical care, and provide staff education in common palliative care situations including, but not limited to a patient's right to decline care, use of high dose medications, withdrawal of technology (e.g., ventilators, dialysis, antibiotics) palliative sedation, futile care, and cessation of artificial and oral nutrition and hydration.

> ** Preferred Practice Example for APRN under DOMAIN/GUIDELINE 8.2**

PP37—The APRN assures establishment of/or access to ethics committees or ethics consultation across care settings to address ethical conflicts at the end of life.

Guideline 8.3—The provision of palliative care occurs in accordance with professional, state, federal laws and regulations and current accepted standards of care.

Criteria

1. The APRN is knowledgeable about legal and regulatory aspects of palliative care and has access to legal and regulatory experts to provide care in accordance with legal and regulatory aspects of palliative care.

2. The APRN models his/her palliative care practice on existing professional codes of ethics, scopes of practice, and standards of care for consistency.

3. The APRN is knowledgeable about federal and state statutes, regulations, and laws regarding disclosure of medical records and health information; medical decision-making; advance care planning and directives; the roles and responsibilities of surrogate decision-makers; appropriate prescribing of controlled substances; death pronouncement and certification processes; autopsy requests, organ and anatomical donation; and healthcare documentation.

4. The adherence to legal and regulatory requirements is expected for disclosure, decision-making capacity assessment, confidentiality, informed consent, as well as assent and permission for people not of legal age to consent.

5. The palliative care program establishes and implements policies outlining staff responsibility in regard to state and federal legal and regulatory requirements regarding patient and family care issues such as abuse, neglect, suicidal ideation, and potential for harm to others.

6. The APRN recognizes the role of cultural variation in the application of professional obligations, including information around diagnosis, disclosure, decisional authority, care, acceptance of and decisions to forgo therapy. The APRN attends to the role of children and adolescents in decision-making.

7. Legal counsel is accessible to the APRN particularly in common palliative care situations including but not limited to decision-making capacity, use of high dose medications, withdrawal of technology (e.g., ventilators, dialysis), palliative sedation, futile care, and cessation of artificial and oral nutrition and hydration.

> ** Preferred Practice Example for APRN under DOMAIN/GUIDELINE 8.3**

36

PP38—The APRN participates in the development of policies on medical decision-making, role of surrogate decision-makers, legal requirements for use of controlled substances, death pronouncement, requests for autopsy, and organ transplantation consistent with federal and state statutes and regulations.

CITED REFERENCES

1. National Consensus Project for Quality Palliative Care. *Clinical Practice Guidelines for Quality Palliative Care.* 3rd ed. Pittsburgh, PA: National Consensus Project for Quality Care; 2013.
2. National Quality Forum. *A National Framework and Preferred Practices for Palliative and Hospice Care Quality.* Washington, DC: National Quality Forum; 2006.
3. U.S. Department of Health and Human Services. *Report to Congress: National Strategy for Quality Improvement in Health Care.* 2011. Available at: www.healthcare.gov/law/resources/reports/quality03212011a.html#na. Accessed October 17, 2012.

CHAPTER 37

PERFORMANCE AND PROGNOSTIC TOOLS

Constance M. Dahlin, APRN-BC, ACHPN®, FPCN, FAAN
Maureen T. Lynch, MS, ANP-BC, AOCN, ACHPN®, FPCN

Performance status is a measure of the patient's functional capacity. It has been strongly correlated to survival in cancer and palliative care with poorer performance linked to shorter survival.[1] Two commonly used performance tools in adults are the Karnofsky Performance score[1] and the Eastern Oncology Cooperative Group's (ECOG) Performance Scale.[2] The Palliative Performance Scale[3] is valid for cancer patients. The Lansky Play Performance scale is used in children under age 16.[4]

The Palliative Prognostic Score (PaP) can be of assistance in prognosticating 30 day survival.[5]

Karnofsky Performance Score[1,6]
Instructions—select the value that best describes the patient. Compare percents over time.

Percent	Level of Functional Capacity
100	Normal, no complaints, no evidence of disease
90	Able to carry on normal activity, minor signs or symptoms of disease
80	Normal activity with effort, some signs or symptoms of disease
70	Cares for self, unable to carry on normal activity or to do active work
60	Requires occasional assistance, but is able to care for most needs
50	Requires considerable assistance and frequent medical care
40	Disabled, requires special care and assistance
30	Severely disabled, hospitalization is indicated although death is not imminent
20	Hospitalization is necessary, very sick, active supportive treatment necessary
10	Moribund, fatal processes progressing rapidly
0	Dead

Eastern Cooperative Oncology Group (ECOG) Performance Scale[2,7]
Instructions—Select the grade that best describes the patient's functional ability. Compare grades over time.

Grade	Definition
0	Fully active; no performance restrictions
1	Strenuous physical activity restricted; fully ambulatory and able to carry out light work
2	Capable of all self-care but unable to perform any work activities. Up and about > 50% of waking hours
3	Capable of only limited self-care; confined to bed or chair > 50% of waking hours
4	Completely disabled; cannot carry out any self-care; totally confined to bed or chair

37

Palliative Performance Scale (PPS)[3]

Instructions—Select the functional status in each of the 5 observer-rated domains (ambulation, activity level/evidence of disease, self-care, intake, level of consciousness) to determine the patient's percent of functional status and the estimated median survival if applicable.

%	Ambulation	Activity Level Evidence of Disease	Self-Care	Intake	Level of Consciousness	Estimated Median Survival in Days		
						(a)	(b)	(c)
100	Full	Normal *No Disease*	Full	Normal	Full			
90	Full	Normal *Some Disease*	Full	Normal	Full	N/A		
80	Full	Normal with Effort *Some Disease*	Full	Normal or Reduced	Full		N/A	
70	Reduced	Can't do normal job or work *Some Disease*	Full	As above	Full	145		108
60	Reduced	Can't do hobbies or housework *Significant Disease*	Occasional Assistance Needed	As above	Full or Confusion	29	4	
50	Mainly sit/lie	Can't do any work *Extensive Disease*	Considerable Assistance Needed	As above	Full or Confusion	30	11	
40	Mainly in Bed	As above	Mainly Assistance	As above	Full or Drowsy or Confusion	18	8	41
30	Bed Bound	As above	Total Care	Reduced	As above	8	5	
20	Bed Bound	As above	As above	Minimal	As above	4	2	
10	Bed Bound	As above	As above	Mouth Care Only	Drowsy or Coma	1	1	6
0	Death	-	-	-	--			

a. Survival post-admission to an inpatient palliative unit, all diagnoses.[8]
b. Days until inpatient death following admission to an acute hospice unit, diagnoses not specified.[9]
c. Survival post admission to an inpatient palliative unit, cancer patients only.[10]

37

Modified Lansky Play-Performance Scale (for use with persons ages 1 through 16 years)[4,11]

Instructions—Select the percent of play-performance that best describes the patient. Compare percents over time.

100%	Fully active, normal
90	Minor restrictions in physically strenuous activity
80	Active, but tires more quickly
70	Both greater restriction of, and less time spent in, play activities
60	Up and around, but minimal active play; keeps busy with quieter activities
50	Gets dressed, but lies around much of the day; no active play; able to participate in all quiet play and activities
40	Mostly in bed; participates in quiet activities
30	In bed; needs assistance even for quiet play
20	Often sleeping; play entirely limited to very passive activities
10	No play; does not get out of bed
5	Unresponsive
0	Dead

PALLIATIVE PROGNOSTIC SCORE (PaP)[5]

Palliative Prognostic Score was developed for use in patients with cancer but has been validated in non-cancer diagnoses to predict 30 day survival. Higher score predicts shorter survival.

Instructions—Select the assessment that best describes the patient for each criterion, then add the associated score. Compare the total score with the risk groups for possible prognostication of 30 day survival.

CRITERION	ASSESSMENT	PARTIAL SCORE
Dyspnea	No Yes	0 1
Anorexia	No Yes	0 1.5
Karnofsky Performance Status	>30 10 - 20	0 2.5
Clinical Prediction of Survival (weeks)	>12 11-12 7-10 5-6 3-4 1-2	0 2 2.5 4.5 6 8.5
Total WBC (x10^9/L)	<8.5 8.6 - 11 >11	0 0.5 1.5
Lymphocyte Percentage	20 - 40% 12 - 19.9% < 12%	0 1 2.5

RISK GROUP	30 DAY SURVIVAL	TOTAL SCORE
A	>70%	0 - 5.5
B	30 - 70%	5.6 - 11
C	< 30%	11.1 - 17.5

37

CITED REFERENCES

1. Lamont EB, Christakis NA. Survival estimated in advanced cancer. *UpToDate.* 2012. Available at: www.uptodate.com/contents/image?imageKey=PC%2F58785&topicKey=PALC%2F2206&rank=1%7E51 &source=see_link&search=karnofsky+performance+scale&utdPopup=true. Accessed August 24, 2012.

2. Eastern Cooperative Oncology Group, Comis R, Group Chair. *ECOG Performance Status.* 2006. Available at: ecog.dfci.harvard.edu/general/perf_stat.html. Accessed August 24, 2012.

3. Wilner LS, Arnold R. *The Palliative Performance Score. Fast Facts and Concepts.* End of Life Education and Resource Center (EPERC). 2009. Available at: www.eperc.mcw.edu/EPERC/FastFactsIndex/ff_125.htm. Accessed August 26, 2012

4. Lansky LL, List MA, Lansky SB, Cohen ME, Sinks LF. Toward the development of a play performance scale for children (PPSC). *Cancer.* 2006;56(7 Suppl):1837-1840.

5. Wilner LS, Arnold R. *The Palliative Prognostic Score. Fast Facts and Concepts.* End of Life Education and Resource Center (EPERC). 2009. Available at: www.eperc.mcw.edu/EPERC/FastFactsIndex/ff_124.htm Accessed August 26, 2012.

6. Karnofsky DA, Burchenal JH. The clinical evaluation of chemotherapeutic agents in cancer. In: MacLeod CM, ed. *Evaluation of Chemotherapeutic Agents.* New York, NY: Columbia University Press; 1949:196.

7. Oken MM, Creech RH, Tormey DC, et al. Toxicity and response criteria of the Eastern Cooperative Oncology Group. *Am J Clin Oncol.* 1982;5:649-655.

8. Virik K, Glare P. Validation of the Palliative Performance Scale for inpatients admitted to a palliative care unit in Sydney, Australia. *J Pain Symp Manage.* 2002;23(6):455-457.

9. Anderson F, Downing GM, Hill J. Palliative Performance Scale (PPS): a new tool. *J Palliat Care.* 1996;12(1):5-11.

10. Morita T, Tsunoda J, Inoue S, et al. Validity of the Palliative Performance Scale from a survival perspective. *J Pain Symp Manage.* 1999;18(1):2-3.

11. Modified Lansky Play – Performance Scale. Available at: www.kfshrc.edu.sa/oncology/files/BMT%20Lansky%20Pay-Performance%20Scale.pdf. Accessed September 2, 2012.

CHAPTER 38

PALLIATIVE CARE AND RELATED RESOURCES

Constance M. Dahlin, APRN-BC, ACHPN®, FPCN, FAAN

PALLIATIVE NURSING TEXTS

Ferrell BR, Coyle N, eds. *Oxford Textbook of Palliative Nursing.* 3rd ed. New York, NY: Oxford University Press; 2010.

Hospice and Palliative Nurses Association, American Nurses Association. *Hospice and Palliative Nursing: Scope and Standards of Practice.* Silver Spring, MD: nursebooks.org; 2007.

Hospice and Palliative Nurses Association. *Competencies for Advance Practice Hospice and Palliative Care Nurses.* Dubuque, IA: Kendal/Hunt Publishing Company; 2002.

Matzo M, Sherman DW, eds. *Palliative Care Nursing: Quality Care to the End of Life.* 3rd ed. New York, NY: Springer Publishing Company; 2010.

Panke J, Coyne P, eds. *Conversations in Palliative Care.* 2nd ed. Pittsburgh, PA; Hospice and Palliative Nurses Association; 2011.

PALLIATIVE CARE EDUCATION

American Association of Colleges of Nursing. Peaceful Death: Recommended Competencies and Curricular Guidelines for End-of-Life Nursing Care. American Association of Colleges of Nursing/Robert Wood Johnson Foundation, 2004. (apps.aacn.nche.edu/Publications/deathfin.htm)

Education in Palliative and End-of-life Care and End-of-life Care (previously Education for Physicians in End of Life Care)—this project is a train-the-trainer program geared at teaching both the content of the curriculum and educational approaches to improve palliative care (www.epec.net/)

End-of-Life Nursing Education Consortium (ELNEC)—the project provides undergraduate and graduate nursing faculty, CE providers, staff development educators, specialty nurses in pediatrics, oncology, critical care and geriatrics, and other nurses with training in palliative care so they can teach this essential information to nursing students and practicing nurses (www.aacn.nche.edu/elnec)

PALLIATIVE CARE JOURNALS

American Journal of Hospice and Palliative Medicine (www.sagepub.com/journals/Journal201797)

European Journal of Palliative Care (www.haywardpublishing.co.uk/ejpc_.aspx)

International Journal of Palliative Nursing (www.ijpn.co.uk/)

Journal of Hospice And Palliative Nursing (www.jhpn.com)

Journal of Pain and Symptom Management (www.jpsmjournal.com/)

38

Journal of Palliative Care (www.criugm.qc.ca/journalofpalliativecare/

Journal of Palliative Medicine (www.liebertpub.com/jpm)

Pain (www.painjournalonline.com/)

Palliative Medicine (pmj.sagepub.com/)

Supportive Care in Cancer (www.springer.com/medicine/oncology/journal/520)

QUALITY GUIDELINES

Center to Advance Palliative Care. *Policies and Tools for Hospital Palliative Care Programs: A Cross Walk of National Quality Forum Preferred Practices.* New York, NY: CAPC; 2009. (www.capc.org/capc-resources/capc_publications/nqf-crosswalk.pdf)

Institute for Healthcare Improvement (www.ihi.org/Pages/default.aspx)

Morrison S, Center to Advance Palliative Care (CAPC), National Palliative Care Research Center (NPCRC). *America's Care of Serious Illness: A State-by-State Report Card on Access to Palliative Care in Our Nation's Hospitals.* New York, NY: CAPC, NPCRC; 2011. (reportcard-live.capc.stackop.com/pdf/state-by-state-report-card.pdf)

National Comprehensive Cancer Network—numerous guidelines in multiple areas including cancer by site, supportive care, and age related recommendations (www.nccn.org/clinical.asp)

National Consensus Project for Quality Palliative Care (2009). *Clinical Practice Guidelines for Quality Palliative Care.* 3rd ed. Pittsburgh, PA: NCP; 2013. (www.nationalconsensusproject.org)

National Quality Forum. *A National Framework and Preferred Practices for Palliative and Hospice Care Quality: A Consensus Report.* Washington, DC: NQF; 2006. (www.qualityforum.org/Publications/2006/12/palliative_hospice_full.aspx)

The Joint Commission: Advanced Certification for Palliative Care Programs. (www.jointcommission.org/certification/palliative_care.aspx)

PALLIATIVE NURSING RELATED ORGANIZATIONS

Hospice and Palliative Nurses Association (www.HPNA.org)

National Board for Certification of Hospice and Palliative Nurses: Certification for Advanced Practice Registered Nurses (www.NBCHPN.org)

OTHER PROFESSIONAL ORGANIZATIONS

American Academy of Hospice and Palliative Medicine (www.AAHPM.org)

Center to Advance Palliative Care (www.CAPC.org)

European Association for Palliative Care (www.eapcnet.eu/)

National Hospice and Palliative Care Organization (www.NHPCO.org)

National Palliative Care Research Center (www.NPCRC.org)

Social Work Hospice and Palliative Care Network. (www.SWHPN.org)

REIMBURSEMENT

Billing Hospice Physician and NP Service
(www.cgsmedicare.com/hhh/education/materials/pdf/Physician_and_NP.pdf)

NHIC, Corp. Part B: Physician Assistant, Nurse Practitioner, Clinical Nurse Specialist, Certified Nurse-Midwife Billing Guide. J14 A/B MAC. 2010. (www.medicarenhic.com/providers/pubs/nonphyguide.pdf)

FEDERAL HEALTHCARE ACTS

Balanced Budget Act of 1997. Public Law 105-33. (frwebgate.access.gpo.gov/cgi-bin/getdoc.cgi?dbname=105_cong_public_laws&docid=f:publ33.105.)

Centers for Medicare and Medicaid Services (CMS). Medicare Benefit Policy Manual: Covered Medical and Other Health Services. Pub 100-02 (www.cms.gov/Regulations-and-Guidance/Guidance/Manuals/downloads/bp102c15.pdf)

Centers for Medicare and Medicaid Services (CMS). Medicare Claims Processing Manual: Physician/Nonphysician Practitioners. Pub 100-04. (www.cms.gov/Regulations-and-Guidance/Guidance/Manuals/downloads/clm104c12.pdf)

Evaluation and Management Documentation Guidelines. (www.cms.gov/Outreach-and-Education/Medicare-Learning-Network-MLN/MLNProducts/downloads/eval_mgmt_serv_guide-ICN006764.pdf)

Medicare Prescription Drug, Improvement, and Modernization Act of 2003. Public Lay 108-173. (www.medicare.gov/medicarereform/108s1013.htm)

The Patient Protection and Affordable Care Act. 2010. Public Law 111-148. (www.gpo.gov/fdsys/pkg/PLAW-111publ148/pdf/PLAW-111publ148.pdf)

REPORTS ON PALLIATIVE CARE AND NURSING

Report of the 2008 Alliance for Excellence in Hospice and Palliative Nursing Summit: The Alliance White Paper (www.theallianceforexcellence.org/DisplayPage.aspx?Title=About%20Us)

The Alliance for Excellence in Hospice and Palliative Nursing (www.theallianceforexcellence.org/)

INSTITUTE OF MEDICINE CONSENSUS REPORTS

Approaching Death: Improving Care at the End of Life (www.iom.edu/Reports/1998/Approaching-Death-Improving-Care-at-the-End-of-Life.aspx)

Crossing the Quality Chasm: A New Health System for the 21st Century (www.iom.edu/Reports/2001/Crossing-the-Quality-Chasm-A-New-Health-System-for-the-21st-Century.aspx)

Improving Palliative Care for Cancer (www.iom.edu/Reports/2003/Improving-Palliative-Care-for-Cancer.aspx)

The Future Of Nursing: Leading Change, Advancing Health (www.iom.edu/Reports/2010/The-Future-of-Nursing-Leading-Change-Advancing-Health.aspx)

When Children Die: Improving Palliative and End-of-Life Care for Children and Their Families (www.iom.edu/Reports/2002/When-Children-Die-Improving-Palliative-and-End-of-Life-Care-for-Children-and-Their-Families.aspx)

NATIONAL STATE BOARDS OF NURSING

Consensus Model for APRN Regulation: Licensure, Accreditation, Certification & Education (www.ncsbn.org/7_23_08_Consensue_APRN_Final.pdf)

PROMOTING EXCELLENCE

A Position Statement from American Nursing Leaders (www.promotingexcellence.org/apn/pe3673.html)

Advanced Practice Nursing: Pioneering Practices in Palliative Care (www.promotingexcellence.org/apn/)

ROBERT WOOD JOHNSON FOUNDATION

Addressing Racial and Ethnic Disparities in Health Care (www.ahrq.gov/research/disparit.htm)

Care at the End of Life Still Not What It Could Be (www.rwjf.org/en/research-publications/find-rwjf-research/2009/04/care-at-the-end-of-life-still-not-what-it-could-be.html)

LAST Acts: Precepts of Palliative Care (www.aacn.org/WD/Palliative/Docs/2001Precep.pdf)

Meier D, Isaacs SL, Hughes R. Palliative Care: Transforming the Care of Serious Illness. Hoboken, NJ: Jossey-Bass; 2010. (rwjf.org/en/research-publications/find-rwjf-research/2009/05/the-robert-wood-johnson-foundation-health-policy-series/palliative-care.html)

RELATED EDUCATIONAL WEBSITES

Education in Palliative and End of Life Care (EPEC) (www.epec.net)

End of Life/Palliative Education Resource Center (EPERC) Over 200 one-page synopsis on topics important to palliative and end-of-life care. For a complete listing of Fast Facts and Concepts (www.eperc.mcw.edu)

ADVANCE CARE PLANNING

Five Wishes. Aging with Dignity (www.agingwithdignity.org/five-wishes.php)

Take Charge of Your Life (www.takechargeofyourlife.org/)

CANCER
American Cancer Society (www.cancer.org)

American Society of Clinical Oncology (www.asco.org/)

CARDIAC

American Heart Association (www.americanheart.org)

CAREGIVERS

Caregiver Network Inc.(caregiver.ca/)

GeriPal: A Geriatrics and Palliative Care Blog (www.geripal.org/)

CAREGIVERS—continued

GeroNurse Online
(www.geronurseonline.org)

HPNA Patient/Family Teaching Sheets
(www.hpna.org/DisplayPage.aspx?Title
=Patient/Family Teaching Sheets)

Fibromyalgia Network
(www.fmnetnews.com)

Institute for Healthcare Improvement
(www.ihi.org)

Leukemia & Lymphoma Society®
(www.leukemia.org)

Make a Wish Foundation® (www.wish.org)

National Family Caregivers Association
(www.nfcacares.org/)

CENSUS AND POPULATION DATA

U.S. Census Bureau: Poverty Reports
(www.census.gov/hhes/www/poverty/)

DEMENTIA

Alzheimer's and Dementia Association
(www.alz.org)

DIABETES

American Diabetic Association
(www.diabetes.org)

HEALTHCARE CHAPLAINCY

Association of Professional Chaplains
(www.professionalchaplains.org/index.a
spx?id=95)

HIV/AIDS

National Association of People with AIDS
(www.napwa.org)

HOMELESSNESS AND POVERTY

Center on Budget and Policy Priorities
(www.cbpp.org/)

Spotlight on Poverty and Opportunity:
Focus on Health
(www.spotlightonpoverty.org/health_an
d_poverty.aspx)

HOSPICE CRITERIA FOR NON CANCERS

LMRP Hospice Determining Terminal Status
2002
(www.nhpco.org/files/public/Draft_CAH
ABA_UniPolicy.pdf)

KIDNEY

National Kidney Foundation
(www.kidneyfoundation.org)

LIVER

American Liver Foundation
(www.liverfoundation.org)

NEUROLOGICAL

ALS Society (www.alsa.org)

Brain Injury Association of America
(www.biausa.org/)

National Stroke Association
(www.stroke.org)

PULMONARY DISEASE

American Lung Association (www.lung.org)

OLDER ADULTS

Aging with Dignity
(www.agingwithdignity.org)

The American Geriatrics Society
(www.americangeriatrics.org)

PAIN

American Chronic Pain Association
(www.theacpa.org/)

American Pain Foundation
(www.painfoundation.org)

American Pain Society
(www.ampainsoc.org/)

Association of Oncology Social Work
(AOSW) (www.aosw.org)

Association of Pediatric Oncology Nurses
(APON) (www.apon.org)

American Society of Pain Management
Nurses (www.aspmn.org)

38

PAIN—continued

City of Hope Pain/Palliative Care Resource
Center (prc.coh.org/)

Center for Pediatric Pain Research
(pediatric-pain.ca/)

Oncology Nursing Society (www.ons.org)

PainLink (www.edc.org/PainLink)

Pain Net, Inc. (www.painnet.com)

Partners Against Pain®
(www.partnersagainstpain.com)

Patient Education Institute (www.patient-
education.com)

Pediatric Pain Education for Patients &
Families (pedspain.nursing.uiowa.edu)

VETERANS ISSUES

Pharmacological Management of Persistent
Pain in Older Adults
(www.americangeriatrics.org/files/docu
ments/2009_Guideline.pdf)

U.S. Department of Veterans Affairs
(www.va.gov)

U.S. Department of Veterans Affairs—
Homeless Veterans: About the Initiative
(www.va.gov/HOMELESS/about_the_in
itiative.asp)

SUBJECT INDEX